Vitamin D

Edited by Öner Özdemir

Published in London, United Kingdom

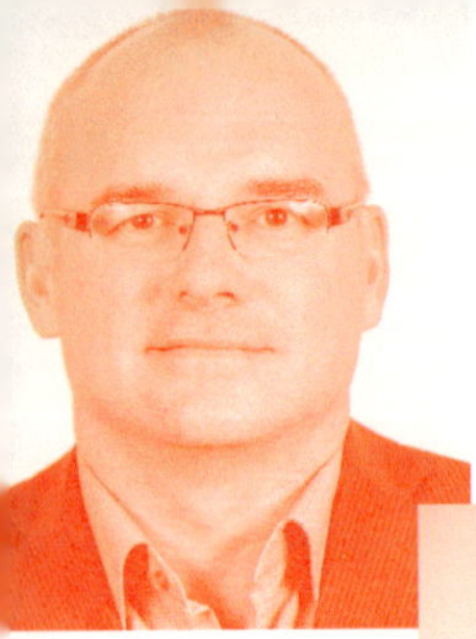
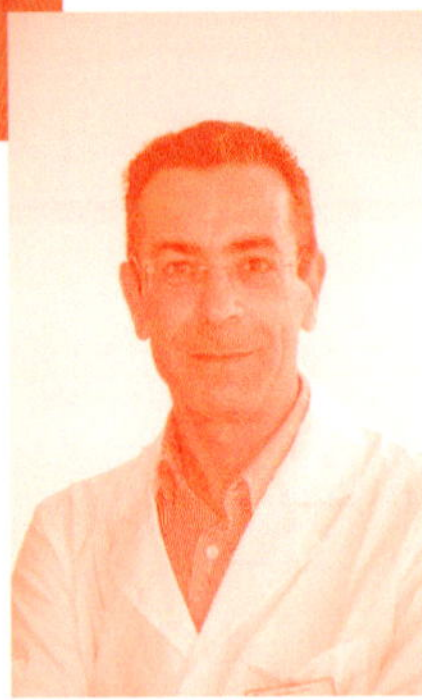
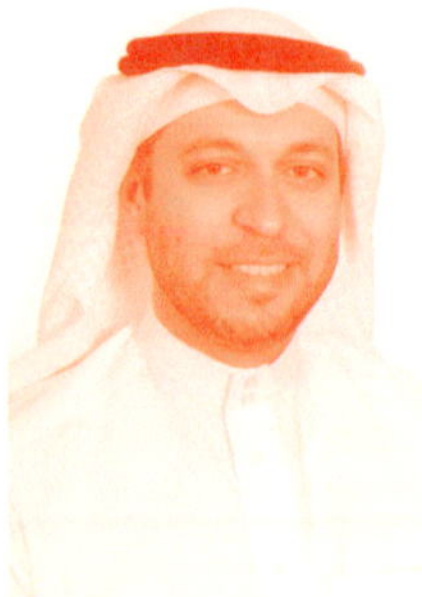
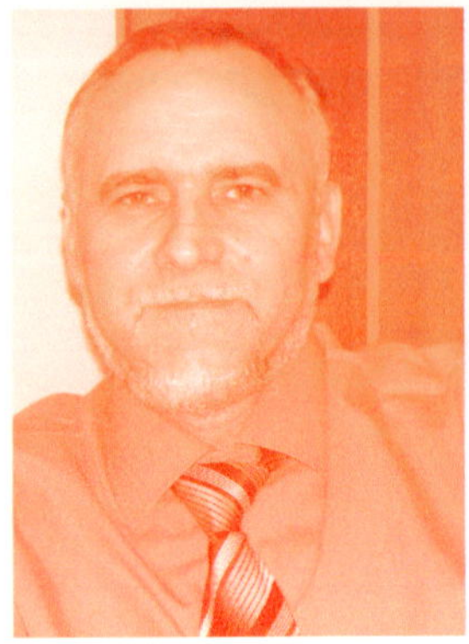
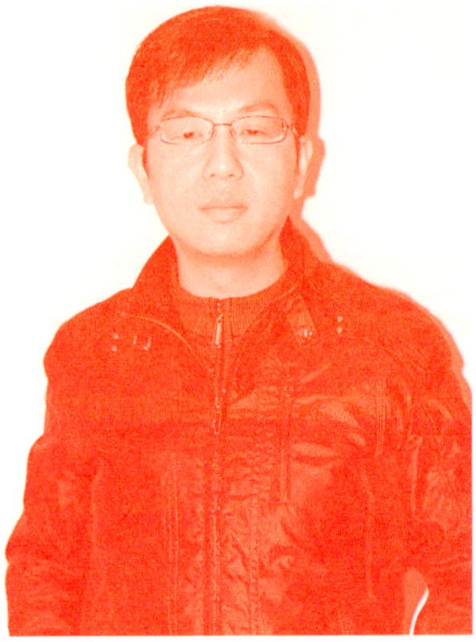
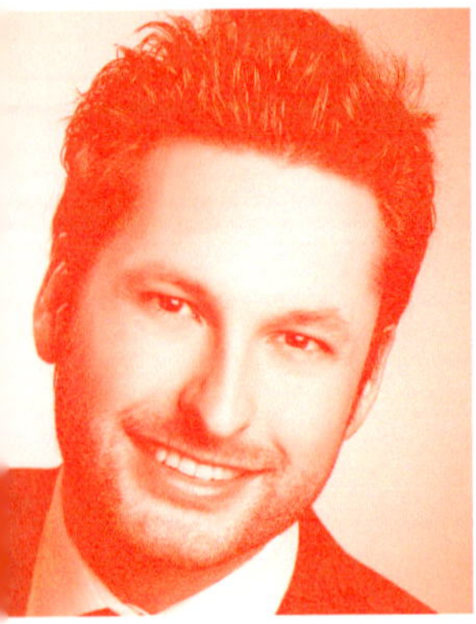
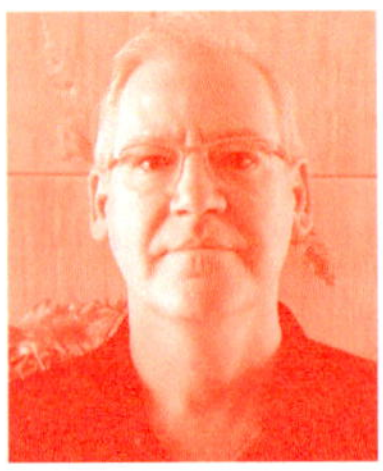

IntechOpen

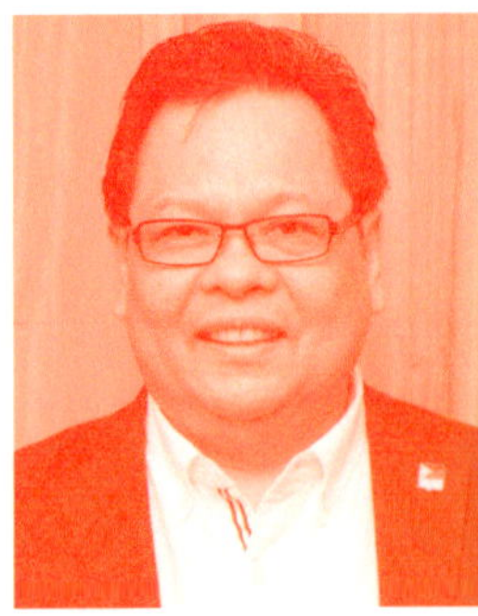
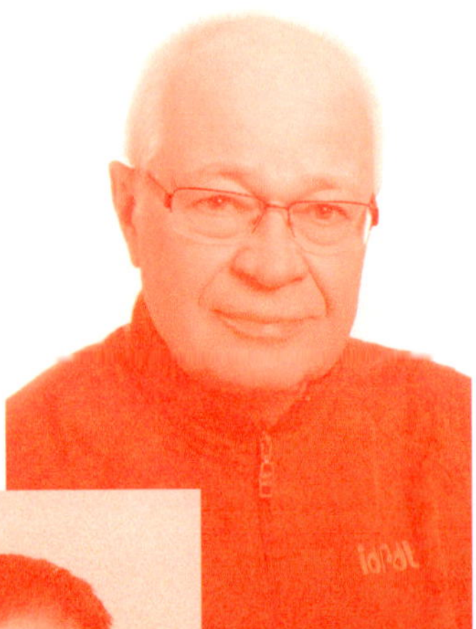
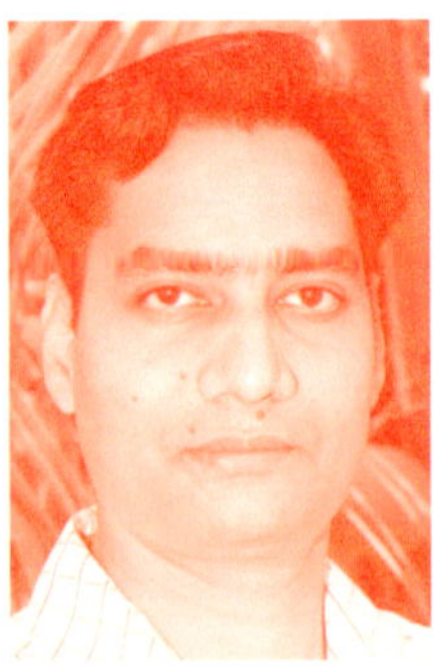
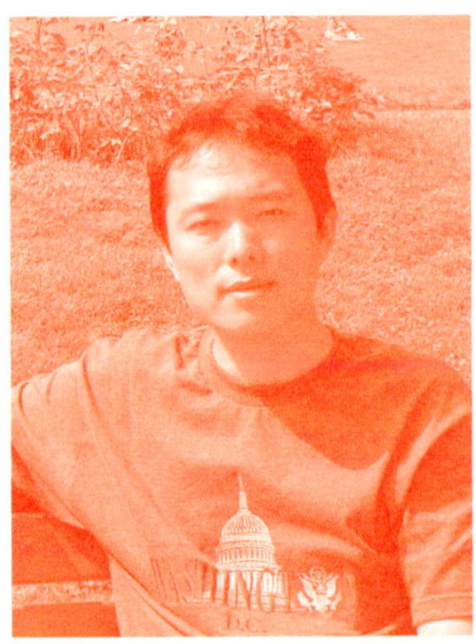
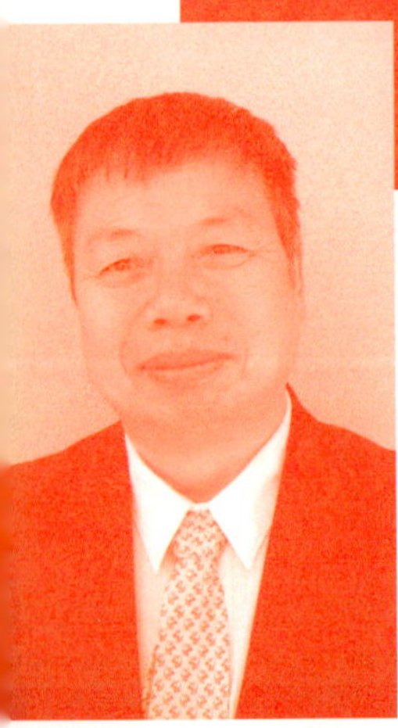
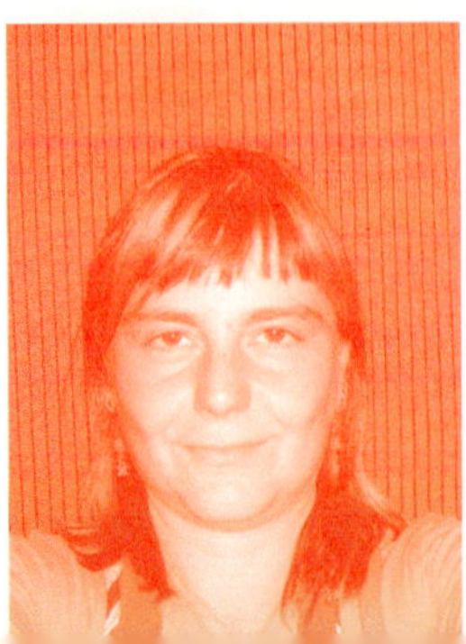

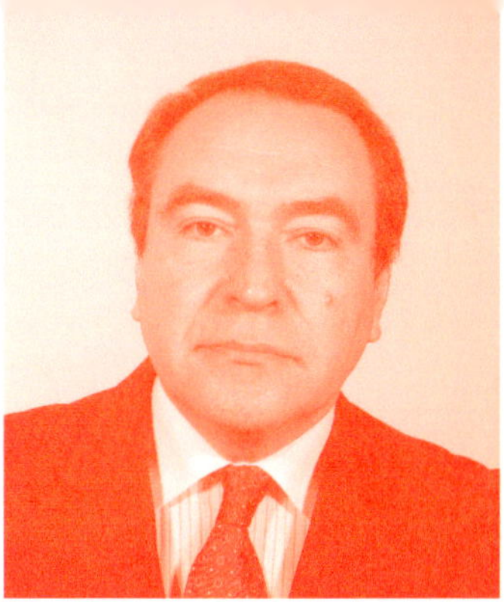

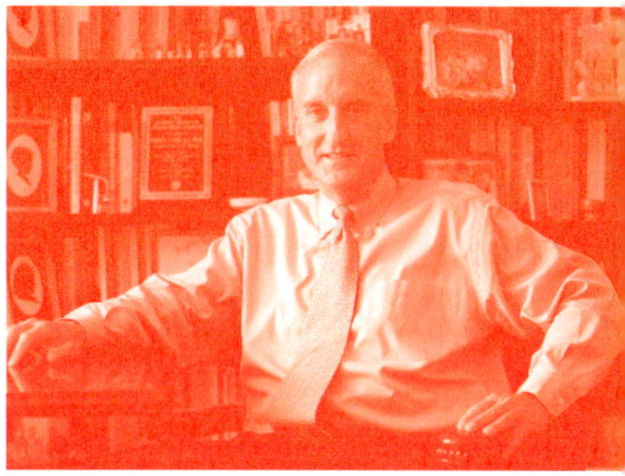

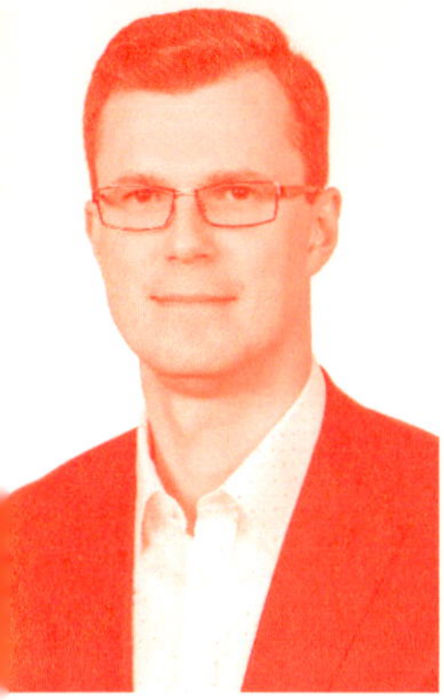

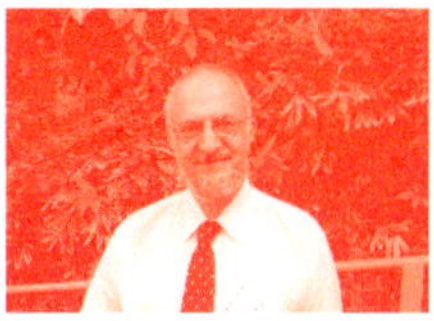

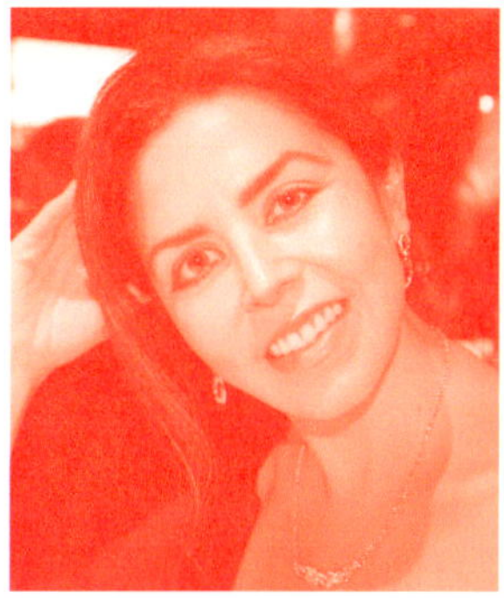

Supporting open minds since 2005

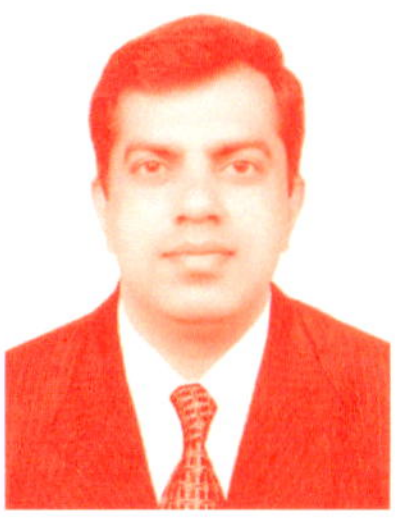

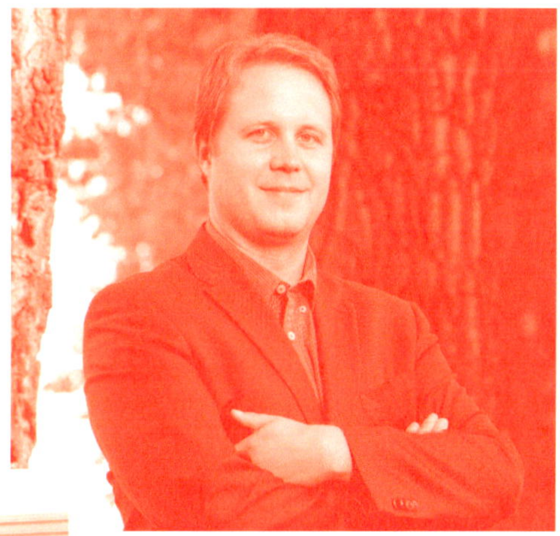

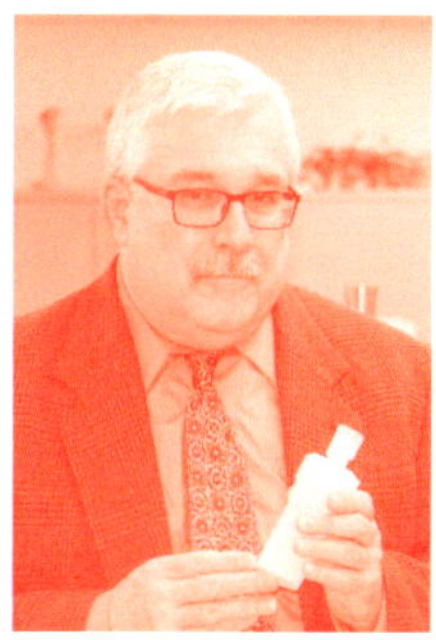

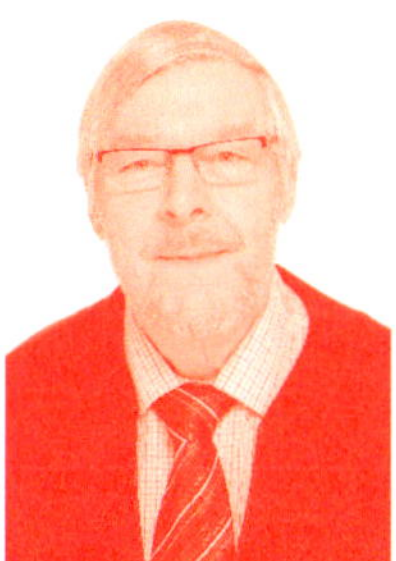

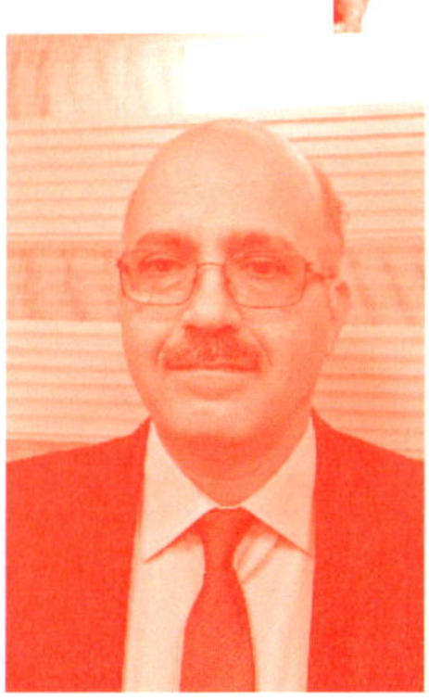

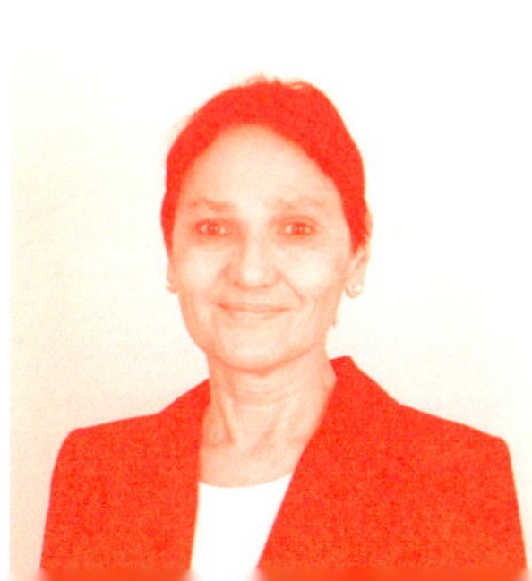

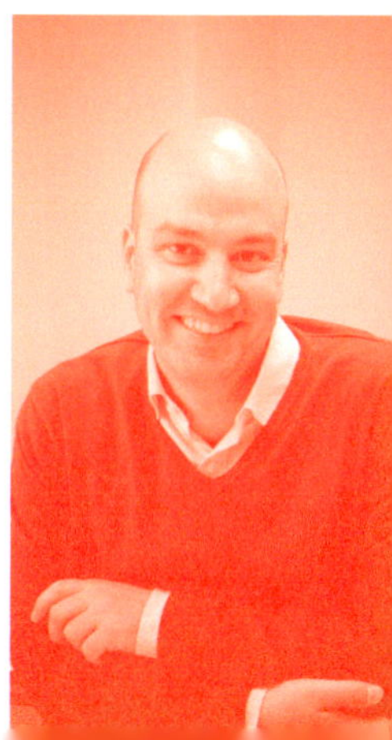

Vitamin D
http://dx.doi.org/10.5772/intechopen.93580
Edited by Öner Özdemir

Contributors
Behzat Özkan, Sezer Acar, Srđana Čulić, Małgorzata Kupisz-Urbańska Kupisz-Urbańska, Ewa Marcinowska-Suchowierska, Jacek Łukaszkiewicz, Egle Jagelaviciene, Neelakanta Kanike Kanike, Jenny Camacho, Naveen Kannekanti, Antony Macido, Öner Özdemir, Elif Gül Aydin, Vikram Singh Chauhan, Mohammad Zahid Ashraf, Syed Mohd, Aastha Mishra, Swati Sharma, Huub F.J Savelkoul, Gosia Teodorowicz, Maud Vegelin, Carl Nikolaus Homann

First published in London, United Kingdom, 2021 by IntechOpen
IntechOpen is the global imprint of INTECHOPEN LIMITED, registered in England and Wales, registration number: 11086078, 5 Princes Gate Court, London, SW7 2QJ, United Kingdom
Printed in Croatia

British Library Cataloguing-in-Publication Data
A catalogue record for this book is available from the British Library

Additional hard and PDF copies can be obtained from orders@intechopen.com

Vitamin D
Edited by Öner Özdemir
p. cm.
Print ISBN 978-1-83969-349-6
Online ISBN 978-1-83969-350-2
eBook (PDF) ISBN 978-1-83969-351-9

For EU product safety concerns:
IN TECH d.o.o., Prolaz Marije Krucifikse Kozulić 3, 51000 Rijeka, Croatia, info@intechopen.com or visit our website at intechopen.com.

Meet the editor

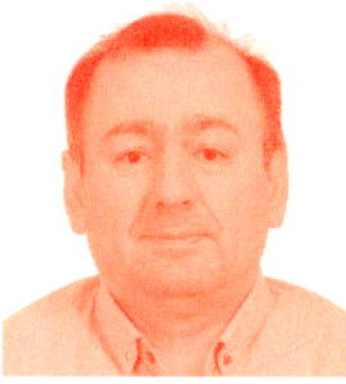

Prof. Dr. Öner Özdemir was born in Alaplı, Zonguldak, Turkey, in 1965. He graduated from İstanbul Medical School, İstanbul University, Turkey, and became a medical doctor in 1989. Dr. Ozdemir did his pediatric residency at the Department of Pediatrics, Children's Hospital, İstanbul Medical School, İstanbul, Turkey. He completed his clinical fellowship training at the Pediatric Allergy/Immunology Division, Louisiana State University, Health Sciences Center, New Orleans, LA. Dr. Ozdemir's clinical research interests are in hereditary angioedema and chronic urticaria. He has published more than 100 international and 86 national publications, 200 international and 150 national presentations, and more than 12 book chapters. He has also served as editor for five books.

Contents

Preface

This book examines the importance and role of vitamin D in health and different diseases. It is divided into four sections that cover vitamin D metabolism and deficiency; vitamin D, immune system and infections; vitamin D and dental medicine; and vitamin D and other diseases.

The first section includes three chapters. The first, by Özkan et al., examines vitamin D metabolism and deficiency; the second, by Kanike et al., discusses vitamin D deficiency in women and newborns; and the third, by Kupisz-Urbanska et al., covers vitamin D in the elderly.

The second section includes three chapters. The first chapter by Vikram et al. describes the function and relation of vitamin D in the immune system, while the second chapter by Čulić and the third by Ashraf et al. discuss the role of vitamin D in viral infections and the human coagulation system including influenza and, conventional coronaviruses, and specifically SARS-CoV-2 and its thrombotic complications.

In the third section, the chapters by Jagelaviciene and Aydın discuss the role and importance of vitamin D in periodontal diseases and dentistry.

In the fourth section, the chapter by Macido describes how vitamin D plays a role in modern diseases such as diabetes and diabetic foot ulcers. The chapter by Homann examines the role of vitamin D in central nervous system pathological processes such as different types of brain injuries and encephalopathies, stroke, meningitis, and autoimmunity including neurodegeneration. The final chapter in this section by Savelkoul et al. describes the role of vitamin D in autism spectrum disorder.

The editor is grateful to his daughter Berrin Nikâme and his wife Seval Hülya for their moral support and patience during the preparation of this book, especially during this difficult time of the COVID-19 pandemic. He also wishes to thank Author Service Manager Ms. Marijana Francetic at IntechOpen for her service.

Öner Özdemir, MD
Faculty of Medicine,
Department of Pediatrics,
Division of Allergy/Immunology,
Sakarya University,
Adapazarı, Turkey

Section 1

Vitamin D Metabolism and Deficiency

Chapter 1

Vitamin D Metabolism

Sezer Acar and Behzat Özkan

Abstract

Vitamin D plays an important role in bone metabolism. Vitamin D is a group of biologically inactive, fat-soluble prohormones that exist in two major forms: ergocalciferol (vitamin D2) produced by plants in response to ultraviolet irradiation and cholecalciferol (vitamin D3) derived from animal tissues or 7-dehydrocholesterol in human skin by the action of ultraviolet rays present in sunlight. Vitamin D, which is biologically inactive, needs two-step hydroxylation for activation. All of these steps are of crucial for Vitamin D to show its effect properly. In this section, we will present vitamin D synthesis and its action steps in detail.

Keywords: Vitamin D, Vitamin D characteristics

1. Introduction

Vitamin D plays an important role in calcium and phosphorus metabolism, which are essential for bone health and various biological functions. In vitamin D deficiency, clinical and biochemical rickets characterized by hypocalcemia (irritability, fatigue, muscle cramps, seizures), hypophosphatemia and skeletal manifestations (delayed closure of fontanelles, craniotabes, frontal bossing, bowed legs, enlarged wrists, bone pain, and short stature) in children and adolescents or osteomalacia in adults may occur. Over the past several decades, it has been reported that the efficiency of vitamin D is not limited only to maintaining bone health by managing the calcium homeostasis, but also seems to have anti-inflamatory, immune-modulating and pro-apopitothic properties [1]. There are two different precursor molecules of vitamin D. The first is vitamin D3, or cholecalciferol, which is the main source of vitamin D in the body and is synthesized from the skin by exposure to sun. Vitamin D3 can also be obtained from dietary animal foods (fish, egg yolks) or medicines (vitamin supplements). The second precursor is vitamin D2, or ergocalciferol, which can be used as a source of vitamin D via oral medication or through enriched foods. Vitamin D3 differs in molecular structure from vitamin D2 in that it has a double bond between the 22nd and 23rd carbon atoms and a methyl group on the 24th carbon atom [2]. These structural differences in vitamin D2 affect its catabolism. Compared to vitamin D3, vitamin D2 has a lower affinity for vitamin D-binding protein (VDBP), which leads to its easy removal from the circulation, a reduced formation of 25-hydroxy vitamin D2 (25OHD2) by the 25-hydroxylase enzyme, and increased inactivation by the action of 24-hydroxylase [3–5]. Although both vitamin D2 and D3 are used as drugs, studies have shown that a higher serum 25OHD2 vitamin level is obtained when vitamin D3 is used in treatment compared to vitamin D2 [6]. In addition, it has been shown that active vitamin D obtained from vitamin D3 has a higher affinity for the vitamin D receptor (VDR) [4]. Despite these differences, vitamins D2 and D3 are both metabolized in substantially the same way and are commonly referred to as vitamin D. Vitamin D is a prohormone and inactive, and to be activated, it must go through a series of enzymatic and non-enzymatic steps.

2. Vitamin D synthesis

2.1 The synthesis of vitamin D3 from the skin and the factors affecting this synthesis

Formation of vitamin D3, which is the first step of vitamin D synthesis, takes place in the epidermis by a non-enzymatic process (**Figure 1**). Vitamin D3 is the most important source of vitamin D in the body. 90–95% of vitamin D3 in the human body is produced from the skin with the effect of sunlight. Therefore, sunlight is the main source of vitamin D synthesis, and if there is sufficient exposure to sunlight, there is no need to take additional vitamin D. The mechanism of non-enzymatic photolysis of vitamin D by ultraviolet B (UVB) rays with wavelengths in the range of 290–315 nm involves the breaking of a bond in the B ring of 7-dehydrocholesterol (pro-vitamin D3), resulting in pre-vitamin D3 formation in the epidermis. Subsequently, two different double bonds are formed between the broken carbon atoms in the B ring by thermo-sensitive non-enzymatic process, and the formation of vitamin D3 from pre-vitamin D3 is completed (**Figure 2**) [7].

The synthesis of vitamin D3 from pro-vitamin D3 in the skin is adjusted according to the needs of the organism. In a period of just fifteen minutes, pre-vitamin D3 is synthesized from pro-vitamin D3 with the effect of ultraviolet light. Conversion from pre-vitamin D3 to vitamin D3 occurs by isomerization in a rather slow and thermo-sensitive manner. In the case of exposure to UV rays or solar radiation for a long period, pre-vitamin D3 converts to a number of photolyzed inactive by-products, such as lumisterol (irreversible) or tachysterol (which can be converted back to pre-vitamin D3). These by-products have no biological effects (**Figure 2**). In other words, once pre-vitamin D3 is formed in the skin, it turns into either vitamin D3 or inactive metabolites. This is a physiological control mechanism that protects the body from vitamin D intoxication by preventing unnecessary vitamin D synthesis [8, 9].

Some conditions that prevent UVB rays from reaching the skin cause a decrease in vitamin D production. One of these reasons is the ozone (O3) layer surrounding the atmosphere, which reflects some of the sun's rays, preventing them from reaching the Earth and their harmful carcinogenic effects on the skin.

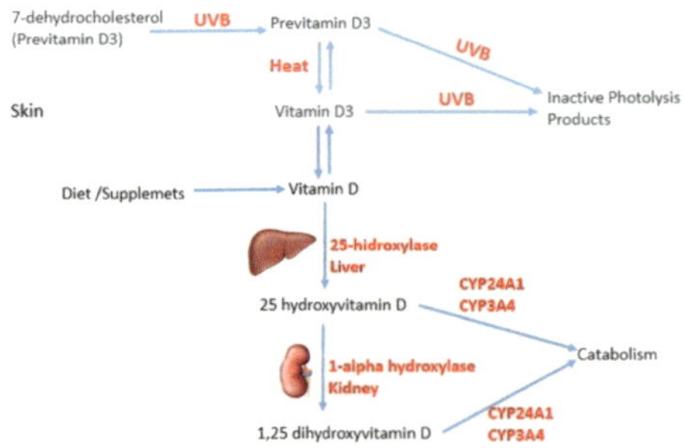

Figure 1.
Vitamin D metabolism.

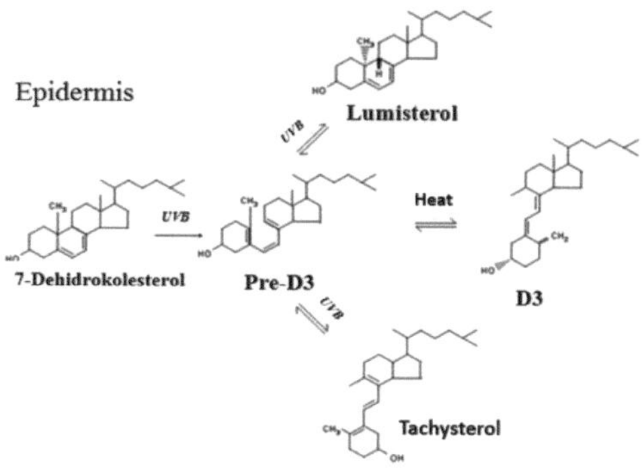

Figure 2.
Vitamin D3 synthesis from 7-dehydrocholesterol in the epidermis.

The peak UVB wavelength required for optimal vitamin D synthesis from the skin is 297 (290–315) nm [1, 8]. In addition, air pollution, aerosols, water vapors, and increased nitrogens in the air also play a role in preventing sunlight reaching the Earth, and consequently result in a potential reduced synthesis of vitamin D [8]. Another factor affecting the effectiveness of UVB rays in the synthesis of vitamin D in the skin is the solar zenith angle, which affects how UVB rays reach the world quantifiably. When the sun moves in a path closer to the horizon, which occurs in the northern latitudes in the winter season, vitamin D synthesis is more adversely affected (or reduced). In the summer time in the northern latitudes, a normal biosynthesis is more propitious or favorable. The narrowing of this angle indicates that the sun rays reach the Earth more steeply and intensely. The solar zenith angle is closely related to sunbathing time during the day, the seasons and the geographic region (latitude). Sunlight reaches the Earth most intensely in the "mid-day" when it is summer in the northern latitudes and the weather is clear. Finally, it is thought that sunlight exposure is sufficient for vitamin D synthesis in all geographic regions below 35 degrees north or south latitude all year round. In regions beyond this latitude toward the poles, especially in winter, sunlight is not sufficient for vitamin D synthesis. For example, UVB rays are not sufficient for vitamin D synthesis between October and April in Rome, which is located on 41.9 degrees north latitude, and between November and February in Berlin and Amsterdam, which are located on 52 degrees north latitude. For the reasons mentioned above, it is difficult to predict how much UVB rays reach the skin and how much of this increases serum vitamin D levels. In experimental studies, it has been reported that UVB rays that will cause minimal erythema in 25% of the skin are equivalent to 1000 units of oral vitamin D intake [2, 3, 8].

UVB rays are also affected by the individual's clothing style, use of sunscreen, and skin colour determined by pigmentation with melanin. In dressing style, especially the type of the clothing fabric used is of great importance [10]. Non-synthetic, light-colored, and linen garments play a less preventive role in UV rays reaching the skin than do garments made of silk, nylon, polyester, and wools. For example, black-dyed cotton clothing prevents 98.6% of UVB rays from reaching the skin compared to white (undyed) cotton clothing, which blocks 47.7% of UVB. Topical sunscreens also prevent UVB rays from reaching the skin by absorbing, reflecting or dispersing them. Topical creams with a sun protection factor of 8 or higher block vitamin D synthesis above 95% [11]. Melanin is a large, opaque polymer synthesized by melanocytes in the skin through the stimulus of exposure to UVB rays. Melanin competes with dehydrocholesterol 7 in the skin to absorb UVB photons and thus inhibits vitamin D synthesis [12]. Individuals with dark skin colour have more melanin pigment in their epidermis than light-skinned individuals and require higher concentrations of sunlight for the same amount of vitamin D synthesis [12]. In addition, the 7-dehydrocholesterol level (provitamin D) in the epidermis can also affect the serum vitamin D concentration. For example, 7-dehydrocholesterol levels in scar tissue caused by the burn are reduced by 42.5% of normal. In these cases, progressive vitamin D deficiency develops, especially if supplemental dietary vitamin D is not provided. Moreover, the content of pro-vitamin D in the skin decreases with age. Skin temperature is also important for vitamin D synthesis. Vitamin D from pre-vitamin D by isomerization whose rate of formation is temperature- dependent. The rate decreases as the skin temperature decreases. In a healthy person, the skin temperature is lower than the central body temperature and varies between 29 and 35 degrees Celcius. When the skin temperature is 37 degrees Celcius, the isomerization of vitamin D from pre-vitamin D occurs within 2.5 hours [13, 14].

2.1.1 Biosynthesis of 25OHD3 (25-hydroxylase) in liver

Vitamin D3 synthesized in the skin is released into the systemic circulation and all forms are transported by binding to VDBP in serum. A portion of vitamin D, a fat-soluble vitamin, is stored in adipose tissue for use when necessary. The ability of vitamin D to be stored in adipose tissue extends its total half-life in the body up to approximately 2 months. When vitamin D3 is transported to the liver, it is first converted into 25OHD3 by the cytochrome P450 25-hydroxylase enzyme. 25OHD3 is the main circulating form of vitamin D, and it is the parameter that provides the best estimation about the body's vitamin D pool [15]. Various enzymes that show 25-hydroxylase properties have been described in the body. Among these, the first one is CYP27A1 located in mitochondria, and the second is microsomally located CYP2R1 [1, 6, 16]. CYP27A1 also exerts 27-hydroxylase effect and is involved in bile acid synthesis. Although CYP27A1 is expressed in different tissues of the body, the tissues where it is most commonly found are liver and skeletal muscle tissues [1, 2]. In experimental studies, it was reported that the serum 25OHD3 levels were increased in mice which possess an inactivated CYP27A1 gene, and that rickets did not occur in these mice [17]. Interestingly, in this study, it was shown that CYP2R1 expression increased after CYP27A1 gene inactivation, and consequently 25-hydroxylation activity increased [17]. In addition, individuals with a CYP27A1-inactivating mutation develop a cerebrotendinous xanthomatosis disease with bile and cholesterol synthesis disorders, but without rickets manifestation [18]. Besides CYP27A1, different CYP-450 enzymes with 25-hydroxylase activity (CYP2D25, CYP2J2, CYP2J3, and CYP2C11) have been identified in humans and animals, with the most important one in human being CYP2R1. It is assumed that enzymes other than CYP2R1 have effects only on serum 25OHD3 levels [2].

Studies have suggested that CYP2R1 is the major enzyme responsible for 25-hydroxylation in the human body. This enzyme is expressed in many tissues, mainly liver, skin, and testis [1, 2, 17]. The 25-hydroxylase encoded by the CYP2R1 gene was first described by Cheng et al. [19]. It was first reported by Chen et al. [20] that homozygous inactivating mutations of this gene lead to clinically observed rickets (vitamin D-dependent rickets type IB) in Nigerian families. It has been reported that these cases gave suboptimal response to standard vitamin D (inactive vitamin D2 or D3 forms) treatment [21]. The CYP2R1 enzyme has equal affinity for the different forms of vitamin D precursors (D2 or D3) [19]. Studies have shown that 25-hydroxylase effect increased in male rats given estrogen, whereas this activity decreased in female rats given testosterone [21]. Despite experimental studies, the effect of sex steroids on 25-hydroxylase enzyme activity in humans is unknown.

It has been shown that in CYP2R1-null mice, the level of 25OHD3 decreases by 50%, when both CYP2R1 and CYP27A1 are inactivated, and that serum 25OHD3 levels decrease by 70%, and serum 25OHD3 level remains at a measurable level in both cases [2, 17]. This supports the view that serum vitamin D level is compensated by other enzymes with recruitable 25-hydroxylase enzyme activity.

2.1.2 Formation of active vitamin D [1,25 (OH) 2D3] by 1-alpha hydroxylase (CYP27B1) in the kidney

The final step of active vitamin D formation takes place in the proximal tubules of the kidney, led by the enzyme 1-alpha hydroxylase. 25OHD3, which is bound to VDBP, is taken into tubule cells and metabolized (1-alpha hydroxylation) through megalin and cubilin, which are transmembrane proteins located in renal tubules and act as surface receptors for VDBP in tubules. 25OHD3, which then undergoes 1-alpha hydroxylation [1, 2]. The 1-alpha hydroxylase enzyme hydroxylates the first carbon atom in the A ring of 25OHD3, resulting in the formation of 1,25 (OH) 2D3 [1]. CYP27B1 is the only enzyme that has 1-alpha hydroxylase activity. This enzyme, which belongs to the cytochrome P-450 enzyme system, is located in the inner mitochondrial membrane and carries out electron transport to NADPH via ferrodoxin-ferrodoxin reductase [1, 2]. The gene for the enzyme consists of nine exons and is located 12q14.1 chromosomal region. Four different groups reported the cloning and sequencing of the gene from rats, mice and humans [22–26]. In biallelic inactivating mutations of this enzyme, which is highly homologous to some mitochondria located cytochrome P-450 enzymes (CYP27A1 and CYP24A1), 25OHD3 cannot be converted to 1.25 (OH) 2D3, which is the active vitamin D form. In this case, the clinical picture of vitamin D-dependent rickets type 1A (also called pseudo-vitamin D deficiency rickets) occurs [23]. This disease is typically characterized by rickets, with clinically observed very low 1.25 (OH) 2D3, low serum calcium/phosphorus, and high parathyroid hormone (PTH) levels. CYP27B1 is expressed mainly in the renal proximal tubules and in the placenta during pregnancy [27]. While the expression of the gene encoding this enzyme increases with the effect of PTH, it decreases with FGF23 (fibroblast growth factor 23) and 1.25 (OH) 2D3. CYP27B1 gene is also expressed in lung, brain, breast and intestinal system epithelial cells, immune system cells (macrophage, T/B lymphocytes and dendritic cells), osteoblasts, chondrocytes, and some tumor cell types [1, 2]. The regulation of the extra-renal localized 1-alpha hydroxylase enzyme differs. In some granulomatous diseases where monocyte/macrophage cells play an important role (sarcoidosis, tuberculosis, Chron's disease, etc.), with the effect of IL-1, TNF-α, IFN-γ, 1-alpha hydroxylase enzyme activity increases and 1,25 (OH) 2D3 is synthesized in greater quantities than normal, and consequently, hypercalcemia and hypercalciuria emerge [28–30]. Additionally, since cells in these tissues do not have PTH receptors, it is not yet understood how PTH exerts its enhancing effect on the 1-alpha hydroxylase enzyme activity in these cells. In one study, it has been suggested that this enhancing effect of PTH may have occurred through post-transcriptional effects [31]. Moreover, 1-alpha hydroxylase enzyme in these cells is not inhibited by 1,25 (OH) 2D3 or hypercalcemia, unlike the renal tubules.

2.1.3 Inactivation of vitamin D by 24-hydroxylase (CYP24A1)

The 24-hydroxylase enzyme is located in the mitochondrial inner membrane of the cells located in the proximal kidney and, like CYP27B1, uses the electron transport system that enables electron transport to NADPH via ferrodoxine-ferrodoxin reductase. It is known that CYP24A1, which is the only enzyme showing

24-hydroxylase enzyme activity in humans, can also exhibit 23-hydroxylase enzyme activity [2]. Which enzyme will be more prominent varies according to the species [32]. The 23-hydroxylase, another enzyme that degrades vitamin D, is the first step activity in the conversion of 1,25 (OH) 2D3 to 1,25 (OH) 2D3-23,26-lactone.

The CYP24A1 enzyme, encoded in 20q13 chromosomal region and having 24-hydroxylase enzyme activity, initiates catabolic processes that lead to the inactivation of vitamin D by hydroxylating the 24th carbon atom. This enzyme can use both 25OHD3 and 1.25 (OH) 2D3 as substrates, but has a higher affinity for 1.25 (OH) 2D3. As a result of a series of enzymatic reactions, calcitroic acid is formed, which becomes biologically inactive. On the other hand, it has been suggested that the 1,25 (OH) 2D3-23,26-lactone, which is formed in the 23-hydroxylase pathway, lowers serum calcium level, inhibits bone resorption induced by 1.25 (OH) 2D3, and stimulates the formation of collagen tissue in bone tissue [33]. In addition, it has been suggested that 24,25 (OH) 2D3 is not only a degradation product, but has an important role in bone metabolism, especially in endochondral bone formation [34].

There are two vitamin D response elements (VDRE) in the promoter region of the CYP24A1 gene [35]. When active vitamin D is bound to the these one of VDRE after heterodimerization with various molecules, thus initiates the inactivation process of vitamin D. In addition, it has been shown that CYP24A1 gene expression decreases with the effect of PTH, whereas it increases with increased FGF23 concentrations [1, 32, 36, 37]. Inactivating mutations in CYP24A1 lead to an idiopathic infantile hypercalcemia clinic characterized by hypercalcemia, hypercalciuria, nephrocalcinosis, low PTH, low 24.25 (OH) 2D3 and high 1.25 (OH) 2D3 levels [37]. As a result, CYP24A1 is a critical enzyme that protects the body from excessive accumulation and possible intoxication of vitamin D.

2.1.4 3-epimerization of Vitamin D

3-epimerase activity was first demonstrated in 2001, with the detection of the 3-epi form of 1,25 (OH) 2D3 in keratinocytes [38]. In the following years, epimer forms of 25OHD3 and other vitamin D metabolites were discovered. However, the enzyme or enzymes involved in epimerization has not yet been identifiedpurified or cloned. This enzyme changes the hydroxyl group in the 3rd carbon of the A ring from the alpha orientation to the beta orientation, causing the three-dimensional structure to change and consequently alter the activity of CYP27B1 and CYP24A1 enzymes on vitamin D metabolism. These epimers can be detected by special liquid chromatography-mass spectroscopy (LC-MC) measurement methods [2]. C-3 epimer forms of 25OHD3 and 1,25 (OH) 2D3 have been shown to have lower affinity for VDR and VDBP compared to non-epimer forms [38]. The C-3 epimer form of 1,25 (OH) 2D3 has been shown to cause PTH suppression similar to the non-epimer form, but its effects on bone tissue are not clear. In addition, epimer forms have also been shown to have non-calcium effects (anti-proliferative effect, surfactant synthesis) [39]. It has been shown that the serum levels of vitamin C-3 epimer forms are found to be 60% higher in the period between the neonatal period and one year old, and decrease after one year of age and decrease to very low levels in adulthood [2, 38]. The reason why epimer forms with limited biological activity are important is that they cause interference and false high results in serum 25OHD3 and 25OHD2 measurement. Therefore, it is important to prefer the method (especially LC–MS / MS) that can exclude this effect of epimer forms that cause serum vitamin D measurement interference. However, the use of LC–MS/MS method in the measurement of vitamin D has not become widespread in the world, and the use of this method is only recommended in selected cases.

2.1.5 Transport of Vitamin D

The largest part of the circulating vitamin D is in the form of 25OHD3, and its serum concentration is in equilibrium with the level of vitamin D stored in muscle and adipose tissues. The parameter that gives the best information about the whole vitamin D pool in the body is 25OHD3 and its known half-life of 15–20 days. Most of all forms of vitamin D in circulation (85–88%) are transported by binding to VDBP and the remaining part (12–15%) to albumin [2, 40]. The serum concentration of VDBP is 4–8 nM and only 2% of it is bound with vitamin D metabolites [2]. Moreover, the affinity of VDBP to 25OHD3 is 20 times higher than 1.25 (OH) 2D3 [3]. 0.03% of 25OHD3 and 0.4% of 1.25 (OH) 2D3 are in free form [2]. In chronic liver disease or nephrotic syndrome, VDBP and albumin levels and thus total serum 25OHD3 and 1.25 (OH) 2D3 levels decrease, but the levels of free forms are not affected [41]. Likewise, since the VDBP level may decrease during the acute disease period, evaluating the body's vitamin D pool by measuring the serum 25OHD3 level with standard immunoassays may lead to misinterpretations [42]. In conclusion, while the total levels of vitamin D forms are affected by the VDBP level, there is no relationship between VDBP and free vitamin D forms, which are essential for biological activity. It was shown that both 25OHD3 and 1.25 (OH) 2D3 levels in VDBP-null mice were lower than wild type mice, but serum PTH and calcium levels were similarly normal in both groups [43]. This supports the view that serum vitamin D level measured by the standard method may not be an indicator of biologically active vitamin D pool. In addition, the predisposition of VDBP-null mice to the development of osteomalacia after a vitamin D-restricted diet suggests that VDBP may play a role in maintaining the existing vitamin D pool [44]. In addition, some single nucleotide polymorphisms (GC1F, GC1S, GC2) in the *VDBP* gene have been shown to impact the affinity of VDBP on vitamin D metabolites [1, 45, 46].

3. The mechanism of Vitamin D actions

Vitamin D provides its biological effect in two different ways. The first is by directly affecting gene transcription (genomic effect) as other steroid hormones. This effect is relatively slow and usually occurs within hours or days. The second is the non-genomic pathway whose biological effect is relatively faster (within minutes). Vitamin D exerts its non-genomic effect by directly altering the transmembrane passage of some ions (Ca, Cl) or by affecting intracellular signaling pathway activities (cAMP, PKA, PLC, PI-3 kinase and MAP kinase) [1, 2]. Genetic studies on vitamin D support that active vitamin D directly or indirectly regulates 0.8–5% of the total genome, suggesting the role of active vitamin D in many actions such as regulation of cellular growth, DNA repair, differentiation, apoptosis, membrane transport, cellular metabolism, adhesion and oxidative stress [1–3, 47].

3.1 Genomic effect of Vitamin D

The active form of vitamin D displays this effect through the vitamin D receptor (VDR). VDR is a member of the nuclear hormone receptor superfamily, which includes steroid, thyroid hormone, and retinoic acid receptors [48]. The VDR gene located on chromosome 12 consists of 427 amino acids encoded by. The structure of the VDR consists of a relatively short N-terminal domain compared to other nuclear receptors, two zinc-fingers that allow the receptor to bind to DNA, and a highly

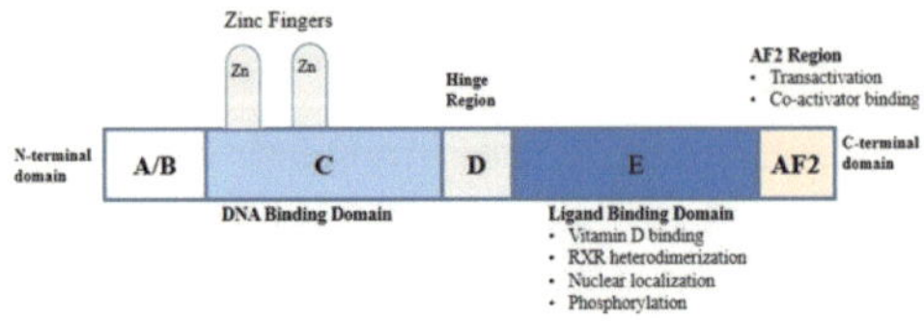

Figure 3.
The structure of the Vitamin D receptor (VDR).

variable C-terminal region, and the hinge region connecting binding these domains (**Figure 3**) [2]. The DNA-binding region of the receptor is rich in cysteine, and the sequence of this region is largely conserved between species. The zinc-finger structure close to the C-terminal part of VDR determines the specificity for the VDRE (vitamin D response element), which is the binding site on the DNA. The other zinc-finger structure is involved in the heterodimerization of VDR with RXR (retinoid X receptor) [1, 2]. The ligand-binding part of the receptor consists of 12 α-helix structures (H1-12; the H12 part is also called AF2) and 3 β-sheet structures (S1-3) [49]. The AF-2 region located at the end of the C-terminal is the binding site of co-activator complex structures such as SRC (steroid receptor coactivator) and DRIP (vitamin D receptor interacting protein). Transcription is initiated by binding co-activators to this region [50]. Apart from these functional domains, there are NLS (nuclear localization signal) regions within the DNA binding region of VDR, which are necessary for maintaining transcriptional activity [2]. In addition, there is a hinge region between the ligand-binding and DNA-binding domains of the VDR that ensures molecule stabilization.

After active vitamin D crosses the target cell membrane, it interacts with the ligand-binding domain of its own receptor (VDR) in the cytoplasm of the cell. Vitamin D is embedded in the ligand-binding domain, and subsequently, in the H12 alpha-helix H12 (AF-2) region, which is located at the end of the ligand binding part [51]. This critical conformational change of AF-2 facilitates the binding of co-activators in later stages [52]. In the next step, vitamin D-bound VDR binds to RXRα to form a VDR/RXR heterodimer structure that binds to cognate VDR elements (VDRE) in the promoter region in the target genes with a high affinity to initiate gene activation or inhibition. There are many gene-specific VDREs associated with bone metabolism, xenobiotic detoxification, drug resistance, cell growth and differentiation, angiogenesis, mammalian hair growth cycle, lipid synthesis regulation, apoptosis, and immune functions, suggesting that vitamin D has numerous regulatory roles in various organs or tissues in the body [53].

After active vitamin D-VDR-RXR-VDRE interaction, the progression of transcription is controlled by co-activator and co-repressors. The best known co-activators are the p160 co-activator family (eg CBP/p300 and p/CAF) and SRC 1,2,3. Both bind to the AF-2 part and have histone acetyl transferase (HAT) activity, which enables the opening of the histone structure and thus facilitates gene expression [54]. The SRC complex has three NR regions that facilitate binding and contain LxxLL (L, leucine; x, any amino acid) motifs. Likewise, the DRIP complex (Mediator) also has NR regions with LxxLL motifs consisting of 15 or more amino acids [55]. Unlike SRC, DRIP complex does not have HAT activity. This suggests the fact that both protein complexes play a complementary role in the initiation of transcription. The mediator multi-protein complex DRIP205/MED1 (also known as MED1) accumulates around RNA polymerase 2of the initiation complex. This complex then interacts with the TATA region in the promoter region and enables transcription to be initiated [56]. Co-repressors (eg SMRT and NCoR) have histone de-acetylase activity and inhibit transcription by preventing unfolding of the histone core.

3.2 Non-genomic effects of vitamin D

Some of the hormones that act on the nuclear hormone receptor can also exert their biological effects on the membrane receptor without the need for additional gene regulation [2]. The non-genomic effect occurs through messenger-mediated pathways. Estrogen, progesterone, testosterone, corticosteroids and thyroid hormones have been reported to exert their effects by using both genomic and non-genomic pathways [2]. Vitamin D has been shown to directly regulate the activation or distribution of various ion-transport channel proteins (for calcium and chloride) and of enzymes (protein kinase C and phospholipase C) through the membrane receptor in osteoblast, liver, muscle, and intestinal cells (**Figure 4**) [57–62]. In order to demonstrate the non-genomic effect of vitamin D, many studies have been conducted on intestinal calcium absorption. Rapid vesicular calcium absorption (also called transcaltachia) has been shown in the chick intestinal tract [63]. Further experimental studies have shown that intestinal calcium transport cannot be blocked by the administration of actinomycin D (which inhibits the genomic effect) [64], whereas calcium absorption can be blocked by inhibition of voltage-gated L-type calcium channel proteins [65] or by protein kinase C [66].

Apart from the intestinal system, it has been suggested that the non-genomic effect also occurs in chondrocytes in the growth plate and keratinocytes in the skin [67, 68]. Vitamin D is believed to exert its non-genomic effects through VDR analog and MARRS (also known as ERp57/GRp58/ERp60) receptors located on the cell membrane [69, 70]. These membrane receptors are located within the caveolar lipid layer [71]. In addition, research findings indicate that VDR is also necessary for the expression of membrane receptors that involve in the emergence of non-genomic effect [1, 2]. In studies evaluating the effects of vitamin D analogs (6-s-cis or 6-s-trans conformations), the 6-s-cis form can activate intestinal rapid calcium entry even though the VDR affinity is very low, whereas the 6-s-trans form has been shown to be ineffective in calcium metabolism [67].

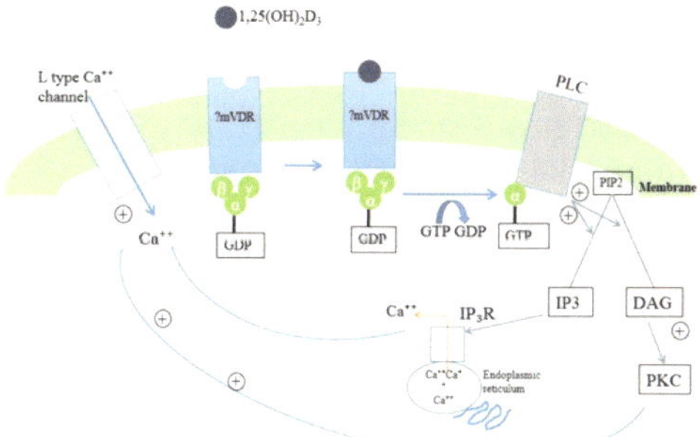

Figure 4.
Representation of the signal transduction pathways where Vitamin D has its non-genomic effect (2). After vitamin D binds to the membrane receptor, GDP in the G protein α-subunit turns into GTP and activation occurs. The α-subunit of the G protein is separated from other subunits and binds to phospholipase C (PLC). The PLC is then activated to convert phosphoinositol bisphosphate (PIP2) to inositol triphosphate (IP3) and diacylglycerol (DAG). Calcium release from the endoplasmic reticulum via the IP3 receptor (IP3R); DAG activates PKC. PKC, on the other hand, provides calcium entry into the cell via the L-type calcium channel in the membrane.

4. Effects of Vitamin D on calcium and phosphorus

4.1 Intestinal calcium absorption

One of the most important functions of vitamin D is to increase calcium absorption from the intestines. Calcium absorption from the intestinal tract occurs trans-cellular and para-cellular processes mediated through genomic and non-genomic effects. Among these, the trans-cellular pathway largely utilized by the intestinal system, which is regulated by vitamin D [2]. The absorption effect of vitamin D with non-genomic effect of calcium occurs directly on the membrane (transcaltachia). The channel-mediated calcium absorption effect of vitamin D occurs more slowly [2].

Calcium enters the epithelian cell by the effect of an electrical and chemical gradient via calcium channel protein TRPV6 (which has significant sequence homology to TRPV5 in the kidney), the transmembrane protein at the lumenal brush border edge of the intestinal epithelial cell. The expression of TRPV6 is activated by vitamin D [72]. Reduced intestinal calcium transport is observed in TRPV6 null mice [73]. Calcium entering the cell binds to calmodulin (CaM), which is bound with myosin 1A (also known as brush border myosin I). This formed complex allows calcium to be transported across the microvilli. Subsequently, the transport of calcium up to the basolateral membrane occurs inside the vesicle via calbindin-D9k (CaBP). The affinity of calcium for calbindinin is greater than for calmodulin, and better facilitates calcium transport inside the cell [74]. The calcium reaching the basolateral membrane is pumped out of the cell to systemic circulation via the Ca-ATPase (PMCA1b) pump located on the membrane [1, 2]. In addition, although it is less important, NCX (sodium/calcium exchanger), located in the basolateral region, also plays a role in excretion of calcium [2, 75]. Vitamin D shows its increasing effect on intestinal calcium absorption by inducing expression of TRPV6, CaBP and PMCAb and increasing the binding affinity of CaM to myosin 1A [1, 2].

Intestinal calcium absorption, serum calcium level and bone mineral content in Kalbindin D9k null mice (regardless of dietary calcium level) have been shown to be similar to normal mice [76]. Intestinal calcium absorption was found to be normal in calbindin D9k and TRPV6 null mice when a diet containing the daily requirement for calcium was given [77]. These findings indicate there is a mechanism other than the genomic effect through which vitamin D exerts its action (a non-genomic effect) in calcium absorption in the intestines when the amount of calcium in the diet is sufficient.

While trans-cellular calcium absorption is effective in compensating for a low-calcium diet, para-cellular calcium transport becomes important with the increase in calcium content in the diet [1]. Paracellular transport occurs through the extracellular space between the layer of the epithelial cells in the intestine. Although it was previously thought that vitamin D does not affect para-cellular calcium absorption, studies conducted in recent years indicate otherwise, with vitamin D still affecting calcium absorption by increasing levels of various transmembrane and adhesion proteins that control the extracellular space between cells [78, 79]. However, it is not clear at what stage of the paracellular pathway these proteins are involved.

Phosphate, another important molecule for bone mineralization, is actively absorbed mostly in the jejunum, with absorption influenced by vitamin D [2]. This absorption is provided by sodium-phosphate co-transporter IIb (NaPi IIb). In experimental studies, it has been shown that phosphate absorption is blocked when cycloheximide, which inhibits protein synthesis, is given [80]. This situation supports that phosphate absorption occurs by genomic effect. Vitamin D increases NaPi-IIb expression and thus phosphate absorption [2].

4.2 The effect of vitamin D on the kidneys

Most of the calcium that reaches the kidney tubules is absorbed from the proximal and distal tubules and approximately 1–2% of it is excreted through urine. Approximately 65% of calcium absorption in the kidney is passively absorbed paracellularly from the proximal tubules with the sodium gradient and independent of vitamin D direct action [1]. The rest of the calcium is absorbed from the ascending limb of the loop of Henle (20%), the distal tubules (15–20%), and the collecting ducts (5%) [81]. Vitamin D plays an important role in calcium absorption in the distal tubules and provides active calcium absorption via the trans-cellular pathway with the help of an electrochemical gradient [1]. Calcium is taken into the cell by TRPV5 channel on the surface of the tubular cell and is transported inside the cell by calbindin-D9k and D28k. Transported to the basolateral part of the cell, calcium is released into the systemic circulation by NCX1 (sodium/calcium exchanger) and PMCA1b. This mechanism is similar to that in the intestinal tract. Vitamin D increases the expression of TRPV5, calbindin, NCX and PMCA1b.

Phosphate is reabsorbed by sodium-dependent phosphate carrier proteins (NaPi-IIa and NaPi-IIc) in proximal tubular cells under vitamin D control. In addition, for phosphate reabsorption, a Na/K-ATPase channel located in the basolateral membrane is also needed [1, 2]. The impact of vitamin D on transport channels is not clearly known. While PTH increases the lysosomal degradation of phosphate transport channels, FGF23 causes a decrease in the expression of these channels [1, 2, 82].

4.3 The effect of vitamin D on bone tissue

Calcium, phosphorus and vitamin D are important molecules for bone metabolism and health. Calcium is one of the most abundant minerals in the body and is obtained entirely from dietary sources. In addition to its various biological effects in the body, it is also essential for bone metabolism [83]. More than 99% of the total body calcium is found in the bone tissue as a calcium-phosphate mineral complex, while the remaining <1% is distributed between the intracellular and extracellular compartments [83]. While 40% of calcium outside bone tissue is bound to protein, 9% forms ionic complexes, and the remaining 51% is found as free ions [84, 85]. Ionized calcium balances the calcium pool in the intracellular-extracellular area and plays an important role in bone metabolism. This balance is provided by the cooperation of various hormones (PTH, vitamin D) and the organs they affect (kidney, bone and intestinal system) [83–85]. Where there is vitamin D deficiency (nutritional or genetic) or VDR-inactivating mutations, serum levels of calcium and phosphate, which play an important role in bone development and growth, are reduced and thus rickets/osteomalacia emerge. Rickets is a disease characterized by excessive osteoid tissue accumulation and defective mineralization of the epiphyseal plate, which occurs as a result of insufficient mineralization in the epiphyseal plates of growing bones [1, 2]. Osteomalacia is a disease characterized by a deterioration in the mineralization of the newly formed osteoid and a decrease in bone turnover.

There is a continuous remodeling cycle consisting bone tissue resorption and mineralization. When calcium, phosphorus, and vitamin D are sufficient, this cycle continues in a balanced manner. In the case of negative calcium balance caused by insufficient calcium intake with diet or increased renal calcium loss, vitamin D increases bone resorption in osteoblasts through VDR signaling, resulting in calcium passage from bone to blood, which leads to impaired bone mineralization. Vitamin D increases the expression of RANKL (receptor activator of NF-κB ligand), which is an osteoclastogenic factor from osteoblasts [86, 89]. RANKL stimulates osteoclastogenesis and increases osteoclast formation by binding to its related receptor, RANK [87]. In conclusion, in the case of negative calcium balance, vitamin D tries to keep the serum calcium level in a certain balance by increasing resorption and decreasing mineralization [1].

In the case of a positive calcium balance, the osteoblastogenic activity of vitamin D is prominent. In this situation where anti-resorbtive effect is in the predominant, bone mineral density increases. The occurrence of this effect has been associated with a decrease in the RANKL/OPG (osteoproteogerin) ratio and an increase in LRP-5 (LDL receptor related protein 5) expression [1]. LRP-5 is controlled by the VDR and is a necessary co-receptor for the anabolic effect of osteoblasts [88]. In addition, vitamin D plays a role in the proliferation of chondrocytes in the growth plate through genomic action.

5. Regulation of vitamin D metabolism

Pro-vitamin-D3, pre-vitamin D3 and then vitamin D3 (cholecalciferol) conversion in the skin is under the control of UV radiation. Serum vitamin D concentration reaches its highest level 24–48 hours after exposure to UV radiation and then shows a gradual decrease. The half-life of serum vitamin D is 36–72 hours. Vitamin D, which is a fat-soluble vitamin, is stored in adipose tissue for later use. The ability of vitamin D to be stored in adipose tissue extends its total half-life in the body up to approximately 2 months.

5.1 Regulation of 25-hydroxylase

There is little information on how this enzyme is regulated because of the few studies performed. What is known is that serum vitamin D level is inversely related to the rate of 25-hydroxylation in the liver, and the synthesis of 25OHD3 from vitamin D (cholecalciferol) is regulated by the 25-hydroxylase enzyme. This activity of the enzyme is directly inhibited by 25OHD3. Consequently, serum 25OHD3 levels can be kept at a physiological window ranging from 75 to 220 nmol/L (30–88 ng/mL). However, when an overdose of vitamin D is taken orally, this inhibitory mechanism in 25OHD3 synthesis cannot prevent vitamin D intoxication [2].

5.2 Regulation of renal 1-alpha hydroxylation

Serum active vitamin D levels in healthy adults vary within extremely narrow ranges, so that even in cases of vitamin D intoxication, serum levels may remain normal. 1-alpha hydroxylation activity in the kidney is controlled by PTH, calcium and phosphorus. Hypocalcemia, increased PTH, and hypophosphatemia will stimulate increases in active vitamin D production through renal 1-alpha hydroxylase enzyme activation, while hypercalcemia, FGF-23 secreted from osteoblasts, and active vitamin D itself have an inhibitory effect on active vitamin D synthesis through the renal 1-alpha hydroxylase enzyme. Active vitamin D increases FGF23 synthesis from osteoblasts. FGF23 suppresses the 1-alpha hydroxylase enzyme and increases the activity of 24 hydroxylase enzymes. In addition, hypercalcemia suppressing PTH and hyperphosphatemia by increasing FGF23 levels results in 1-alpha hydroxylase enzyme activity inhbition [1–3]. It is also suggested that calcium and phosphate have a direct regulatory effect on 1-alpha hydroxylase enzyme [89].

Calcitonin is known to reduce serum calcium levels through osteoclast inhibition. In addition, this hormone has been shown to increase the expression of

CYP27B1, the gene encoding the 1-alpha hydroxylase enzyme, in normocalcemic pregnant women due to the increase in calcium need. In this way, active vitamin D synthesis and consequently intestinal calcium absorption is increased [1, 90]. Apart from calcitonin, it has been suggested that prolactin also increases CYP27B1 expression, especially during lactation, and thus contributes to the increased calcium demand of the body [1, 91].

CYP3A4 enzyme in the liver and intestinal system has also been shown to be effective in the inactivation of 25OHD3 and reduction of active vitamin D [92]. Long-term use of drugs such as phenytoin, rifampicin, and carbamazepine may lead to up-regulation of the CYP3A4 enzyme and thus to a decrease in serum 25OHD3 and active vitamin D levels.

5.3 Regulation of 24-alpha hydroxylase

When serum calcium, phosphate and PTH levels are within normal levels, 25OHD3 and 1–25 (OH) 2 D3 are metabolized into biologically inactive forms by activation of 24-alpha hydroxylase enzyme in the kidneys (24–25 dihydroxy vitamin D3 and 1,24, 25 trihydroxy vitamin D3). This enzyme preferably binds to 1–25 (OH) 2 D3, thus limiting the effect of active vitamin D in tissues through inactivation [2]. The low level of 24-hydroxylase enzyme activity leads to high levels of 1–25 (OH) 2D3 and thus hypercalcemia. In addition, it has been suggested that a decrease in this enzyme activity may lead to impairment in intra-membranous bone mineralization [1, 2]. On the other hand, when 1–25 (OH) 2 D3 synthesis decreases, 1-alpha hydroxylase enzyme activity increases and 24-hydroxylase enzyme activity decreases. It is also known that FGF23 increases the activity of 24 hydroxylase enzymes [1, 2].

5.4 Regulation of active vitamin D synthesis in extra-renal tissues

Numerous studies have shown active vitamin D synthesis by 1-alpha hydroxylase enzyme is not only a renal feature [2, 93]. The gene encoding the 1-alpha hydroxylase enzyme and the vitamin D receptor gene can be expressed in many cells or tissues such as skin, placenta, prostate, parathyroid, bone tissue, colon, lung, breast tissue, monocytes and macrophages, as well as renal cells. It has been reported that active vitamin D synthesized in the aforementioned tissues functions mostly as an intracrine or paracrine factor in the tissues where they are located, and does not contribute to the active vitamin D levels in the circulation, except for some special cases [1, 2]. Since PTH and FGF-23 receptors are not found in these tissues, they are not directly involved in controlling active vitamin D synthesis. However, it is propable that PTH increases the effect of vitamin D through posttranscriptional modification [31]. Unlike in other tissues, in activated macrophages, there is also no negative feedback of active vitamin D on 1-alpha hydroxylase enzyme [91]. Moreover, although the 24-hydroxylase enzyme is expressed in these cells, its function is not fully understood. Cytokines such as IL-1, TNF-α, IFN-γ induce the synthesis of active vitamin D in keratinocytes. Unlike macrophages, keratinocytes have a fully functional 24-hydroxylase enzyme activity and is induced by active vitamin D. In this way, active vitamin D limits its own synthesis in the epidermis through alternative catabolism [1, 2, 93].

6. Vitamin D measurement methods

Measurement of serum levels of vitamin D, which plays an important role in calcium and phosphorus metabolism and bone mineralization, is routinely performed worldwide. For this, it is preferred to measure the 25OHD level, which has a longer half-life (24–36 hours), can be taken exogenously, and can be synthesized endogenously. The half-life of the 1–25 (OH) 2D3 form is short (4–6 hours), and its serum levels are 1000 times lower than 25OHD. For these reasons, the active form is not preferred for routine measurement. In this section, the measurement methods of 25OHD vitamin are discussed.

To date, many methods have been developed for measuring serum vitamin D levels. These methods are basically divided into two groups. One methodology is the use of competitive binding and immunoassays: radioimmunoassay (RIA), enzyme immunoassay (EIA/ELISA), chemiluminescent immunoassay (CLIA), electrochemiluminescence assay (ECLIA), and competitive protein binding assay. The other methodology involves chemical methods. Chemical methods are based on the non-immunological direct detection methods typically after preparative chromatographic separation. Chemical methods include high performance liquid chromatography (HPLC) and LC/MS (liquid chromatography-mass spectrometer).

The first method used in the measurement of vitamin D is the competitive binding method in which VDBP binds. This method was first reported in 1971 and identifies 25OHD2 and 25OHD3 forms equally [94]. Limitations of this method include the incubation period of 10 days and its inability to separate some polar vitamin D metabolites [24,25(OH)2D, 25,26 (OH)2D ve 25,26 (OH)2D-26,23--lactone] [94]. In the late 1970s, the HPLC method was developed that can exclude the effect of polar vitamin D metabolites causing interference to the chromatographic method [95]. The advantages of this method, which uses a UV absorption technique, include the absence of lipid and polar vitamin D metabolite interference, the ability to measure 25OHD2 and 25OHD3 separated at high resolution, and a high specificity and reliability. Its disadvantages include the use of excess sample amounts, equipment cost, a need for preparative chromatography, and interference by other UV-absorbing compounds, and that the method is somewhat complex and not easily practical. It would not be considered a routine diagnostic test, as it is used in only about 2% of laboratories in the world) [94, 95]. With the later development of the RIA method, the value of quantifying vitamin levels improved. The advantages of this method type are that sample amount can be small and not pre-analytical preparative purification process is required. The assay is economical and easily applicable, and results reliable. As to the disadvantages, chemical and radioactive (with the RIA) waste are issues, and there is cross-reactivity with polar vitamin D metabolites as in the earlier competitive binding type assays. The RIA also is 100% specific for 25OHD3 and 75% specific for 25OHD2, so the final calculation requires an adjustment [94, 96]. Nonetheless automated immunoassay methods are widely used in our country and all over the world (approximately 76% of laboratories in the world) [97]. Requiring less sample volume, not requiring sample preparation, easy equipment supply, easy application, fast results, no cross-reactivity with C3-epimer forms, and low user error are among the reasons why this method is used more widely in the world [97, 98]. Despite its widespread use, this method has some significant disadvantages. In this method, 25OHD2 and 25OHD3 cannot be distinguished and both are measured as total of 25OHD. This may lead to misinterpretation in countries that use ergocalciferol in treatment (eg America) [97]. In addition, automated immunoassay results can be affected by pregnancy, whether sampled from intensive care patients, the presence of chronic disease and liver diseases, all of which affect the amount of VDBP synthesized from the liver [99, 100]. In addition, it has been reported that there is a high probability of interferences involving automated immunoassay measurement methods [97, 101].

Due to the low reliability of immunoassay measurements, this method has begun to be replaced by LC–MS/MS, which is considered to be the "gold standard" method. This method is used in approximately 18% of laboratories around the world, and it is estimated that its prevalence will increase due to its more accurate and precise results [97]. This method provides distinguishing quantitative measurements of both 25OHD2 and 25OHD3 forms in both serum and plasma [102]. Hence, 25OHD2 can be easily monitored in countries where ergocalciferol is widely used. In addition, with this method, C-3 epimer forms of vitamin D, which are present in high levels in serum in the first year, can be separated from other forms, and these metabolites are prevented from causing vitamin D measurement interference [97, 102].

In recent years, instead of measuring the level of vitamin D bound to VDBP, there is a strong belief in the need to measure free vitamin D levels as that is the form that accounts for the principal bioactivity. Routine methods measure the level of 25OHD vitamin bound to VDBP and provide information about the total body pool. In parallel with this, if the total body pool is sufficient, free vitamin D level is estimated to be sufficient. However, the situation is somewhat complex in obese patients, where a negative correlation between the amount of adipose tissue and serum vitamin D levels has been reported. In these cases, it has been reported that serum 25OHD level is lower than those with normal body weight, since large adipose tissue creates a larger pool for vitamin D sequestration [101–105]. In other words, serum 25OHD level in obese patients may not provide information about the body pool of vitamin D. It is thought that it would be more valuable to measure vitamin D levels that are not bound to binding protein in these cases. However, there is a serious standardization problem in the measurement of free 25OHD [103]. Also, Bikle et al. [106] proposed a method by which free 25OHD vitamin can be calculated. However, studies have shown that the results obtained with this method are not reliable [107]. Finally, direct measurement or indirect calculations of free forms of vitamin D are not yet suitable for routine use.

Author details

Sezer Acar and Behzat Özkan*
Division of Pediatric Endocrinology, University of Health Science, Dr. Behçet Uz Child Disease and Pediatric Surgery Training and Research, Izmir, Turkey

*Address all correspondence to: ozkan.behzat@gmail.com

References

[1] Christakos S, Dhawan P, Verstuyf A, Verlinden L, Carmeliet G. Vitamin D: Metabolism, Molecular Mechanism of Action, and Pleiotropic Effects. Physiol Rev 2016;96(1):365-408.

[2] Bikle DD. Vitamin D metabolism, mechanism of action, and clinicalapplications. Chem Biol. 2014;21(3):319-29.

[3] Houghton LA, Vieth R. The case against ergocalciferol (vitamin D2) as a vitamin supplement. Am J Clin Nutr. 2006; 84(4):694-7.

[4] Hollis BW. Comparison of equilibrium and disequilibrium assay conditions for ergocalciferol, cholecalciferol and their major metabolites. J Steroid Biochem. 1984;21(1):81-6.

[5] Horst RL, Reinhardt TA, Ramberg CF, Koszewski NJ, Napoli JL. 24-Hydroxylation of 1,25-dihydroxyergocalciferol. An unambiguous deactivation process. J Biol Chem. 1986; 261(20):9250-6.

[6] Tripkovic L, Lambert H, Hart K, et al. Comparison of vitamin D2 and vitamin D3supplementation in raising serum 25-hydroxyvitamin D status: a systematic review and meta-analysis. Am J Clin Nutr. 2012;95(6):1357-64.

[7] Bikle D. Vitamin D: Production, Metabolism, and Mechanisms of Action. [Updated 2017 Aug 11]. In: Feingold KR, Anawalt B, Boyce A, et al., editors. Endotext [Internet]. South Dartmouth (MA): MDText.com, Inc.; 2000-. Available from: https://www.ncbi.nlm.nih.gov/books/NBK278935/ (accessed on 20 January 2020)

[8] Holick MF. The cutaneous photosynthesis of previtamin D3: a unique photoendocrine system. J Invest Dermatol. 1981;77(1):51-8.

[9] Holick MF, MacLaughlin JA, Clark MB, et al. Photosynthesis of previtamin D3 in human skin and the physiologic consequences. Science. 1980;210(4466):203-5.

[10] Matsuoka LY, Wortsman J, Dannenberg MJ, Hollis BW, Lu Z, Holick MF. Clothing prevents ultraviolet-B radiation-dependent photosynthesis of vitamin D3. J Clin Endocrinol Metab. 1992;75(4):1099-103.

[11] Matsuoka LY, Ide L, Wortsman J, MacLaughlin JA, Holick MF. Sunscreens suppress cutaneous vitamin D3 synthesis. J Clin Endocrinol Metab. 1987;64(6):1165-8.

[12] Bell NH, Greene A, Epstein S, Oexmann MJ, Shaw S, Shary J. Evidence for alteration of the vitamin D-endocrine system in blacks. J Clin Invest. 1985;76(2):470-3.

[13] Holick MF. Environmental factors that influence the cutaneous production of vitamin D. Am J Clin Nutr. 1995;61 (3 Suppl):638-45.

[14] Holick MF. Vitamin D: A D-lightful solution for health. J Investig Med. 2011;59(6):872-80.

[15] Heaney RP, Horst RL, Cullen DM, Armas LA. Vitamin D distribution and status in the body. J Am Coll Nutr. 2009;28(3):252-6.

[16] Zhu J, DeLuca HF. Vitamin D 25-hydroxylase: four decades of searching, are we there yet? Arch Biochem Biophys. 2012;523(1):30-6.

[17] Zhu JG, Ochalek JT, Kaufmann M, Jones G, Deluca HF. CYP2R1 is a major, but not exclusive, contributor to 25-hydroxyvitamin D production in vivo. Proc Natl Acad Sci 2013;110(39):15650-5.

[18] Moghadasian MH. Cerebrotendinous xanthomatosis: clinical course, genotypes and metabolic backgrounds. Clin Invest Med. 2004; 27(1):42-50.

[19] Cheng JB, Motola DL, Mangelsdorf DJ, Russell DW. De-orphanization of cytochrome P450 2R1: a microsomal vitamin D 25-hydroxilase. J Biol Chem. 2003;278(39):38084-93.

[20] C Cheng JB, Levine MA, Bell NH, Mangelsdorf DJ, Russell DW. Genetic evidence that the human CYP2R1 enzyme is a key vitamin D 25-hydroxylase. Proc Natl Acad Sci U S A. 2004;101(20):7711-5.

[21] Saarem K, Pedersen JI. Sex differences in the hydroxylation of cholecalciferol and of 5 beta-cholestane-3 alpha, 7 alpha, 12 alpha-triol in rat liver. Biochem J. 1987;247(1):73-8.

[22] Fu GK, Portale AA, Miller WL. Complete structure of the human gene for the vitamin D 1alpha-hydroxylase, P450c1alpha. DNA Cell Biol. 1997;16(12):1499-507.

[23] Fu GK, Lin D, Zhang MY, et al. Cloning of human 25-hydroxyvitamin D-1 alpha-hydroxylase and mutations causing vitamin D-dependent rickets type 1. Mol Endocrinol. 1997;11(13):1961-70.

[24] Shinki T, Ueno Y, DeLuca HF, Suda T. Calcitonin is a major regulator for the expression of renal 25-hydroxyvitamin D3-1alpha-hydroxylase gene in normocalcemic rats. Proc Natl Acad Sci U S A. 1999;96(14):8253-8.

[25] Takeyama K, Kitanaka S, Sato T, Kobori M, Yanagisawa J, Kato S. 25-Hydroxyvitamin D3 1alpha-hydroxylase and vitamin D synthesis. Science. 1997;277(5333):1827-30.

[26] St-Arnaud R, Messerlian S, Moir JM, Omdahl JL, Glorieux FH. The 25-hydroxyvitamin D 1-alpha-hydroxylase gene maps to the pseudovitamin D-deficiency rickets (PDDR) disease locus. J Bone Miner Res. 1997;12(10):1552-9.

[27] DeLuca HF 2. Evolution of our understanding of vitamin D. Nutr Rev. 2008;66(10 Suppl 2): 73-87.

[28] Adams JS, Sharma OP, Gacad MA, Singer FR. Metabolism of 25-hydroxyvitamin D3 by cultured pulmonary alveolar macrophages in sarcoidosis. J Clin Invest. 1983;72(5):1856-60.

[29] Barbour GL, Coburn JW, Slatopolsky E, Norman AW, Horst RL. Hypercalcemia in an anephric patient with sarcoidosis: evidence for extrarenal generation of 1,25-dihydroxyvitamin D. N Engl J Med. 1981;305(8):440-3.

[30] Bosch X. Hypercalcemia due to endogenous overproduction of 1,25-dihydroxyvitamin D in Crohn's disease. Gastroenterology. 1998;114(5):1061-5.

[31] Flanagan JN, Wang L, Tangpricha V, Reichrath J, Chen TC, Holick MF. Regulation of the 25- hydroxyvitamin D-1alpha-hydroxylase gene and its splice variant. Recent Results Cancer Res. 2003;164:157-167.

[32] Jones G, Prosser DE, Kaufmann M. 25-Hydroxyvitamin D-24-hydroxylase (CYP24A1): its important role in the degradation of vitamin D. Arch Biochem Biophys. 2012;523(1):9-18.

[33] Shima M, Tanaka H, Norman AW, et al. 23(S),25(R)-1,25-dihydroxyvitamin D3-26,23-lactone stimulates murine bone formation in vivo. Endocrinology. 1990;126(2):832-6.

[34] Plachot JJ, Du Bois MB, Halpern S, Cournot-Witmer G, Garabedian M,

Balsan S. In vitro action of 1,25-dihydroxycholecalciferol and 24,25-dihydroxycholecalciferol on matrix organization and mineral distribution in rabbit growth plate. Metab Bone Dis Relat Res. 1982;4(2):135-42.

[35] Zierold C, Darwish HM, DeLuca HF. Two vitamin D response elements function in the rat 1,25-dihydroxyvitamin D 24-hydroxylase promoter. J Biol Chem. 1995;270(4):1675-8.

[36] Inoue Y, Segawa H, Kaneko I, et al. Role of the vitamin D receptor in FGF23 action on phosphate metabolism. Biochem J. 2005;390(Pt 1):325-31.

[37] Schlingmann KP, Kaufmann M, Weber S, et al. Mutations in CYP24A1 and idiopathic infantile hypercalcemia. N Engl J Med. 2011 Aug 4;365(5):410-21.

[38] ailey D, Veljkovic K, Yazdanpanah M, Adeli K. Analytical measurement and clinical relevance of vitamin D(3) C3-epimer. Clin Biochem. 2013 Feb;46(3):190-6.

[39] Kamao M, Tatematsu S, Hatakeyama S, et al. C-3 epimerization of vitamin D3 metabolites and further metabolism of C-3 epimers: 25-hydroxyvitamin D3 is metabolized to 3-epi-25-hydroxyvitamin D3 and subsequently metabolized through C-1alpha or C-24 hydroxylation. J Biol Chem. 2004;279(16):15897-907.

[40] Cooke NE, Haddad JG. Vitamin D binding protein (Gc-globulin). Endocr Rev. 1989;10(3):294-307.

[41] Bikle DD, Halloran BP, Gee E, Ryzen E, Haddad JG. Free 25-hydroxyvitamin D levels are normal in subjects with liver disease and reduced total 25-hydroxyvitamin D levels. J Clin Invest. 1986;78(3): 748-52.

[42] Madden K, Feldman HA, Chun RF, et al. Critically Ill Children Have Low Vitamin DBinding Protein, Influencing Bioavailability of Vitamin D. Ann Am Thorac Soc. 2015;12(11):1654-61.

[43] Zella LA, Shevde NK, Hollis BW, Cooke NE, Pike JW. Vitamin D-binding protein influences total circulating levels of 1,25-dihydroxyvitamin D3 but does not directly modulate the bioactive levels of the hormone in vivo. Endocrinology. 2008;149(7):3656-67.

[44] Safadi FF, Thornton P, Magiera H, et al. Osteopathy and resistance to vitamin D toxicity in mice null for vitamin D binding protein. J Clin Invest. 1999;103(2):239-51.

[45] Arnaud J, Constans J. Affinity differences for vitamin D metabolites associated with the genetic isoforms of the human serum carrier protein (DBP). Hum Genet. 1993;92(2):183-8.

[46] Bouillon R, van Baelen H, de Moor P. Comparative study of the affinity of the serum vitamin D-binding protein. J Steroid Biochem. 1980;13(9):1029-34

[47] Cantorna MT. Vitamin D and its role in immunology: multiple sclerosis, and inflammatory bowel disease. Prog Biophys Mol Biol. 2006;92(1):60-4.

[48] Margolis RN, Christakos S. The nuclear receptor superfamily of steroid hormones and vitamin D gene regulation. An update. Ann N Y Acad Sci. 2010;1192:208-14.

[49] Rochel N, Wurtz JM, Mitschler A, Klaholz B, Moras D. The crystal structure of the nuclear receptor for vitamin D bound to its natural ligand. Mol Cell. 2000;5(1):173-9.

[50] Rachez C, Gamble M, Chang CP, Atkins GB, Lazar MA, Freedman LP. The DRIP complex and SRC-1/p160 coactivators share similar nuclear

receptor binding determinants but constitute functionally distinct complexes. Mol Cell Biol. 2000;20(8):2718-26.

[51] Orlov I, Rochel N, Moras D, Klaholz BP. Structure of the full human RXR/VDR nuclear receptor heterodimer complex with its DR3 target DNA. EMBO J. 2012;31(2):291-300.

[52] Chen S, Cui J, Nakamura K, Ribeiro RC, West BL, Gardner DG. Coactivator-vitamin D receptor interactions mediate inhibition of the atrial natriuretic peptide promoter. J Biol Chem. 2000;275(20):15039-48.

[53] Haussler MR, Whitfield GK, Haussler CA, et al. 1,25-Dihydroxyvitamin D and Klotho: A Tale of Two Renal Hormones Coming of Age. Vitam Horm. 2016;100:165-230.

[54] Haussler MR, Whitfield GK, Kaneko I, et al. Molecular mechanisms of vitamin D action. Calcif Tissue Int. 2013;92(2):77-98.

[55] Essa S, Denzer N, Mahlknecht U, et al. VDR microRNA expression and epigenetic silencing of vitamin D signaling in melanoma cells. J Steroid Biochem Mol Biol. 2010;121(1-2):110-3.

[56] Yin JW, Wang G. The Mediator complex: a master coordinator of transcription and cell lineage development. Development. 2014;141(5):977-87.

[57] Caffrey JM, Farach-Carson MC. Vitamin D3 metabolites modulate dihydropyridine-sensitive calcium currents in clonal rat osteosarcoma cells. J Biol Chem. 1989;264(34):20265-74.

[58] Baran DT, Sorensen AM, Honeyman TW, Ray R, Holick MF. 1 alpha,25-dihydroxyvitamin D3-induced increments in hepatocyte cytosolic calcium and lysophosphatidylinositol: inhibition by pertussis toxin and 1 beta,25-dihydroxyvitamin D3. J Bone Miner Res. 1990;5(5):517-24.

[59] Morelli S, de Boland AR, Boland RL. Generation of inositol phosphates, diacylglycerol and calcium fluxes in myoblasts treated with 1,25-dihydroxyvitamin D3. Biochem J. 1993 Feb 1;289 (Pt 3):675-9.

[60] Wali RK, Baum CL, Sitrin MD, Brasitus TA. 1,25(OH)2 vitamin D3 stimulates membrane phosphoinositide turnover, activates protein kinase C, and increases cytosolic calcium in rat colonic epithelium. J Clin Invest. 1990;85(4):1296-303.

[61] Khare S, Bolt MJ, Wali RK, et al. 1,25 dihydroxyvitamin D3 stimulates phospholipase C-gamma in rat colonocytes: role of c-Src in PLC-gamma activation. J Clin Invest. 1997;99(8):1831-41.

[62] Revelli A, Massobrio M, Tesarik J. Nongenomic effects of 1alpha,25-dihydroxyvitamin D(3). Trends Endocrinol Metab. 1998;9(10):419-27.

[63] Nemere I, Yoshimoto Y, Norman AW. Calcium transport in perfused duodena from normal chicks: enhancement within fourteen minutes of exposure to 1,25-dihydroxyvitamin D3. Endocrinology. 1984;115(4):1476-83.

[64] Nemere I, Norman AW. Rapid action of 1,25-dihydroxyvitamin D3 on calcium transport in perfused chick duodenum: effect of inhibitors. J Bone Miner Res.1987;2(2):99-107.

[65] de Boland AR, Norman AW. Influx of extracellular calcium mediates 1,25-dihydroxyvitamin D3-dependent transcaltachia (the rapid stimulation of duodenal Ca2+ transport). Endocrinology. 1990;127(5):2475-80.

[66] de Boland AR, Norman A. Evidence for involvement of protein kinase C and cyclic adenosine 3',5'

monophosphate-dependent protein kinase in the 1,25-dihydroxy-vitamin D3-mediated rapid stimulation of intestinal calcium transport, (transcaltachia). Endocrinology. 1990;127(1):39-45.

[67] Norman AW, Okamura WH, Hammond MW, et al. Comparison of 6-s-cis- and 6-s-trans-locked analogs of 1alpha,25-dihydroxyvitamin D3 indicates that the 6-s-cis conformation is preferred for rapid nongenomic biological responses and that neither 6-s-cis- nor 6-s-trans-locked analogs are preferred for genomic biological responses. Mol Endocrinol. 1997;11(10):1518-31.

[68] Sequeira VB, Rybchyn MS, Tongkao-On W, et al. The role of the vitamin D receptor and ERp57 in photoprotection by 1α,25-dihydroxyvitamin D3. Mol Endocrinol. 2012;26(4):574-82.

[69] Mizwicki MT, Norman AW. The vitamin D sterol-vitamin D receptor ensemble model offers unique insights into both genomic and rapid-response signaling. Sci Signal. 2009;2(75):re4.

[70] Nemere I, Farach-Carson MC, Rohe B, et al. Ribozyme knockdown functionally links a 1,25(OH)2D3 membrane binding protein (1,25D3-MARRS) and phosphate uptake in intestinal cells. Proc Natl Acad Sci U S A. 2004;101(19):7392-7.

[71] Huhtakangas JA, Olivera CJ, Bishop JE, Zanello LP, Norman AW. The vitamin D receptor is present in caveolae-enriched plasma membranes and binds 1 alpha,25(OH)2-vitamin D3 in vivo and in vitro. Mol Endocrinol. 2004;18(11):2660-71.

[72] Song Y, Peng X, Porta A, et al. Calcium transporter 1 and epithelial calcium channel messenger ribonucleic acid are differentially regulated by 1,25 dihydroxyvitamin D3 in the intestine and kidney of mice. Endocrinology. 2003;144(9):3885-94.

[73] Bianco SD, Peng JB, Takanaga H, et al. Marked disturbance of calcium homeostasis in mice with targeted disruption of the Trpv6 calcium channel gene. J Bone Miner Res. 2007;22(2):274-85.

[74] Glenney JR Jr, Glenney P. Comparison of Ca++-regulated events in the intestinal brush border. J Cell Biol. 1985;100(3):754-63.

[75] Ghijsen WE, De Jong MD, Van Os CH. ATP-dependent calcium transport and its correlation with Ca2+ -ATPase activity in basolateral plasma membranes of rat duodenum. Biochim Biophys Acta. 1982;689(2):327-36.

[76] Lee GS, Lee KY, Choi KC, et al. Phenotype of a calbindin-D9k gene knockout is compensated for by the induction of other calcium transporter genes in a mouse model. J Bone Miner Res. 2007;22(12):1968-78.

[77] Benn BS, Ajibade D, Porta A, et al. Active intestinal calcium transport in the absence of transient receptor potential vanilloid type 6 and calbindin-D9k. Endocrinology. 2008;149(6):3196-205.

[78] Fujita H, Sugimoto K, Inatomi S, et al. Tight junction proteins claudin-2 and -12 are critical for vitamin D-dependent Ca2+ absorption between enterocytes. Mol Biol Cell. 2008;19(5):1912-21.

[79] Karbach U. Paracellular calcium transport across the small intestine. J Nutr. 1992;122(3 Suppl):672-7.

[80] Peterlik M, Wasserman RH. Regulation by vitamin D of intestinal phosphate absorption. Horm Metab Res. 1980;12(5):216-9.

[81] Friedman PA, Gesek FA. Cellular calcium transport in renal epithelia:

measurement, mechanisms, and regulation. Physiol Rev. 1995;75(3):429-71.

[82] Yu X, Ibrahimi OA, Goetz R, et al. Analysis of the biochemical mechanisms for the endocrine actions of fibroblast growth factor-23. Endocrinology. 2005;146(11):4647-56.

[83] Wang L, Nancollas GH, Henneman ZJ, Klein E, Weiner S. Nanosized particles in bone and dissolution insensitivity of bone mineral. Biointerphases. 2006;1(3):106-11.

[84] Peacock M. Calcium metabolism in health and disease. Clin J Am Soc Nephrol. 2010;5(Suppl 1):23-30.

[85] Robertson WG, Marshall RW. Calcium measurements in serum and plasma--total and ionized. CRC Crit Rev Clin Lab Sci. 1979;11(3):271-304.

[86] Kim S, Yamazaki M, Zella LA, Shevde NK, Pike JW. Activation of receptor activator of NF-kappaB ligand gene expression by 1,25-dihydroxyvitamin D3 is mediated through multiple long-range enhancers. Mol Cell Biol. 2006;26(17):6469-86.

[87] Suda T, Takahashi N, Udagawa N, Jimi E, Gillespie MT, Martin TJ. Modulation of osteoclast differentiation and function by the new members of the tumor necrosis factor receptor and ligand families. Endocr Rev. 1999;20(3):345-57.

[88] Fretz JA, Zella LA, Kim S, Shevde NK, Pike JW. 1,25-Dihydroxyvitamin D3 regulates the expression of low-density lipoprotein receptor-related protein 5 via deoxyribonucleic acid sequence elements located downstream of the start site of transcription. Mol Endocrinol. 2006;20(9):2215-30.

[89] Bikle DD, Murphy EW, Rasmussen H. The ionic control of 1,25-dihydroxyvitamin D3 synthesis in isolated chick renal mitochondria. The role of calcium as influenced by inorganic phosphate and hydrogen-ion. J Clin Invest. 1975;55(2):299-304.

[90] Shinki T, Ueno Y, DeLuca HF, Suda T. Calcitonin is a major regulator for the expression of renal 25-hydroxyvitamin D3-1alpha-hydroxylase gene in normocalcemic rats. Proc Natl Acad Sci U S A. 1999;96(14):8253-8.

[91] Robinson CJ, Spanos E, James MF, et al. Role of prolactin in vitamin D metabolism and calcium absorption during lactation in the rat. J Endocrinol. 1982;94(3):443-53.

[92] Wang Z, Schuetz EG, Xu Y, Thummel KE. Interplay between vitamin D and the drug metabolizing enzyme CYP3A4. J Steroid Biochem Mol Biol. 2013;136:54-8.

[93] Weisman Y. Non-classic unexpected functions of vitamin D. Pediatr Endocrinol Rev. 2010;8(2):103-7.

[94] Holick MF. Vitamin D status: measurement, interpretation, and clinical application. Ann Epidemiol. 2009;19(2):73-8.

[95] Jones G. Assay of vitamins D2 and D3, and 25-hydroxyvitamins D2 and D3 in human plasma by high-performance liquid chromatography. Clin Chem. 1978;24(2):287-98.

[96] Hollis BW. Editorial: The determination of circulating 25-hydroxyvitamin D: no easy task. J Clin Endocrinol Metab. 2004;89(7):3149-51.

[97] Dirks NF, Ackermans MT, Lips P, et al. The When, What & How of Measuring Vitamin D Metabolism in Clinical Medicine. Nutrients. 2018;10(4). pii: E482

[98] Pearce SH, Cheetham TD. Diagnosis and management of vitamin D deficiency. BMJ. 2010;340:b5664.

[99] Heijboer AC, Blankenstein MA, Kema IP, Buijs MM. Accuracy of 6 routine 25-hydroxyvitamin D assays: influence of vitamin D binding protein concentration. Clin Chem. 2012;58(3):543-8.

[100] Elsenberg EHAM, Ten Boekel E, Huijgen H, Heijboer AC. Standardization of automated 25-hydroxyvitamin D assays: How successful is it? Clin Biochem. 2017;50(18):1126-1130.

[101] Le Goff C, Peeters S, Crine Y, Lukas P, Souberbielle JC, Cavalier E. Evaluation of the cross-reactivity of 25-hydroxyvitamin D2 on seven commercial immunoassays on native samples. Clin Chem Lab Med. 2012;50(11):2031-2.

[102] Carter GD, Jones JC, Shannon J, et al. 25-Hydroxyvitamin D assays: Potential interference from other circulating vitaminD metabolites. J Steroid Biochem Mol Biol. 2016;164:134-138.

[103] Saggese G, Vierucci F, Prodam F, et al. Vitamin D in pediatric age: consensus of the Italian Pediatric Society and the Italian Society of Preventive and Social Pediatrics, jointly with the Italian Federation of Pediatricians. Ital J Pediatr. 2018;44(1):51.

[104] Dong Y, Pollock N, Stallmann-Jorgensen IS, et al. Low 25-hydroxyvitamin D levels in adolescents: race, season, adiposity, physical activity, and fitness. Pediatrics. 2010;125(6):1104-11.

[105] Earthman CP, Beckman LM, Masodkar K, Sibley SD. The link between obesity and low circulating 25-hydroxyvitamin D concentrations: considerations and implications. Int J Obes (Lond). 2012;36(3):387-96.

[106] Bikle DD, Gee E, Halloran B, Kowalski MA, Ryzen E, Haddad JG. Assessment of the free fraction of 25-hydroxyvitamin D in serum and its regulation by albumin and the vitamin D-binding protein. J Clin Endocrinol Metab. 1986; 63(4):954-9.

[107] Schwartz JB, Lai J, Lizaola B, et al. A comparison of measured and calculated free 25(OH) vitamin D levels in clinical populations. J Clin Endocrinol Metab. 2014;99(5):1631-7.

Chapter 2

Vitamin D Deficiency in Pregnant Women and Newborn

Neelakanta Kanike, Naveen Kannekanti and Jenny Camacho

Abstract

Vitamin-D is not only an essential element in bone health, but it is also a pro-hormone. Deficiency of vitamin D is the most common cause of rickets and is also known to increase the risk of respiratory distress syndrome, lower respiratory infections, food sensitivities, asthma, type I diabetes, autism and schizophrenia. Vitamin D deficiency limits the effective absorption of dietary calcium and phosphorus. Vitamin D status in newborns is entirely dependent on maternal supply during pregnancy. Low maternal vitamin D status during pregnancy is a major risk factor for rickets in infants. Rickets in children is caused by severe, chronic vitamin D deficiency with apparent skeletal abnormalities, but neonates with vitamin D insufficiency have no overt skeletal or calcium metabolism defects. Rickets was a global disease in the early twentieth century. It has nearly disappeared in developed countries after its causal pathway was understood and fortification of milk with the hormone vitamin D was introduced at the population level. Surprisingly, rickets is re-emerging per recent evidence. Vitamin D deficiency is prevalent in both developed and developing countries. The chapter will review the prevalence of vitamin D deficiency in pregnant women and newborn population and its adverse effects on pregnancy and infant's health. The chapter also describes evidence-based recommendations to prevent vitamin D deficiency in these vulnerable population.

Keywords: Vitamin D, deficiency, newborn, preterm, rickets, pregnancy

1. Introduction

Vitamin D is a fat-soluble secosteroid. It is a prohormone that can be ingested or derived from body sterols by the photolytic activity of ultraviolet rays on human skin. Vitamin-D is not only an essential element in bone health, but it is also a pro-hormone that plays a well-recognized role in other organs of body. Vitamin D deficiency is a worldwide health issue that affects more than one billion children and adults globally [1]. Vitamin-D deficiency in neonates has been linked to higher risk of respiratory distress syndrome, lower respiratory infections, food sensitivities, asthma, type I diabetes, autism and schizophrenia [2–9]. Serum 25-hydroxycholecalciferol (25[OH]D) is the main circulating metabolite of vitamin D with a reported half-life of approximately three weeks [10]. It is the best estimator of human body vitamin D stores. During pregnancy it crosses the placenta through passive or facilitated transport according to a concentration gradient [11, 12]. Vitamin-D status in the fetus and newborn infant is largely determined by maternal vitamin-D status [11]. The main risk factor for vitamin-D deficiency in neonates is maternal vitamin-D deficiency [13]. Rickets was a global problem in the early 20th century. It virtually disappeared in developed countries after its causal pathway was identified and fortification of milk with vitamin-D was implemented at population level [14]. Recent reports have suggested that rickets is re-emerging [15, 16] and vitamin-D deficiency is widespread in developed and developing countries [15, 17–21]. Globally, vitamin-D deficiency at birth is prevalent and in general reflects deficient maternal vitamin-D status [10, 22–24].

2. Vitamin D metabolism and biological functions

Vitamin D is unique among vitamins because it can be made in the skin from sunlight exposure. Vitamin D has two forms: Ergocalciferol (D_2) and Cholecalciferol (D_3). D_2 is produced from ultraviolet irradiation of the yeast sterol ergosterol and is naturally found in sun-exposed mushrooms. D3 is synthesized in the skin from the cholesterol precursor 7-dehydrocholesterol which is naturally present in the skin or obtained from lanolin [25]. Vitamin D (in the form of D_2, or D_3, or both) that is ingested is assimilated into chylomicrons, which are absorbed into the lymphatic system and enter the venous blood. Vitamin D that comes from the skin or diet is biologically inert and needs its first hydroxylation in the liver by the vitamin D-25-hydroxylase to 25[OH]D [25, 26]. 25[OH]D undergoes a second hydroxylation in the kidneys by the 25[OH]D-1α-hydroxylase to form the biologically active form of vitamin D 1,25[OH]$_2$D (3, 8). 1,25[OH]$_2$D interacts with its vitamin D nuclear receptor, which is present in the small intestine, kidneys, and other tissues [25, 26].

1,25[OH]$_2$D plays a main physiological role in bone hemostasis. It stimulates intestinal calcium absorption [27]. Without vitamin D, only 10 to 15% of dietary calcium and about 60% of phosphorus are absorbed. Vitamin D sufficiency enhances calcium and phosphorus absorption by 30–40% and 80%, respectively [25, 28]. 1,25[OH]$_2$D interacts with its vitamin D receptor in the osteoblast to stimulate the expression of receptor activator of nuclear factor κB ligand; this, in turn, interacts with receptor activator of nuclear factor κB to induce immature monocytes to become mature osteoclasts, which dissolve the matrix and mobilize calcium and other minerals from the skeleton. In the kidney, 1,25[OH]$_2$D stimulates calcium reabsorption from the glomerular filtrate [25, 29].

The strong correlation between maternal and infant 25[OH]D levels offers further evidence that newborn 25[OH]D levels are dependent on maternal plasma 25[OH]D levels [12, 30, 31]. There is no clear consensus on the cut off levels of serum 25[OH]D levels to define vitamin deficiency. The US Endocrine Society has categorized vitamin D deficiency as 25[OH]D < 20 ng/mL, vitamin D insufficiency as levels 21–30 ng/mL, sufficiency as levels greater than 30 ng/mL, and toxicity as vitamin D levels more than 150 ng/mL [32]. The American Academy of Pediatrics (AAP) and Institute of Medicine define vitamin D deficiency as serum 25[OH]D < 15 ng/mL, mild to moderate deficiency as 5–15 ng/mL, severe deficiency as levels less than 5 ng/mL, and insufficiency as 16–20 ng/mL. They define sufficiency as levels between 21 and 100 ng/mL, excess as 101–149 ng/mL, and intoxication as levels more than 150 ng/mL [33]. The Kidney Disease Outcome Quality Initiative supports the AAP in defining vitamin D deficiency as levels <15 ng/mL. However, it defines insufficiency as levels between 16 and 30 ng/mL and sufficiency as levels of more than 30 ng/mL. An expert committee of the US Food and Nutrition Board (FNB) at the National Academies of Sciences, Engineering, and Medicine (NASEM) concluded that people are at risk of vitamin D deficiency at serum 25[OH]D concentrations less than 12 ng/mL. The same cutoffs were used for both pregnant women and neonates, because experts contend that there is no reason to think the definition of vitamin-D sufficiency varies by age [16].

3. Prevalence of vitamin D deficiency in pregnant women

3.1 Developed countries

An US survey from National Health and Nutrition Examination Survey (NHANES) 2011–2014 on serum 25[OH]D levels found that 5.7% women had vitamin D deficiency (<12 ng/ml) and 17.8% women had vitamin D insufficiency (12–20 ng/mL). Rates of deficiency and insufficiency were 7.6% and 23.8% respectively in adults aged 20–39 years. Rates of deficiency varied by race and ethnicity: 17.5% of non-Hispanic Blacks, 7.6% of non-Hispanic Asians, 5.9% of Hispanics, and 2.1% of non-Hispanic White people were at risk of vitamin D deficiency respectively. Vitamin D status in the United States remained stable in the decade between 2003 and 2004 and 2011–2014 [34].

Boston's cross-sectional study from 2005 to 2007 reported vitamin-D deficiency (25[OH]D < 20 ng/mL) in 35.8% of the mothers and 58% of the neonates, severe deficiency (25[OH]D < 15 ng/mL) in 23.1% of the mothers and 38.0% of the neonates. Risk factors for neonatal vitamin-D deficiency included maternal deficiency (adjusted odds ratio [aOR]: 5.28 [95% CI: 2.90–9.62]), winter birth (aOR: 3.86 [95% CI: 1.74–8.55]), African-American (AA) race (aOR: 3.36 [95% CI: 1.37–8.25]), and maternal body mass index of 35 (aOR: 2.78 [95% CI: 1.18–6.55]) [31].

A Canadian study found a prevalence of 25% vitamin D insufficiency (defined as serum 25-[OH]D < 40 nmol/L) in women aged 18–35 years during the winter season [17]. Vitamin D deficiency is also common in Europe and the Middle East. Vitamin D deficiency defined as serum 25[OH]D < 50 nmol/L or 20 ng/mL, occurs in 6–33% of the population in Northern Europe, in 30–60% in Western, Southern and Eastern Europe and 30–90% in the Middle East countries. Severe deficiency (serum 25(OH)D < 30 nmol/L or 12 ng/mL) is found in >10% of Europeans [35]. Vitamin D deficiency is usually is more prevalent in immigrants from non-Western countries, compared with native European people [36]. This is even worse in pregnant non-Western immigrants, who displayed mean serum 25(OH)D levels around 25 nmol/L [37].

3.2 Developing countries

The major proportion of vitamin D is produced endogenously with skin exposure of the skin to sunlight. In tropical areas like India, Africa and middle east, where there is abundant overhead sun for most or all of the year, deficiency of vitamin D is unexpected. However, despite stable and sufficient sun exposure in countries across equator, high prevalence of vitamin D deficiency in pregnancy ranging 26–95% in such areas was reported [38]. In Africa, Asia and the Middle East, women have been always regarded as "high risk" for vitamin D deficiency [39, 40]. In 2009, the International Osteoporosis Foundation reported that vitamin D deficiency was seen in 84% of pregnant women and 96% of infants in Asia [41]. In India, 50–90% of the population suffers from vitamin D deficiency due to inadequate exposure to sunlight and a lower dietary intake [42–44]. A recent study from northern India reported the prevalence of vitamin D deficiency in 85.5% of mothers and 74% of infants [45]. Vitamin D deficiency, defined as <50 nmol/L of 25[OH]D and severe vitamin D deficiency defined as <30 nmol/L of 25[OH]D was reported in 34% and 18% of the population respectively in African countries [46].

Vitamin D deficiency is even worse in mainland China with deficiency seen in 72% and severe deficiency seen in 37% of pregnant women [47].

4. Effects of vitamin D deficiency on pregnancy

Despite the wide intake of prenatal vitamins, Vitamin D deficiency in pregnancy is still common worldwide. The adverse outcomes of pregnancy secondary to vitamin D deficiency include miscarriages, preeclampsia, intrauterine growth restriction (IUGR), increased risk for gestational diabetes, preterm birth and low birth weight infants [48–50]. Vitamin D deficiency in pregnant women may affect fetal growth, tooth enamel formation and bone ossification [13]. Decreased vitamin D levels in general is associated with increased mortality and vitamin D supplementation reduces mortality [51]. The reasons behind increased mortality include diabetes mellitus, cardiovascular disease and cancer [52]. Vitamin D deficiency has been associated with several autoimmune diseases, including rheumatoid arthritis (RA), systemic lupus erythematosus (SLE), antiphospholipid syndrome (APS), Hashimoto Thyroiditis (HT), and multiple sclerosis (MS). Autoimmune diseases are more commonly seen in females than males. Pregnant women with these autoimmune disorders are at increased risk for poor pregnancy outcomes [48, 53].

Animal studies showed that vitamin D deficiency causes placental inflammation which leads to placental insufficiency and potentially fetal IUGR [53]. In both pregnancy and lactation it is important to have adequate vitamin D levels to avoid disturbances in bone and mineral metabolism [54]. The fetal and neonatal status of vitamin D is entirely dependent on the mother's vitamin D levels. This confirms the correlation of mother and cord blood 25[OH]D concentrations. While 25[OH]D crosses the placenta, 1,25[OH]2D is produced by the fetal kidneys [54]. Research regarding the exact physiological role of vitamin D in pregnancy and lactation is ongoing. There is convincing data that vitamin D is important for the immunomodulation of the maternal-fetal interface [54–58]. Vitamin D is also crucial for the prevention of pre-eclampsia by stabilizing the endothelium through non-genomic mechanisms [54]. Other functions of vitamin D may include stimulation of sex hormone secretion, implantation/placentation and respiratory epithelium maturation. Vitamin D may also induce epigenetic changes in expressing vitamin D receptors and enzymes involved in vit D metabolism throughout the male and female reproductive tracts [54–58].

5. Etiology of vitamin D deficiency in pregnant women

Vitamin D deficiency is prevalent worldwide in pregnant women and infants. In pregnancy, maternal vitamin D physiology is altered to facilitate the transfer of calcium to the fetus. In pregnancy there is a significant increase in 1,25[OH]2 D concentrations with a two-fold increase in the first trimester followed by a 2–3-fold increase during the second and third trimesters of pregnancy. Then there is a rapid decrease after delivery. PTH-related peptide may also regulate serum 1,25[OH]2D concentrations in pregnancy. 1,25[OH]2D synthesis is dependent up the levels of 25[OH]D. There is a positive correlation between serum 1,25[OH]2D and 25[OH]D concentrations and it is stronger in pregnant women compared to non-pregnant women [54].

Eating foods fortified with vitamin D as well as adequate exposure to sunlight are needed for upholding a normal vitamin D status. The most common reasons for vitamin D deficiency are low sun exposure, decreased vitamin D intake, obesity, and low socio-economic conditions. Various factors influence vitamin D synthesis from sunlight, such as latitude, pigmentation, and area of skin exposed. Many prevalent social and cultural practices in Asia and middle east that prevent the adequate exposure of young women and adolescent girls to sunlight contribute to vitamin D deficiency [59]. Increasing urbanization resulting in greater pollution and decreased time spent outdoors coupled with greater skin pigmentation contribute to vitamin D deficiency [60]. When women in these circumstances become pregnant with already low serum 25 [OH]D levels, this contributes to vitamin D deficiency or insufficiency in their offspring. These children at increased risk for developing rickets [49]. Furthermore, vitamin D supplementation is not part of antenatal care programs in developing countries like India [59].

Diets low in vitamin D are more common in people who have milk allergy or lactose intolerance and those who consume an ovo-vegetarian or vegan diet. Women who are homebound, have occupations that limit sun exposure, or who wear long dresses, robes, or head coverings for religious reasons are at risk for vitamin D deficiency due to limited exposure to sunlight [61]. The use of sunscreen also limits vitamin D synthesis from sunlight. Obese women have lower vitamin D levels than nonobese individuals. The skin's capacity to produce vitamin D is not affected by obesity. In fact, thick subcutaneous fat sequesters more of vitamin D [62, 63]. Serum levels transiently increase following weight loss possibly due to the release of vitamin D in the circulation. This was noted in obese patients after roux-en-y gastric bypass surgery as well as patients with non-surgical weight loss. However, 1 year after a Roux-en-y gastric bypass surgery, vitamin D levels returned to baseline values [64]. Finally, since vitamin D is fat soluble, its absorption is poor in individuals with fat malabsorption disorders like celiac disease, cystic fibrosis, ulcerative colitis and Crohn's disease [65].

6. Prevalence of vitamin D deficiency in newborn

Due to the bone deposition that mostly occurs in the latter half of the pregnancy, vitamin D requirements for the fetus are higher at this time frame [66]. In early pregnancy the plasma levels of 1,25(OH)2D increase and peak in the third trimester. It is estimated that the fetus accumulates 2–3 mg/day of calcium in the skeleton in the first trimester. This calcium accumulation doubles in the third trimester [67]. When infants are born prematurely, the time required for this transfer of Vitamin D and calcium is truncated [68].

Saraf and et al. conducted a global summary and systematic review of maternal and newborn vitamin D status by looking at studies published between 1959 and 2014. They found that 75% of newborns had vitamin D deficiency (defined as 25[OH]D level < 50 nmol/L) and that severe vitamin D deficiency (defined as 25[OH]D level < 25 nmol/L) occurred in 29% of newborns. In this summary, the average newborn 25[OH]D levels in nmol/L by region is as follows: 35–77 (Americans), 20–50 (European), 5–50 (Mediterranean), 20–22 (South-East Asia), 32–67 (Western Pacific) and 27–35 (African). They also found wide variability in 25[OH]D levels within in each defined region [24]. Both this study and another systemic review by Hilger and colleagues found that the average 25[OH]D levels in the general populations in North America were higher compared to Europe and the Middle East [69]. Furthermore, two other reviews found that vitamin D deficiency and severe vitamin D deficiency were more common in South-East Asia and the Eastern Mediterranean regions for newborns [41, 70]. Racial disparity in serum 25[OH]D levels has been well documented in several studies. AA preterm infants and their mothers have lower serum 25[OH]D levels compared to white infants [71–73].

Seto and colleagues measured cord blood 25 [OH]D levels in 276 AA term infants and 162 term white infants and found that AA infants had a 3.6 greater adjusted odds of vitamin D deficiency [74].

Currently, there continues to be emerging information on the distribution of 25[OH]D levels in preterm neonates. A few studies have documented 25[OH]D levels from neonates at birth with sample sizes ranging from 8 to 278 neonates [2, 75–80] with mean 25[OH]D levels ranging from ~6.5 ng/mL among preterm neonates in the United Arab Emirates [78] to 26.8 ng/mL preterm neonates in Canada [10]. A recent study on 596 preterm infants from Ohio, USA reported median 25[OH]D level of 18.5 ng/mL for infants born at 34–36 weeks and 18.6 ng/mL for infants born <32 weeks [81].

The levels of 25[OH]D between the mother and the fetus are positively correlated [68, 81, 82]. Kassai et al. found that mothers who gave birth to preterm neonates had significantly lower mean 25[OH]D blood levels compared to those mothers who gave birth at term. Also, preterm neonates had significantly lower 25[OH]D levels compared to term neonates [83]. A study by Burris et al. measured umbilical cord plasma levels of 25[OH]D in 471 infants born at <37 weeks. They found that babies born at <32 weeks are at increased risk for vitamin D deficiency (25[OH]D levels <20 ng/dL) compared to infants born between 32 and 37 weeks [79]. Monagni et al. studied 120 mother infant dyads at three children's hospitals in Ohio where neonates were delivered at <32 weeks. They not only found that low serum concentrations of 25[OH]D (defined as <50 nmol/L) was common in preterm neonates at admission (64%), but they also found that maternal 25[OH]D levels were lower in infants born at <28 weeks compared to those that were born between 28 and 32 weeks' gestation. Serum 25[OH]D concentrations in preterm infants directly correlated with maternal vitamin D status at the time of delivery. Low 25[OH]D levels were noted at either 36 weeks post-menstrual age (PMA) or at discharge in 40% of infants <28 weeks and 30% of infants between 28 and 32 weeks PMA. Even though infants received vitamin D supplementation from various sources and intake progressively increased during their hospitalization, only 60% received 400 IU vitamin D daily by 36 weeks PMA or discharge [68].

In contrast to the above studies, a Canadian study and an US study did not show any significant difference in vitamin-D status between term and preterm neonates [10, 81]. A study of 3731 term infants in Jordan revealed that 94% had vitamin D deficiency defined as 25[OH]D level < 50 nmol/L. Shahraki et al. found that 25[OH]D levels in preterm neonates were not significantly lower than term neonates. Over 50% of both the term and preterm infants in this study had vitamin D insufficiency and about 25% had vitamin D deficiency [82]. In a cohort born in Cleveland area in US (latitude 41^0N), Kanike et al. reported a remarkably high proportion of vitamin-D deficiency and insufficiency among neonates at birth, 31% and 49% respectively. Notably, they noted low stores of vitamin D despite 75% of women reporting regular multivitamin intake during pregnancy. Vitamin D deficiency was found to be more common in AA neonates (63%) than Caucasian (27%) neonates [81]. Bodnar et.al studied 400 mother–infant pairs in Pittsburgh. They showed that nearly 50% of AA neonates and 10% of white neonates, had serum 25[OH]D levels at birth less than 15 ng/mL despite adequate compliance with a 400 IU daily vitamin-D intake by 90% of their mothers [22]. A prolonged winter season with limited sun exposure in Cleveland might be a contributing factor to the vitamin-D deficiency found in this population. There has been no significant improvement in the vitamin-D status among neonates born to AA women in the last 3 decades in Cleveland area [12].

7. Consequences of vitamin D deficiency in children

Vitamin-D deficiency is the most common cause of rickets and also increases the risk of respiratory distress syndrome, lower respiratory infections, food sensitivities, asthma, type I diabetes, autism and schizophrenia [2, 3, 6, 8, 15]. Vitamin D deficiency in pregnancy impairs fetal lung development partially through suppressing type II pneumocyte differentiation increasing the risk of respiratory distress syndrome in the newborn period [84]. Furthermore, studies have shown that early onset sepsis and late onset sepsis occurs more frequently in term infants with vitamin D deficiency [85–87]. To highlight, one study by Singh and Chaudari found that vitamin D deficiency was more common in neonates with early onset sepsis and was associated with increased severity of sepsis and mortality [87].

Vitamin D deficiency prevents effective absorption of dietary calcium and phosphorus. Vitamin D stores in newborn are completely dependent on vitamin D supply from the mother [12]. Not surprisingly, poor maternal vitamin D status during pregnancy is a major risk factor for infant rickets [13, 88, 89]. Severe chronic vitamin D deficiency leads to overt skeletal abnormalities in children like rickets [90, 91]. However, neonates who are vitamin-D insufficient have no apparent skeletal or calcium metabolism abnormalities [16]. In developing countries rickets has been ranked among the five most prevalent diseases in children [92]. Poorer outcomes during pregnancy, at birth and during infancy are associated with lower serum 25[OH]D levels [24, 93]. Reduced bone mass at 9 years of age was seen in children born with low serum 25[OH]D concentrations [94].

There is conflicting data about role of vitamin D and neurodevelopmental outcomes. A meta-analysis by Tous and colleauges found that infants born to mothers with vitamin D insufficiency had lower scores in both mental and language development [95]. In contrast, Wang et al. found that vitamin D deficiency was not associated with neurodevelopment in infancy [84]. A prospective cohort study by McCarthy et al. found no association between antenatal 25[OH]D levels and neurodevelopmental outcomes at 5 years. Tous et al. found that maternal vitamin D deficiency is associated with lower birth weights, smaller head circumference, increased risk for small for gestational age (SGA) status, and preterm birth. Maternal vitamin D insufficiency was associated with increased risk for infants with SGA status and preterm birth [95]. Seto and colleagues found that black infants with vitamin D deficiency had 2.4 greater adjusted odds for SGA status at birth. The association between SGA and vitamin D deficiency was not demonstrated in white infants [74]. Furthermore, a systematic review by Pligt et al. found the maternal vitamin D deficiency was associated with low birth weight, SGA status at birth, stunting of growth immediately after delivery, and preterm birth [96].

8. Recommended dietary intake in pregnant women and Newborn at risk for vitamin D deficiency

As per the US federal government's 2020–2025 guidelines, fortified foods and dietary supplements are beneficial when it is impossible to meet needs for one or more nutrients during certain life stages such as pregnancy. Milk, many ready-to-eat cereals, and some brands of yogurt, orange juice and margarines are fortified with vitamin D. Trout, tuna, salmon, and mackerel are fatty fish with a high content of vitamin D. One tablespoon of cod liver oil has 1360 IU of vitamin D. Cheese, beef liver and egg yolks naturally contain small amounts of vitamin D. The United States and Canada mandates the fortification of infant formula with 1–2.5 mcg/100 kcal (40–100 IU) vitamin D and 1–2 mcg/100 kcal (40–80 IU) respectively.

Global consensus recommendations on prevention and management of nutritional rickets states that pregnant women should receive 600 IU/d of vitamin-D, preferably as a combined preparation with other recommended micronutrients such as iron and folic acid [97]. The Endocrine Society clinical practice guidelines also recommend at least 600 IU/d of vitamin D in pregnant and lactating women. They also recognize that 1500–2000 IU/day of vitamin D may be needed to maintain 25[OH]D levels>30 ng/mL [32]. However, the average prenatal supplements contain only 400 IU of vitamin D [97]. There is also mounting evidence of the importance of vitamin D supplementation to achieve serum 25[OH]D level of ≥40 ng/ml [55].

Rostami et al. evaluated the effectiveness of a prenatal screening study for optimizing vitamin-D status during pregnancy. The outcome of this program was the prevention of complications of pregnancy. They observed a > 25-fold increase in the number of pregnant women who were able to accomplish a 25[OH]D that was >20 ng/mL when they were screened for their vitamin-D status and provided supplementation compared with pregnant women who were not screened and consequently were not counseled to take vitamin-D supplements. They observed an outstanding decrease in adverse outcomes in pregnant women who were screened and received vitamin-D supplementation. They reported 60%, 50%, and 40% decreases in preeclampsia, gestational diabetes, and preterm delivery, respectively [98].

A recent Cochrane review on Vitamin D supplementation in pregnancy included 30 clinical studies on 3700 pregnant women and reported that taking vitamin D supplements in pregnancy probably reduces the risk of pre-eclampsia, gestational diabetes, post-partum hemorrhage and low-birthweight infant, but there was no difference in the risk of preterm birth before 37 weeks. They also reported that taking vitamin D and calcium together in pregnancy may increase the risk of preterm birth. These results warrant further research [99]. Prenatal supplementation with 4400 IU daily decreased the incidence of asthma and recurrent wheezing in these children at age 3 years by 6.1% [100].

In the 2020 WHO guidelines, routine oral supplementation of vitamin D is not recommended for pregnant women to improve maternal and perinatal outcomes. Pregnant women should be encouraged to receive adequate nutrition, which is best achieved through consumption of a healthy, balanced diet. Pregnant women should be advised that sunlight is the most important source of vitamin D. The amount of time needed in the sun is not known and depends on many variables, such as the amount of skin exposed, the time of day, latitude and season, skin pigmentation and sunscreen use. For pregnant women with suspected vitamin D deficiency, vitamin D supplements may be given at the current recommended nutrient intake of 200 IU per day. This may include women in populations where direct sun exposure is limited.

9. Conclusion

Vitamin D status is more significant during pregnancy, affecting not only the mother but also her growing fetus, and later, her growing child. There are variations in vitamin D status based on gestation at birth, global region of birth, race, and maternal vitamin D status during pregnancy. The current literature suggests that neonates are at high risk of vitamin-D deficiency, even when mothers are compliant with prenatal vitamins. Current prenatal vitamins may not contain enough vitamin-D to prevent deficiency. There has been substantial debate surrounding the daily requirement of vitamin D and what constitutes sufficiency during pregnancy. Higher-dose supplementation may be needed to improve maternal and neonatal vitamin-D status. Future multicenter studies are needed to determine the minimum dose of vitamin-D requirements during pregnancy to achieve vitamin-D sufficiency. It is time to rethink our approach to ensure vitamin-D sufficiency in pregnant women and their newborn infants.

Conflicts of interest statement

The authors have indicated no financial relationships relevant to this article to disclose. The authors have indicated they have no potential/perceived conflicts of interest to disclose.

Author contributions

N.K and J.C conceptualized and drafted the initial manuscript and reviewed and revised the manuscript. N.KG reviewed and revised the manuscript. All authors approved the final manuscript as submitted and agree to be accountable for all aspects of the work.

Author details

Neelakanta Kanike[1]*, Naveen Kannekanti[2] and Jenny Camacho[1]

1 Department of Pediatrics, Division of Neonatology, Indiana University School of Medicine, The Women's Hospital-Deaconess, Newburgh, IN, USA

2 Department of Pediatrics, Division of Neonatology, Case Western Reserve University, MetroHealth Medical Center, Cleveland, OH, USA

*Address all correspondence to: neelkanike@gmail.com

References

[1] Holick MF: **The vitamin D deficiency pandemic: Approaches for diagnosis, treatment and prevention.** Rev Endocr Metab Disord 2017, **18:**153-165.

[2] Mohamed Hegazy A, Mohamed Shinkar D, Refaat Mohamed N, Abdalla Gaber H: **Association between serum 25 (OH) vitamin D level at birth and respiratory morbidities among preterm neonates.** J Matern Fetal Neonatal Med 2018, **31:**2649-2655.

[3] Camargo CA, Jr., Rifas-Shiman SL, Litonjua AA, Rich-Edwards JW, Weiss ST, Gold DR, Kleinman K, Gillman MW: **Maternal intake of vitamin D during pregnancy and risk of recurrent wheeze in children at 3 y of age.** Am J Clin Nutr 2007, **85:**788-795.

[4] Camargo CA, Jr., Ingham T, Wickens K, Thadhani R, Silvers KM, Epton MJ, Town GI, Pattemore PK, Espinola JA, Crane J, et al: **Cord-blood 25-hydroxyvitamin D levels and risk of respiratory infection, wheezing, and asthma.** Pediatrics 2011, **127:**e180-e187.

[5] Stene LC, Joner G, Norwegian Childhood Diabetes Study G: **Use of cod liver oil during the first year of life is associated with lower risk of childhood-onset type 1 diabetes: a large, population-based, case-control study.** Am J Clin Nutr 2003, **78:**1128-1134.

[6] Sorensen IM, Joner G, Jenum PA, Eskild A, Torjesen PA, Stene LC: **Maternal serum levels of 25-hydroxy-vitamin D during pregnancy and risk of type 1 diabetes in the offspring.** Diabetes 2012, **61:**175-178.

[7] McGrath J, Saari K, Hakko H, Jokelainen J, Jones P, Jarvelin MR, Chant D, Isohanni M: **Vitamin D supplementation during the first year of life and risk of schizophrenia: a Finnish birth cohort study.** Schizophr Res 2004, **67:**237-245.

[8] Vinkhuyzen AAE, Eyles DW, Burne THJ, Blanken LME, Kruithof CJ, Verhulst F, White T, Jaddoe VW, Tiemeier H, McGrath JJ: **Gestational vitamin D deficiency and autism spectrum disorder.** BJPsych Open 2017, **3:**85-90.

[9] Vinkhuyzen AAE, Eyles DW, Burne THJ, Blanken LME, Kruithof CJ, Verhulst F, Jaddoe VW, Tiemeier H, McGrath JJ: **Gestational vitamin D deficiency and autism-related traits: the Generation R Study.** Mol Psychiatry 2018, **23:**240-246.

[10] Morgan C, Dodds L, Langille DB, Weiler HA, Armson BA, Forest JC, Giguere Y, Woolcott CG: **Cord blood vitamin D status and neonatal outcomes in a birth cohort in Quebec, Canada.** Arch Gynecol Obstet 2016, **293:**731-738.

[11] Kovacs CS: **Vitamin D in pregnancy and lactation: maternal, fetal, and neonatal outcomes from human and animal studies.** Am J Clin Nutr 2008, **88:**520S-528S.

[12] Hollis BW, Pittard WB, 3rd: **Evaluation of the total fetomaternal vitamin D relationships at term: evidence for racial differences.** J Clin Endocrinol Metab 1984, **59:**652-657.

[13] Specker BL: **Do North American women need supplemental vitamin D during pregnancy or lactation?** *Am J Clin Nutr* 1994, **59:**484S-490S; discussion 490S-491S.

[14] Harrison HE: **A tribute to the first lady of public health (Martha M. Eliot). V. The disappearance of rickets.** Am J Public Health Nations Health 1966, **56:**734-737.

[15] Wharton B, Bishop N: **Rickets.** Lancet 2003, **362:**1389-1400.

[16] Holick MF: **Resurrection of vitamin D deficiency and rickets.** J Clin Invest 2006, **116:**2062-2072.

[17] Calvo MS, Whiting SJ: **Prevalence of vitamin D insufficiency in Canada and the United States: importance to health status and efficacy of current food fortification and dietary supplement use.** Nutr Rev 2003, **61:**107-113.

[18] Hanley DA, Davison KS: **Vitamin D insufficiency in North America.** J Nutr 2005, **135:**332-337.

[19] Holick MF: **Vitamin D: A millenium perspective.** J Cell Biochem 2003, **88:**296-307.

[20] Holick MF: **The vitamin D epidemic and its health consequences.** J Nutr 2005, **135:**2739S-2748S.

[21] Kumar J, Muntner P, Kaskel FJ, Hailpern SM, Melamed ML: **Prevalence and associations of 25-hydroxy vitamin D deficiency in US children: NHANES 2001-2004.** Pediatrics 2009, **124:**e362-e370.

[22] Bodnar LM, Simhan HN, Powers RW, Frank MP, Cooperstein E, Roberts JM: **High prevalence of vitamin D insufficiency in black and white pregnant women residing in the northern United States and their neonates.** J Nutr 2007, **137:**447-452.

[23] Johnson DD, Wagner CL, Hulsey TC, McNeil RB, Ebeling M, Hollis BW: **Vitamin D deficiency and insufficiency is common during pregnancy.** Am J Perinatol 2011, **28:**7-12.

[24] Saraf R, Morton SM, Camargo CA, Jr., Grant CC: **Global summary of maternal and newborn vitamin D status - a systematic review.** Matern Child Nutr 2016, **12:**647-668.

[25] Holick MF: **Vitamin D deficiency.** N Engl J Med 2007, **357:**266-281.

[26] DeLuca HF: **Overview of general physiologic features and functions of vitamin D.** Am J Clin Nutr 2004, **80:**1689S-1696S.

[27] Christakos S, Dhawan P, Liu Y, Peng X, Porta A: **New insights into the mechanisms of vitamin D action.** J Cell Biochem 2003, **88:**695-705.

[28] Heaney RP: **Functional indices of vitamin D status and ramifications of vitamin D deficiency.** Am J Clin Nutr 2004, **80:**1706S-1709S.

[29] Dusso AS, Brown AJ, Slatopolsky E: **Vitamin D.** Am J Physiol Renal Physiol 2005, **289:**F8-28.

[30] Lee JM, Smith JR, Philipp BL, Chen TC, Mathieu J, Holick MF: **Vitamin D deficiency in a healthy group of mothers and newborn infants.** Clin Pediatr (Phila) 2007, **46:**42-44.

[31] Merewood A, Mehta SD, Grossman X, Chen TC, Mathieu JS, Holick MF, Bauchner H: **Widespread vitamin D deficiency in urban Massachusetts newborns and their mothers.** Pediatrics 2010, **125:**640-647.

[32] Holick MF, Binkley NC, Bischoff-Ferrari HA, Gordon CM, Hanley DA, Heaney RP, Murad MH, Weaver CM, Endocrine S: **Evaluation, treatment, and prevention of vitamin D deficiency: an Endocrine Society clinical practice guideline.** J Clin Endocrinol Metab 2011, **96:** 1911-1930.

[33] Gartner LM, Greer FR, Section on B, Committee on Nutrition. American Academy of P: **Prevention of rickets and vitamin D deficiency: new**

guidelines for vitamin D intake. Pediatrics 2003, **111:**908-910.

[34] Herrick KA, Storandt RJ, Afful J, Pfeiffer CM, Schleicher RL, Gahche JJ, Potischman N: **Vitamin D status in the United States, 2011-2014.** Am J Clin Nutr 2019, **110:**150-157.

[35] Lips P, Cashman KD, Lamberg-Allardt C, Bischoff-Ferrari HA, Obermayer-Pietsch B, Bianchi ML, Stepan J, El-Hajj Fuleihan G, Bouillon R: **Current vitamin D status in European and Middle East countries and strategies to prevent vitamin D deficiency: a position statement of the European Calcified Tissue Society.** Eur J Endocrinol 2019, **180:**P23-P54.

[36] Cashman KD, Dowling KG, Skrabakova Z, Gonzalez-Gross M, Valtuena J, De Henauw S, Moreno L, Damsgaard CT, Michaelsen KF, Molgaard C, et al: **Vitamin D deficiency in Europe: pandemic?** Am J Clin Nutr 2016, **103:**1033-1044.

[37] van der Meer IM, Karamali NS, Boeke AJ, Lips P, Middelkoop BJ, Verhoeven I, Wuister JD: **High prevalence of vitamin D deficiency in pregnant non-Western women in The Hague, Netherlands.** Am J Clin Nutr 2006, **84:**350-353; quiz 468-359.

[38] Mutlu N, Esra H, Begum A, Fatma D, Arzu Y, Yalcin H, Fatih K, Selahattin K: **Relation of maternal vitamin D status with gestational diabetes mellitus and perinatal outcome.** Afr Health Sci 2015, **15:**523-531.

[39] Tao M, Shao H, Gu J, Zhen Z: **Vitamin D status of pregnant women in Shanghai, China.** J Matern Fetal Neonatal Med 2012, **25:**237-239.

[40] Palacios C, De-Regil LM, Lombardo LK, Peña-Rosas JP: **Vitamin D supplementation during pregnancy: Updated meta-analysis on maternal outcomes.** J Steroid Biochem Mol Biol 2016, **164:**148-155.

[41] Mithal A, Wahl DA, Bonjour JP, Burckhardt P, Dawson-Hughes B, Eisman JA, El-Hajj Fuleihan G, Josse RG, Lips P, Morales-Torres J, Group IOFCoSANW: **Global vitamin D status and determinants of hypovitaminosis D.** Osteoporos Int 2009, **20:**1807-1820.

[42] Balasubramanian S, Dhanalakshmi K, Amperayani S: **Vitamin D deficiency in childhood-a review of current guidelines on diagnosis and management.** Indian Pediatr 2013, **50:**669-675.

[43] Joiner TA, Foster C, Shope T: **The many faces of vitamin D deficiency rickets.** Pediatr Rev 2000, **21:**296-302.

[44] Harinarayan CV, Joshi SR: **Vitamin D status in India--its implications and remedial measures.** J Assoc Physicians India 2009, **57:**40-48.

[45] Chacham S, Rajput S, Gurnurkar S, Mirza A, Saxena V, Dakshinamurthy S, Chaturvedi J, Goyal JP, Chegondi M: **Prevalence of Vitamin D Deficiency Among Infants in Northern India: A Hospital Based Prospective Study.** Cureus 2020, **12:**e11353.

[46] Mogire RM, Mutua A, Kimita W, Kamau A, Bejon P, Pettifor JM, Adeyemo A, Williams TN, Atkinson SH: **Prevalence of vitamin D deficiency in Africa: a systematic review and meta-analysis.** Lancet Glob Health 2020, **8:**e134-e142.

[47] Zhang W, Stoecklin E, Eggersdorfer M: **A glimpse of vitamin D status in Mainland China.** Nutrition 2013, **29:**953-957.

[48] Cyprian F, Lefkou E, Varoudi K, Girardi G: **Immunomodulatory Effects of Vitamin D in Pregnancy and Beyond.** Front Immunol 2019, **10:** 2739.

[49] Kiely ME, Wagner CL, Roth DE: **Vitamin D in pregnancy: Where we are and where we should go.** J Steroid Biochem Mol Biol 2020, **201:**105669.

[50] Aghajafari F, Nagulesapillai T, Ronksley PE, Tough SC, O'Beirne M, Rabi DM: **Association between maternal serum 25-hydroxyvitamin D level and pregnancy and neonatal outcomes: systematic review and meta-analysis of observational studies.** BMJ 2013, **346:**f1169.

[51] Autier P, Gandini S: **Vitamin D supplementation and total mortality: a meta-analysis of randomized controlled trials.** Arch Intern Med 2007, **167:**1730-1737.

[52] Pilz S, Tomaschitz A, Obermayer-Pietsch B, Dobnig H, Pieber TR: **Epidemiology of vitamin D insufficiency and cancer mortality.** Anticancer Res 2009, **29:**3699-3704.

[53] Chen YH, Liu ZB, Ma L, Zhang ZC, Fu L, Yu Z, Chen W, Song YP, Wang P, Wang H, Xu X: **Gestational vitamin D deficiency causes placental insufficiency and fetal intrauterine growth restriction partially through inducing placental inflammation.** J Steroid Biochem Mol Biol 2020, **203:**105733.

[54] Kovacs CS: **Bone development and mineral homeostasis in the fetus and neonate: roles of the calciotropic and phosphotropic hormones.** Physiol Rev 2014, **94:**1143-1218.

[55] Hollis BW, Wagner CL: **New insights into the vitamin D requirements during pregnancy.** Bone Res 2017, **5:**17030.

[56] Karras SN, Wagner CL, Castracane VD: **Understanding vitamin D metabolism in pregnancy: From physiology to pathophysiology and clinical outcomes.** Metabolism 2018, **86:**112-123.

[57] Ganguly A, Tamblyn JA, Finn-Sell S, Chan SY, Westwood M, Gupta J, Kilby MD, Gross SR, Hewison M: **Vitamin D, the placenta and early pregnancy: effects on trophoblast function.** J Endocrinol 2018, **236:**R93-R103.

[58] Carmeliet G, Bouillon R: **How Important Is Vitamin D for Calcium Homeostasis During Pregnancy and Lactation?** J Bone Miner Res 2018, **33:**13-15.

[59] Sachan A, Gupta R, Das V, Agarwal A, Awasthi PK, Bhatia V: **High prevalence of vitamin D deficiency among pregnant women and their newborns in northern India.** Am J Clin Nutr 2005, **81:**1060-1064.

[60] Agarwal KS, Mughal MZ, Upadhyay P, Berry JL, Mawer EB, Puliyel JM: **The impact of atmospheric pollution on vitamin D status of infants and toddlers in Delhi, India.** Arch Dis Child 2002, **87:**111-113.

[61] Sowah D, Fan X, Dennett L, Hagtvedt R, Straube S: **Vitamin D levels and deficiency with different occupations: a systematic review.** BMC Public Health 2017, **17:**519.

[62] Ekwaru JP, Zwicker JD, Holick MF, Giovannucci E, Veugelers PJ: **The importance of body weight for the dose response relationship of oral vitamin D supplementation and serum 25-hydroxyvitamin D in healthy volunteers.** PLoS One 2014, **9:**e111265.

[63] Earthman CP, Beckman LM, Masodkar K, Sibley SD: **The link between obesity and low circulating 25-hydroxyvitamin D concentrations: considerations and implications.** Int J Obes (Lond) 2012, **36:**387-396.

[64] Lin E, Armstrong-Moore D, Liang Z, Sweeney JF, Torres WE, Ziegler TR, Tangpricha V, Gletsu-Miller

N: **Contribution of adipose tissue to plasma 25-hydroxyvitamin D concentrations during weight loss following gastric bypass surgery.** Obesity (Silver Spring) 2011, **19:**588-594.

[65] Pappa HM, Bern E, Kamin D, Grand RJ: **Vitamin D status in gastrointestinal and liver disease.** Curr Opin Gastroenterol 2008, **24:**176-183.

[66] Sotunde OF, Laliberte A, Weiler HA: **Maternal risk factors and newborn infant vitamin D status: a scoping literature review.** Nutr Res 2019, **63:**1-20.

[67] Urrutia-Pereira M, Sole D: **[Vitamin D deficiency in pregnancy and its impact on the fetus, the newborn and in childhood].** Rev Paul Pediatr 2015, **33:**104-113.

[68] Monangi N, Slaughter JL, Dawodu A, Smith C, Akinbi HT: **Vitamin D status of early preterm infants and the effects of vitamin D intake during hospital stay.** Arch Dis Child Fetal Neonatal Ed 2014, **99:**F166-F168.

[69] Hilger J, Friedel A, Herr R, Rausch T, Roos F, Wahl DA, Pierroz DD, Weber P, Hoffmann K: **A systematic review of vitamin D status in populations worldwide.** Br J Nutr 2014, **111:**23-45.

[70] Arabi A, El Rassi R, El-Hajj Fuleihan G: **Hypovitaminosis D in developing countries-prevalence, risk factors and outcomes.** Nat Rev Endocrinol 2010, **6:**550-561.

[71] Taylor SN, Wagner CL, Fanning D, Quinones L, Hollis BW: **Vitamin D status as related to race and feeding type in preterm infants.** Breastfeed Med 2006, **1:**156-163.

[72] Basile LA, Taylor SN, Wagner CL, Quinones L, Hollis BW: **Neonatal vitamin D status at birth at latitude 32 degrees 72': evidence of deficiency.** J Perinatol 2007, **27:**568-571.

[73] Hanson C, Armas L, Lyden E, Anderson-Berry A: **Vitamin D status and associations in newborn formula-fed infants during initial hospitalization.** J Am Diet Assoc 2011, **111:**1836-1843.

[74] Seto TL, Tabangin ME, Langdon G, Mangeot C, Dawodu A, Steinhoff M, Narendran V: **Racial disparities in cord blood vitamin D levels and its association with small-for-gestational-age infants.** J Perinatol 2016, **36:**623-628.

[75] Backstrom MC, Maki R, Kuusela AL, Sievanen H, Koivisto AM, Ikonen RS, Kouri T, Maki M: **Randomised controlled trial of vitamin D supplementation on bone density and biochemical indices in preterm infants.** Arch Dis Child Fetal Neonatal Ed 1999, **80:**F161-F166.

[76] Delmas PD, Glorieux FH, Delvin EE, Salle BL, Melki I: **Perinatal serum bone Gla-protein and vitamin D metabolites in preterm and fullterm neonates.** J Clin Endocrinol Metab 1987, **65:**588-591.

[77] Salle BL, Glorieux FH, Delvin EE, David LS, Meunier G: **Vitamin D metabolism in preterm infants. Serial serum calcitriol values during the first four days of life.** Acta Paediatr Scand 1983, **72:**203-206.

[78] Dawodu A, Nath R: **High prevalence of moderately severe vitamin D deficiency in preterm infants.** Pediatr Int 2011, **53:**207-210.

[79] Burris HH, Van Marter LJ, McElrath TF, Tabatabai P, Litonjua AA, Weiss ST, Christou H: **Vitamin D status among preterm and full-term infants at birth.** Pediatr Res 2014, **75:** 75-80.

[80] Park SH, Lee GM, Moon JE, Kim HM: **Severe vitamin D deficiency in preterm infants: maternal and neonatal clinical features.** Korean J Pediatr 2015, **58:**427-433.

[81] Kanike N, Hospattankar KG, Sharma A, Worley S, Groh-Wargo S: **Prevalence of Vitamin D Deficiency in a Large Newborn Cohort from Northern United States and Effect of Intrauterine Drug Exposure.** Nutrients 2020, **12.**

[82] Shahraki AD, Hasanabadi MS, Dehkordi AF: **The a ssociation of 25-hydroxy Vitamin D level in mothers with term and preterm delivery and their neonates.** J Res Med Sci 2020, **25:**21.

[83] Kassai MS, Cafeo FR, Affonso-Kaufman FA, Suano-Souza FI, Sarni ROS: **Vitamin D plasma concentrations in pregnant women and their preterm newborns.** BMC Pregnancy Childbirth 2018, **18:**412.

[84] Wang P, Tan ZX, Fu L, Fan YJ, Luo B, Zhang ZH, Xu S, Chen YH, Zhao H, Xu DX: **Gestational vitamin D deficiency impairs fetal lung development through suppressing type II pneumocyte differentiation.** Reprod Toxicol 2020, **94:**40-47.

[85] Dhandai R, Jajoo M, Singh A, Mandal A, Jain R: **Association of vitamin D deficiency with an increased risk of late-onset neonatal sepsis.** Paediatr Int Child Health 2018, **38:**193-197.

[86] Agrawal A, Gupta A, Shrivastava J: **Role of Vitamin-D Deficiency in Term Neonates with Late-Onset Sepsis: A Case-Control Study.** J Trop Pediatr 2019, **65:**609-616.

[87] Singh P, Chaudhari V: **Association of Early-Onset Sepsis and Vitamin D Deficiency in Term Neonates.** Indian Pediatr 2020, **57:**232-234.

[88] Zeghoud F, Vervel C, Guillozo H, Walrant-Debray O, Boutignon H, Garabedian M: **Subclinical vitamin D deficiency in neonates: definition and response to vitamin D supplements.** Am J Clin Nutr 1997, **65:**771-778.

[89] Wagner CL, Greer FR, American Academy of Pediatrics Section on B, American Academy of Pediatrics Committee on N: **Prevention of rickets and vitamin D deficiency in infants, children, and adolescents.** Pediatrics 2008, **122:**1142-1152.

[90] Markestad T, Halvorsen S, Halvorsen KS, Aksnes L, Aarskog D: **Plasma concentrations of vitamin D metabolites before and during treatment of vitamin D deficiency rickets in children.** Acta Paediatr Scand 1984, **73:**225-231.

[91] Pettifor JM: **Rickets and vitamin D deficiency in children and adolescents.** Endocrinol Metab Clin North Am 2005, **34:**537-553, vii.

[92] Glorieux FH: **Rickets, the continuing challenge.** N Engl J Med 1991, **325:**1875-1877.

[93] Hossein-nezhad A, Holick MF: **Vitamin D for health: a global perspective.** Mayo Clin Proc 2013, **88:**720-755.

[94] Javaid MK, Crozier SR, Harvey NC, Gale CR, Dennison EM, Boucher BJ, Arden NK, Godfrey KM, Cooper C, Princess Anne Hospital Study G: **Maternal vitamin D status during pregnancy and childhood bone mass at age 9 years: a longitudinal study.** Lancet 2006, **367:**36-43.

[95] Tous M, Villalobos M, Iglesias L, Fernandez-Barres S, Arija V: **Vitamin D status during pregnancy and offspring outcomes: a systematic review and meta-analysis of observational studies.** Eur J Clin Nutr 2020, **74:** 36-53.

[96] van der Pligt P, Willcox J, Szymlek-Gay EA, Murray E, Worsley A, Daly RM: **Associations of Maternal Vitamin D Deficiency with Pregnancy and Neonatal Complications in Developing Countries: A Systematic Review.** Nutrients 2018, **10**.

[97] Munns CF, Shaw N, Kiely M, Specker BL, Thacher TD, Ozono K, Michigami T, Tiosano D, Mughal MZ, Makitie O, et al: **Global Consensus Recommendations on Prevention and Management of Nutritional Rickets.** J Clin Endocrinol Metab 2016, **101**:394-415.

[98] Rostami M, Tehrani FR, Simbar M, Bidhendi Yarandi R, Minooee S, Hollis BW, Hosseinpanah F: **Effectiveness of Prenatal Vitamin D Deficiency Screening and Treatment Program: A Stratified Randomized Field Trial.** J Clin Endocrinol Metab 2018, **103**:2936-2948.

[99] Palacios C, Kostiuk LK, Pena-Rosas JP: **Vitamin D supplementation for women during pregnancy.** Cochrane Database Syst Rev 2019, **7**:CD008873.

[100] Litonjua AA, Carey VJ, Laranjo N, Harshfield BJ, McElrath TF, O'Connor GT, Sandel M, Iverson RE, Jr., Lee-Paritz A, Strunk RC, et al: **Effect of Prenatal Supplementation With Vitamin D on Asthma or Recurrent Wheezing in Offspring by Age 3 Years: The VDAART Randomized Clinical Trial.** JAMA 2016, **315**:362-370.

Chapter 3

Vitamin D in Elderly

Malgorzata Kupisz-Urbańska, Jacek Łukaszkiewicz and Ewa Marcinowska-Suchowierska

Abstract

Vitamin D deficiency is common in elderly people, especially in patients with comorbidity and polypharmcy. In this group, low vitamin D plasma concentration is related to osteoporosis, osteomalacia, sarcopenia and myalgia. Vitamin D status in geriatric population is an effect of joint interaction of all vitamin D metabolic pathways, aging processes and multimorbidity. Therefore, all factors interfering with individual metabolic stages may affect 25-hydroxyvitamin D plasma concentration. The known factors affecting vitamin D metabolism interfere with cytochrome CYP3A4 activity. The phenomenon of drugs and vitamin D interactions is observed first and foremost in patients with comorbidity. This is a typical example of the situation where a lack of "hard evidence" is not synonymous with the possible lack of adverse effects. Geriatric giants, such as sarcopenia (progressive and generalized loss of skeletal muscle mass and strength) or cognitive decline, strongly influence elderly patients. Sarcopenia is one of the musculoskeletal consequences of hypovitaminosis D. These consequences are related to a higher risk of adverse outcomes, such as fracture, physical disability, a poor quality of life and death. This can lead not only to an increased risk of falls and fractures, but is also one of the main causes of frailty syndrome in the aging population. Generally, Vitamin D plasma concentration is significantly lower in participants with osteoporosis and muscle deterioration. In some observational and uncontrolled treatment studies, vitamin D supplementation led to a reduction of proximal myopathy and muscle pain. The most positive results were found in subjects with severe vitamin D deficiency and in patients avoiding high doses of vitamin D. However, the role of vitamin D in muscle pathologies is not clear and research has provided conflicting results. This is most likely due to the heterogeneity of the subjects, vitamin D doses and environmental factors.

Keywords: Vitamin D, pleiotropic effect, elderly, aging

1. Introduction

Vitamin D is a fat-soluble vitamin mainly produced by the skin after sun exposure (cholecalciferol - vitamin D3) and can also be obtained from food (ergocalciferol-vitamin D2 and vitamin D3) or supplementation. In the liver, vitamin D (the term "vitamin D" refers both vit.D2 and vit.D3") is converted to 25-hydroxyvitamin D [25(OH)D]), also known as "calcidiol", the major circulating metabolite of vitamin D which can be measured in the blood. In the kidney, [25(OH)D] is converted by 1-alfa-hydroxylase into its active form called 1,25-dihydroxyvitamin D [1,25(OH)2D], also known as "calcitriol", that plays a vital role in maintaining bone homeostasis by regulating calcium metabolism. This action of [1,25(OH)2D] is referred to as endocrine action. The other area where [25(OH)D] is converted by peripheral 1-alfa-hydroxylase to [1,25(OH)2D] are cells in various tissues. There, [1,25(OH)2D] regulation by autocrine or paracrine actions have been observed.

Vitamin D deficiency and insufficiency is one of the major world-wide health problems and its consequences seem to be more serious in the elderly population than in younger adults. It has been associated with a wide range of diseases including autoimmune diseases (among others multiple sclerosis, type 1 diabetes, rheumatoid arthritis), cardiovascular diseases (for example stroke), infectious diseases (bacterial, viral and, fungal), type 2 diabetes and some types of cancers (colorectal, breast and prostate gland). It is also recognized that vitamin D deficiency is associated with some psychiatric disorders including depression, neurocognitive dysfunction and others forms of neurodegenerative disorders (Alzheimer's disease) [1].

This recognition has not only resulted in broadening our knowledge and more conscious vitamin D prescriptions but also led to the crucial question in everyday clinical practice: How can we use our knowledge to improve care for elderly people with vitamin D deficiency and to guide future research studies? Therefore, our publication is focused on distinctive characteristics of vitamin D metabolism, deficiency and drug interaction in the elderly population. As the range of aspects of vitamin D effects in the geriatric population is extremely wide, only chosen elements typical for elderly patients could be presented to emphasise the complexity of the issue.

2. Vitamin D deficiency in the aging population

Available data indicates that in many countries all over the world, the general population (irrespective of the latitude of residence, age, sex and race) and patients considered as otherwise healthy, suffer from vitamin D insufficiency, defined as 25(OH)D < 30 ng/ml. Recent large observational data have suggested that ~40% of Europeans are vitamin D deficient, and 13% are severely deficient [2]. When 25-hydroxyvitamin D levels were analyzed in relation to age (based on 10-year ranges) there were significant differences in the level of 25(OH)D. The level of 25(OH) D was significantly lower in the older population. However, there are conflicting data concerning the subject, for example in a large Japanese study, the adjusted odds ratio for circulating 25OHD > 75 nmol/l (>30 ng/ml) was in men and women aged >70 years (reference group: individuals aged <50 years) 2.55 and 2.26, respectively. In Bergman et all study, patients aged over 65 years had significant lower circulating 25OHD levels than patients over 75 years [3–6].

3. Elderly people are not a homogenic population

Meanwhile, the elderly and the oldest-old are one of the fastest growing populations all over the world. The number of people aged 65 and older is expected to rapidly increase in the next decades. Not only the elderly, but also the oldest old are still increasing in numbers. Globally, the current average annual growth rate of people aged 80 years or older (3.8 per cent) is twice as high as the growth rate of the persons younger than 60 years of age (1.9 per cent) [7]. Despite the same range of biological age, it is not a homogenic population regarding the aging type (successful or unsuccessful). Multimorbidity combined with polypharmacy is common, so functional assessment and mobility determine the quality of life. The role of vitamin D in the prevention and treatment of diseases associated with aging is still being researched. Therefore, during last decade, geriatric medicine has been focused on studies concerning not only vitamin D deficiency in elderly, but especially on its possible impact on Healthy life years (HLY, also called disability-free life expectancy) taking into account the role of vitamin D considered as a potential factor strongly influencing possible elongation of HLY. Vitamin D status has been widely studied in the last decade. Undoubtedly, one of the most important clinical question concerns the possibilities of preventing of unhealthy aging.

4. Factors contributing to vitamin D deficiency in the elderly

Most importantly, [1,25(OH)2D] directly or indirectly regulates over 200 genes including those involved in: rennin production in the kidney, insulin in the pancreas, the release of cytokines from lymphocytes, production of cathelicidin by macrophages, and the growth and proliferation smooth muscle cells and cardiomyocytes. The main cause of aging-associated vitamin D deficiency is low vitamin D production. As we age, there is a reduction in the skin's concentration of 7-dehydrocholesterol [8]. Specifically, for each decade past the age of 40, there is approximately a 10 to 15% decrease in the level of 7-dehydrocholesterol. Furthermore, the character of dressing style makes the sun exposure indispensable as well as short time of outdoor activities, taking into account that a sufficient amount of sunlight radiation for vitamin D production by the skin only occurs between May and September in some latitudes. Additionally, there is about a 35% decrease in intestinal calcium absorption after the age of 70 [9]. This decrease is even greater in women because of reduced fractional calcium absorption and estrogen changes after the menopause with increased urinary calcium losses [10]. Other causes of aging-associated vitamin D deficiency are related to poor vitamin D and calcium nutrition. With age, comorbidity must also be taken into account with a special focus on renal and liver insufficiency.

5. Vitamin D and geriatric giants

With advanced age, people appear to change their health status perception as a range of independence rather than lack of disease. The presence of "geriatric giants" (coined by Bernard Isaacs in 1965 to encompass common impairments) contributes to more serious consequences than in younger groups [11–13]. Recent epidemiological research has shown that the concentration of 25-hydroxyvitamin D may have an impact on various age-related diseases, as well as on geriatric giants. Geriatric giants are common, have multiple contributing factors and their consequences are stronger in older groups of patients. Some geriatric giants, like sarcopenia, falls or cognitive decline, neurodegenerative disease, and depression are likely to have extremely strong impact on independency of individuals and high risk of negative outcomes.

5.1 Sarcopenia

Sarcopenia is known as a new geriatric giant. It is an interdisciplinary and multifactor symptom whose prevalence rises with age. Furthermore, the development of secondary hyperparathyroidism favors a negative calcium balance, high bone turnover and accelerates age-related bone loss and osteoporotic fractures.

According to the consensus of The European Working Group on Sarcopenia in Older People, the diagnosis is based on three criteria: low muscle strength or/and low physical performance, and low muscle mass. Sarcopenia is a progressive process and, as a new geriatric giant, has many contributing factors - not only the aging processes, but also vitamin D deficiency, diet, sedentary lifestyle, diseases, drug treatments and drug interactions [14].

Sarcopenia has strong impact on the outcomes of the risk of falls and osteoporotic fractures, lack of independency and lack of ability to perform activities of daily living. Subjects with sarcopenic obesity in the MrOS study had a 1.9 increased risk of any fracture and 3.1 increased risk of spine fracture [15]. The loss of strength is also an important criteria for a diagnosis of frailty syndrome (FS). Therefore, sarcopenia associated with muscle loss in frailty syndrome is one of the major issues of geriatric medicine. The prevalence of frailty syndrome is growing with age. The key role that vitamin D plays in muscle function and low muscle strength has been described in subjects with osteomalacia. The effects of 1,25(OH)D on the proliferation and differentiation in myogenic cells have also been described [20]. Although it remains highly debated, the action of vitamin D via the VDR receptor seems to play a significant role in muscle development and growth [16–18].

It remains unclear in observational studies if there is a key role in vitamin D interaction with muscle, or rather this is the effect of other factors. In an eight-year longitudinal study, the supplementation of vitamin D was not associated with a decreased risk of frailty, but the average daily dosage of oral vitamin D was lower than 400 IU and probably not enough to achieve the target of serum 25(0H) D concentration of 20 ng/ml. Additionally, the lowest 25(OH)D season-specific quartile correlated with a faster rate of muscle strength loss in men aged over 85 [19, 20]. The process was observed in all subjects, including those who were not supplemented with vitamin D. Some interventional studies have been conducted to describe the role of vitamin D in musculosceletal health. However, only a few of these studies had muscle strength as the endpoint. Vitamin D may affect muscle function, particularly in vulnerable populations such as the oldest old and patients with severe sarcopenia. However, it is difficult to create a homogenic group of subjects with the oldest old due to a large number of cofactors that influence physical performance. Nevertheless, vitamin D supplementation for preventing sarcopenia still requires a controlled, double–blind research design.

Sarcopenia being one of the crucial factors of frailty syndrome constitution provides a significant increase in falls that are one of the many causes of disability and functional decline in elderly people. Despite numerous trials and meta-analyses conducted the efficacy of vitamin D supplementation as a mean to prevent falls remains uncertain. The effectiveness of vitamin D in fall prevention remains an issue of the debate. Authors of publications have underscored the importance of further trials on vitamin D and falls and highlight 3 key characteristics these trials should comprise: vitamin D deficiency, vitamin D administration, and unified falls documentation [21].

5.2 Cognitive decline: dementia, depression

Vitamin D, by direct and indirect regulation of more than 200 genes, exerts bioactivity as a hormone and plays an important role in processes important for the functioning of all systems as well as central nervous system, including calcium absorption, tissue and immune cell growth, and inflammation. However, the crucial role of vitamin D for brain health is supported by the presence of the enzyme that produces its active form 1-hydroxylase in cerebrospinal fluid. The receptor for the active metabolite is found throughout the human brain. Vitamin D has been linked with neuron growth and survival by its regulation of factors such as glutathione, growth factors, neurotrophies and neurotransmitters. Moreover, in animal models, vitamin D supplementation showed reduced inflammatory biomarkers in the hippocampus. Vitamin D receptor (VDR) seems to be one of the most probable genetic factors of Alzheimer disease (AD). VDR polymorphism increases the risk of AD by 2.3 times and in molecular studies, vitamin D treatment prevented amyloid production and enhanced its removal [22].

The pleiotropic aspects of vitamin D action was tested in numerous observational studies suggesting an association between low serum concentration and the increased risk of other geriatric giants such as cognitive decline, dementia and depression and its supplementation has also shown an improvement in the cognitive performance in elderly patients with senile dementia.

5.2.1 Epidemiological studies

A survey was conducted in Norway among patients over 65 years old with depression who were admitted to psychiatric wards. Vitamin D deficiency (below 20 ng/ml) was observed in 71% patients with depression, 50% patients with bipolar affective disorder and in 25% of control group patients. However, in other studies, there exist a wide range of differences between vitamin D deficiency status (from 34,6% in USA to 100% in British research). Because of the existing conflicts in the data, Li et all in 2018 conducted a meta-analysis to extend the knowledge concerning vitamin D deficiency in patients with depression. They assumed that for every 10 ng/ml of vitamin D level, the increase risk of depression decreases 12%. So, vitamin D supplementation could be useful in the reduction of depression risk, but until this time, the data of RCT's are not conclusive [23, 24].

5.2.2 Alzheimer's disease (AD)

Two meta-analysis underscored significantly lower vitamin D concentrations in patients with AD compared to healthy individuals. The risk of AD in patients with vitamin D deficiency was found to be twice higher in an American study and 2.85 times higher in a French study. There exists a correlation between the stage of deficiency and concentration - respectively 19% for concentration below 20 ng/ml and 31% for severe deficiency (<10 ng/ml). However, concentrations >35 ng/ml were not correlated with a of lower risk of AD. Vitamin D pretends to be an independent protective factor reducing Alzheimer diseases processes. For example, in a Spanish study, the dynamics of Alzheimer disease was slower in patients receiving vitamin D. However, the data concerning influence of vitamin D supplementation in AD remains not conclusive [25, 26]. There is also lack of prospective RCT studies.

6. Comorbidity and infections

Notably, several studies have reported an inverse association between 25(OH)D serum levels and the risk of infections (including oral, gastrointestinal, urinary, and respiratory). Many studies underscored the potential immunomodulatory effects as well as the association between the low serum vitamin D levels and many other diseases, such as endocrinal dysfunction leading to increasing insulin resistance, diabetic negative outcomes (for example retinopathy), and cardiovascular disorders. Therefore, all those elements of diseases, typical for elderly patients, create unfavourable background for constitution and progression of geriatric giants. However, in a Lithuanian cross-sectional study (Alekna et al.) of serum 25(OH)D concentrations in relation to activities of daily living (ADL) conducted among octogenarians the regression coefficient for 25(OH)D concentration vs. ADL category was 0.2 (p = 0.01). As highlighted by the authors, it was impossible in this study to determine whether ADL status was a cause or an effect of serum 25(OH)D concentration [27] Complexity of aging processes, age related diseases, geriatric giants and socioeconomic factors influencing elderly patients result in multifactorial, elaborate relation between all this factors to vitamin D status.

The last several months have strongly influenced geriatric medicine. COVID infection has become a clinical example of how important the role of vitamin D is in immunomodulation and anti-inflammatory effect for organisms in particular of aging organs.

7. Vitamin D supplementation and vitamin D treatment in elderly

7.1 Recommendations for general elderly populations

Recommendations for vitamin D intake in asymptomatic healthy individuals and in asymptomatic healthy individuals at high risk of vitamin D deficiency (which was published as the Central European Recommendation; similar to the Endocrine Society in USA) are presented in **Tables 1** and **2**. These guidelines recommend the use of vitamin D supplements to obtain and maintain the optimal target 25(OH)D concentration in range of 30-50 ng/ml (75-125 nmol/m).

As presented in **Tables 1** and **2**, people over the age of 65 should take 800- 2000 IU/d of vitamin D throughout the whole year, but people younger than 65 should take vitamin D in the same doses only when the photosynthesis in the skin is insufficient, during the winter months at latitude of $>40^{\circ}$, little or no UVB radiation reaches the surface of the earth; such as in Poland from October to March (**Table 1**). The recommended vitamin D intake for groups at risk of vitamin D deficiency and requires larger doses of vitamin D (**Table 2**). This includes night-time workers and dark-skinned people (1000-2000 IU/d of vitamin D for the whole year) and obese people (1600 IU/d to 4000 IU/d for the whole year). There are two essential points about supplementation in the healthy population. First, measurements of [25(OH)D] should not be tested before and during supplementation and second, vitamin D doses larger than the tolerable upper intake levels (ULS) to prevent deficiency of vitamin should not be prescribed. The ULS for adults and seniors with normal body weight is 4000 IU/d, but in obese adults and seniors, it is higher (10 000 IU/d.) [28].

It is very important that treatment of vitamin D deficiency is based on 25(OH) D concentration and antecedent prophylactic management. Individual patients with serum 25(OH) < 20 ng/ml that have clinical risk factors for vitamin D deficiency (decreased intake, gastrointestinal diseases, chronic hepatic diseases, renal diseases, medication with antiepileptic drugs and others which disturbing metabolism of vitamin D) with bone diseases (fragility fractures, documented osteoporosis or

		Sufficient skin synthesis		Supplementaion vitamin D IU	
Season in year		**October–March**	**April–September**	**October–March**	**April-September**
Adults	to 65 years	—	+	800-2000	—
	after 65 years	—	—	800-2000	
		Recommendation: do not routinely test 25 (OH)D levels in these groups			

Table 1.
Recommended vitamin D intake in asymptomatic healthy individuals at high risk of vitamin D deficiency.

		Sufficient skin synthesis		Supplementaion vitamin D IU	
Season in year		**October–March**	**April–September**	**October–March**	**April–September**
Adults	Nighttime workers	—	—	1000-2000	
	Dark-skinned	—	—	1000-20000	
	Obese (adults and seniors)	—	—	1600-4000	
Recommendation: do not routinely test 25 (OH)D levels in these groups					

Table 2.
Recommended treatment for individual patients with vitamin D deficiency.

high fracture risk, treated with antiresorptive medication, osteomalacia) should be treated. The primary treatment objectives for vitamin D deficiency are the prescription of adequate doses to ensure correction of vitamin D deficiency (>20 ng/ml), reversing the clinical consequences of vitamin D in a timely manner and avoiding toxicity.

The oral route (intake) of treatment is recommended (vitamin D2 and vitamin D3) and should be taken with food to aid absorption. The dosage should be adjusted on the basis of the baseline deficit and the patient's weight (schematic representation for elderly population presented below in the **Figure 1**). The control level of [25(OH)D] should be attained during treatment at the beginning and after 7-10 weeks.

Treatment of vitamin D deficiency should consist of 2 parts: the initial repletion phase of therapy (loading phase), and after the loading phase, initiating the maintenance.

The loading phase with vitamin D requires 7 to 10 weeks. The aim is to saturate all body compartments so the level of [25(OH)D] is above 30 ng/ml (75 nnom/l. During this time, loading doses of vitamin D (about 300 000 IU) should be given as daily split (divide) doses or intermittent doses every week. Single mega doses (300 000 IU to treat deficiency) are not recommended in the treatment of vitamin D deficiency. Maintenance regiments may be considered after the loading doses.

Example regiments: all loading doses are 300 000 IU and may by administered by a weekly or daily split.

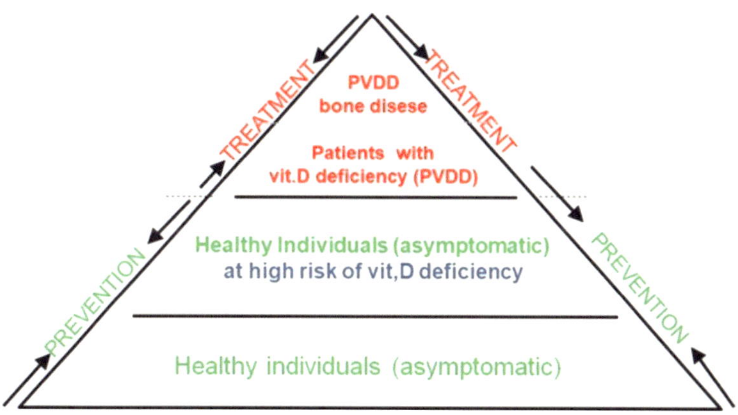

Figure 1.
Schematic representation elderly population vulnerable to vitamin D deficiency that defines broad groups for clinical consideration and decision-making about supplementation or treatment with vitamin D elderly individuals' (PVDD – patients with vitamin D deficiency).

50 000 IU capsules, one given weekly for 6 weeks.
20 000 IU capsules, two given weekly for 7 weeks.
1000 IU capsules, 4 a day for 10 weeks.

Maintenance regiments after loading doses (given either daily (800 – 4000 IU/D) or intermittently at higher equivalent doses (20 000 every 2 weeks).

The rapid correction of vitamin D deficiency may be necessary in some patients. Rapid correction is required in patients with symptomatic disease or those about to start treatment with potent antiresorptive agent, such as zolenndronate or denosumab. In these cases, the recommended treatment is based on split-loading doses (not single large doses) followed by regular maintenance therapy. Regarding the differences between cholecalciferol and calcifediol, including faster intestine absorption of the calcifediol and linear increment uninfluenced by baseline vitamin D level, in elderly patients often this type of therapy should be considered.

Less urgent correction with lower subsequent dosing is required in patients with increased sensitivity to vitamin D therapy because of genetic abnormality in vitamin D metabolism, co-morbidities such as CD, granulomatoforming diseases or hyperparathyreoidismus [29, 30] .

Analogs 1 alfa (OH)D, 1, alfa 25(0H2)D and others should not be used in therapy of vitamin D deficiency or insufficiency. It is worth of mentioning that in the elderly patients, presence of geriatric giants, multimorbidity and drug interactions should be taken into account.

8. Vitamin D intake and polypharmacy

The problem of polypharmacy and drug interaction is common in geriatric patients, as multimorbidity is a typical characteristic of this population. This makes it necessary to take into account assumptions concerning the possible interferences of widely used drugs on vitamin D metabolism. Vitamin D status in humans is an effect of the joint interaction of all vitamin D metabolic pathways. Therefore, all factors that interfere with individual metabolic stages may affect 25-hydroxyvitamin D concentration in the circulation. To date, there is little hard evidence that agents such as lipase inhibitors, statins, antimicrobials, antiepileptics and others affect [25(OH)D] concentration in blood serum. The issue of drug and vitamin D interactions is a clear example of a situation where lack of evidence does not equate to "no harm".

The agents with a potential to influence vitamin D status can be roughly divided into drugs that effect vitamin D intestinal absorption and those that influence vitamin D metabolism [31].

Included in the first category, lipase inhibitors are widely used for obesity treatment. They decrease triglycerides hydrolysis in the gut, causing an incremental rise of excreted fat from the typical 5% up to 30%. This increases fat-soluble vitamin D loss in the feces, at the same time decreasing the vitamin D pool available for absorption in the small intestine. In the second category of drugs that influence vitamin D metabolism, statins are an important class and are widely used as very effective agents in both the primary and secondary prevention of cardiovascular diseases.

Statins are the most widely prescribed cholesterol-lowering drugs in the world, and they are expected to generate a revenue over $1 billion by 2025. All statins function as inhibitors of a rate-limiting enzyme in synthesis of cholesterol, namely hydroxyl-methyl coenzyme A (HMG-CoA) reductase. This action brings statins close to vitamin D metabolism, at the same time suggesting their uniform action and similar side effects. Nevertheless, the results of numerous studies show that the statins/vitamin D interaction give diverse and pleiotropic results. This is evident by a meta-analysis that was "inconclusive on the effects of statins on vitamin D with conflicting directions from interventional and observational studies". Although the fundamental mechanism of action is identical for all the statins, they differ in water solubility, and are catabolized in different ways depending on the statin type, patient's age and vitamin D status, nutritional conditions and insolation. There are two basic ways of the disposition of statins from the human body. One is degradation of some statins in the stomach and excretion as native compounds, the second is an oxidative pathway where the statins undergo modification by a specific cytochrome P450 isoenzymes resulting in an enhanced solubility and subsequent excretion. Some of those enzymes belong to the CYP3A family, and that is the meeting point of the vitamin D and statins catabolic pathways [32].

It is known that atorvastatin, lovastatin and simvastatin are primarily metabolized by CYP3A4, a multi-substrate cytochrome involved also in vitamin D metabolites catabolism. Cytochromes in the CYP3A category are also very important enzymes in the vitamin D catabolic pathways. Therefore, any interference with their activity may cause a disturbance in the vitamin D status of the patient. It is known that some statins may compete for the active centers of the CYP3A enzymes, slowing down the catabolism of the vitamin D metabolites. This results in the vitamin D status increasing, especially in patients who are supplemented with vitamin D. It has been found that atorvastatin treatment significantly increases 25-hydroxyvitamin D concentration in patient's blood serum. This increase is especially visible in patients treated with 800 IU of vitamin D per day. This effect is probably due to inhibitive competition of vitamin D metabolites and the statin for a limited number of active centers available in CYP3A4, and therefore the decrement of the metabolic clearance of the vitamin D metabolites. There are also reports that statins (e.g., rosuvastatin) that are not metabolized by CYP3A4 correlate with the increased 25OHD concentrations in the circulation system of the patient. There is no simple explanation for this finding. One possibility is that statins may act as inducers of the vitamin D 25-hydroxylase activity expressed to a certain extend by the CYP3A4 [33].

Statins are also known to increase the catabolic clearance of vitamin D metabolites. The mechanism of this phenomenon relays on their affinity for nuclear receptors (PXR, CAR) involved in regulating the expression of CYP3A proteins. [34].

Antiepileptics (AEDs) as carbamazepine, oxcarbazepine, phenobarbital, phenytoin, primidone, and valproate have all been associated with bone health problems in epileptic patients. Taking into account that some of them are prescribed as coanalgesics, this type of therapy is widely use in clinical practice among elderly patients. AEDs are known to induce the enzymes from the catabolic pathway of the vitamin D. This action results in a specific sequence of events leading to an increased fracture risk beginning with the induction of hepatic cytochromes and accelerated degradation of the vitamin D metabolites. AEDs can result in decreased vitamin D status and decreased intestinal calcium absorption that has a negative effect on the circulating calcium pool. In turn, this activates a compensatory increase in PTH concentrations resulting in increased bone resorption and an increased risk of fractures. The negative effects of anticonvulsants on fracture risk were confirmed by a population-based analysis. The study had nearly 16,000 participants who had a nontraumatic fracture of the wrist, hip and vertebra with up to 3 matched controls ("n" around 47,000). A significant increase of fracture risk was found for most of the antiepileptic drugs investigated namely for carbamazepine, clonazepam, gabapentin, phenobarbital and phenytoin. OR values ranged from 1,24 for clonazepam to 1,91 for phenytoin. Valproic acid was the only AED not associated with increased fracture risk. These results are consistent with other population-based studies [35, 36].

Research was conducted to determine if vitamin D supplementation improves the bone condition in patients taking anti-epileptic drugs. The results of a systematic review of 9 studies reported that the research was marred by very little uniformity with respect to the vitamin D dosing regimen, sample sizes, the antiepileptic drugs used, study length and design and bone outcomes measured. Nevertheless, the review states that vitamin D supplementation seems to have a positive effect on bone turnover markers, especially alkaline phosphatase and bone mineralization in adults with epilepsy.

The mechanisms of action and observational data suggest that other factors might interfere with the metabolism of vitamin D. This group comprises of glucocorticoids, immunosuppressive agents (cyclosporine, tacrolimus), many chemotherapeutic agents, highly active antiretroviral agents, and histamine H2-receptor antagonists.

Glucocorticoids belong to a widely used class of drugs. Prednisone, hydrocortisone, dexamethasone are used in adrenal replacement, immune suppression and chemotherapy. The well-known side-effect of their application is osteoporosis. Therefore, alterations in vitamin D metabolism have been investigated as a possible mechanism. It has been found that glucocorticoids induce several P450 cytochromes in a way similar to AED, including the vitamin D catabolizing CYP2A4. Although the RCT class studied failed to produce conclusive results, a recent overview of systematic literature revealed that the prevalence range of fractures or osteoporosis in patients taking glucocorticoids is 21 to 30%. The postulated remedy for these problems, save for decreasing the glucocorticoids dose, is vitamin D supplementation [37, 38].

9. Other drugs

One of published metanalysis underscored undoubted need for further research to understand the impact of drugs that inhibit CYP enzyme activity related to vitamin D status. Regarding such treatment as the antimicrobial agent ketoconazole or proton pump inhibitor omeprazole, have been shown to inhibit both CYP3A4 166, 167 and CYP24 168 in vitro, so far, no studies have evaluated the clinical effect of these drugs on human vitamin D status in elderly [39].

10. Vitamin D toxicity in elderly

Vitamin D toxicity (VDT) due to excess of vitamin D is a clinical condition characterized by severe hypercalcemia that may persist for a prolonged period of time and lead to serious health consequences. Hypervitaminosis D with hypercalcemia develops after uncontrolled use of vitamin D mega doses or vitamin D metabolites [25(OH)D, 1,25(OH)2D]. Hypervitaminosis D may develop in some clinical conditions as a result of using vitamin D analogs (exogenous VDT). Hypervitaminosis D with hypercalcemia may also be a manifestation of excessive production of 1,25(OH)2D in granulomatous disorders such as sarcoidosis, tuberculosis, leprosy, fungal diseases, giant cell polymyositis, and berylliosis. In healthy geriatric population, exogenous vitamin D toxicity may be caused by prolonged use (months) of vitamin D mega doses, but not by the abnormally high exposure of skin to the sun or by eating a diversified diet. Exogenous VDT due to vitamin D overdosing is diagnosed in the elderly similar as in younger people (very rare) by markedly elevated 25(OH)D concentrations (>150 ng/ml) accompanied by severe hypercalcemia and hypercalciuria and by very low or undetectable parathyroid hormone (PTH) activity [40, 41].

Exogenous VDT can be the result of patients taking excessive amounts of 1,25(OH)2D or other 1–hydroxylated vitamin D analogs [1(OH)D], for example paricalcitol and doxercalciferol, used to treat hypercalcemic disorders, including hypoparathyroidism, pseudohypoparathyroidism, osteomalacia, and end- stage renal failure. When this occurs, hypercalcemia is a harmful side effect of treatment with a pharmacological vitamin D agent that is not related to 25(OH)D concentration and when the concentration value of 1,25(OH)2D is elevated. The increased risk of endogenous VDT is a serious clinical issue in the elderly with granuloma-forming disorders and in lymphomas. Patients with granuloma-forming disorders and lymphomas are hypersensitive to vitamin D. Elevated 1,25(OH)2D concentration with hypercalcemia may develop after vitamin D supplementation, from dietary products fortified with vitamin D or after sunbathing. In granulomatous diseases (including tuberculosis, sarcoidosis, leprosy, fungal diseases, infantile subcutaneous fat necrosis, giant cell polymyositis, and berylliosis) endogenous VDT is related to the abnormal extrarenal synthesis of 1,25(OH)2D by activated macrophages. In lymphomas, the etiology of VDT is multiple, heterogeneous, and still not fully recognized. In endogenous VDT, hypercalcemia is related to increased 1,25(OH)2D concentration. In contrast, hypercalcemia is a consequence of high 25(OH)D concentration due to an overdose of vitamin D (exogenous VDT) [42, 43].

Over the last decade, the Institute of Medicine (IOM) and the Endocrine Society have both concluded that acute VDT is extremely rare in the literature, that serum 25(OH)D concentrations must exceed 150 ng/ml (375 nmol/l). Other considerations, such as calcium intake, can have an effect the risk of hypercalcemia and VDT. Despite of the risk factors associated with VDT, there is empirical evidence that vitamin D is among the least toxic fat-soluble vitamins, and significantly less toxic than vitamin A. Dudenkov and colleagues researched more than 20,000 serum 25(OH)D measurements performed at the Mayo Clinic from 2002 to 2011 to determine the prevalence of VDT, demonstrated by the presence of hypercalcemia. The number of individuals with a serum 25(OH)D concentration > 50 ng/ml (>75 nmol/l) had increased by 20 times during that period. On the other hand, high 25(OH)D concentrations can coincide with normal concentrations of serum calcium. In this study, only one patient was diagnosed with hypercalcemia with a 25(OH)D concentration of 364 ng/ml (910 nmol/l). Pietras and colleagues [16] reported no evidence of VDT in healthy adults in a clinical setting who received 50,000 IU of vitamin D2 once every 2 weeks (equivalent to approximately 3,300 IU/day) for up to 6 years. These patients maintained 25(OH)D concentrations of 40–60 ng/ml (100–150 nmol/l). Ekwaru and colleagues had similar findings of no evidence of toxicity in Canadian adults who received up to 20,000 IU of vitamin D3 per day and had a significant increase of 25(OH)D concentrations, up to 60 ng/ml (150 nmol/l) [44–47].

11. Conclusions

The world-wide prevalence of vitamin D deficiency and its role in the maintenance of skeletal and non-skeletal health calls for continuing investigation of vitamin D. These actions should take into account a multitude of confounding variables, including age – elderly as well as the oldest-old, presence of geriatric giants and their consequences, evaluation of vitamin D deficiency as symptomatic or asymptomatic, distinction between the need of supplementation or treatment,

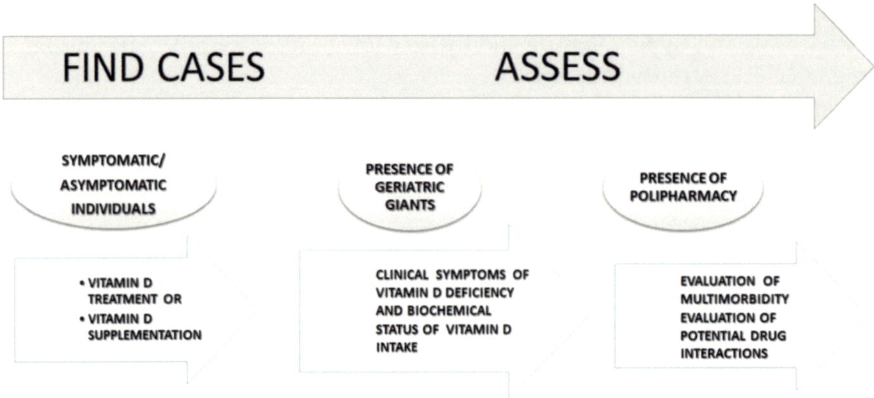

Figure 2.
Proposed strategy for geriatric patient with vitamin D deficiency.

the way of supplementation/treatment, polypharmacy and potential drug interactions. All these factors lead us to define the broad groups for clinical consideration and decision-making regarding the supplementation or treatment with vitamin D in elderly individuals. Heterogeneity of the elderly population contributes to making impossible the creation one, simple algorithm for every patient.

Therefore, the proposed strategy (presented above in the **Figure 2**) to prevent vitamin D deficiency and the negative outcomes in the general elderly population in everyday clinical practice, takes into account multifactorial character of geriatric patient.

Author details

Malgorzata Kupisz-Urbańska[1*], Jacek Łukaszkiewicz[2] and Ewa Marcinowska-Suchowierska[3]

1 Department of Geriatrics, Medical Centre for Postgraduate Education, Warsaw, Poland

2 Warsaw Medical School, Poland

3 Department of Gerontology and Geriatrics, School of Public Health, Medical Centre for Postgraduate Education, Warsaw, Poland

*Address all correspondence to: gosia.kupisz.urbanska@gmail.com

References

[1] Pludowski P, Grant WB, Konstantynowicz J, Holick MF. Editorial: Classic and Pleiotropic Actions of Vitamin D. Front Endocrinol. 2019 May 29;10:341. doi: 10.3389/fendo.2019.00341.

[2] Amrein K, Scherkl M, Hoffmann M, Neuwersch-Sommeregger S, Köstenberger M, Tmava Berisha A, Martucci G, Pilz S, Malle O. Vitamin D deficiency 2.0: an update on the current status worldwide. Eur J Clin Nutr. 2020 Nov;74(11):1498-1513. doi: 10.1038/s41430-020-0558-y. Epub 2020 Jan 20.

[3] Spiro A, Buttriss JL. Vitamin D:an overview of vitamin D status and intake in Europe. Nutr Bull 2014; 39:322-350.

[4] Cashman KD, Dowling KG, Škrabáková Z, Gonzalez-Gross M, et al. Vitamin D deficiency in Europe: pandemic? Am J Clin Nutr. 2016 Apr;103(4):1033-1044.

[5] Nakamura K, Kitamura K, Takachi R, Saito T, Kobayashi R, Oshiki R, Watanabe Y, Tsugane S, Sasaki A, Yamazaki O. Impact of demographic, environmental, and lifestyle factors on vitamin D sufficiency in 9084 Japanese adults. Bone. 2015 May;74:10-7. doi: 10.1016/j.bone.2014.12.064. Epub 2015 Jan 7.

[6] Börgermann J, Lazouski K, Kuhn J, Dreier J, Schmidt M, Gilis-Januszewski T, Knabbe C, Gummert JF, Zittermann A. 1,25-Dihydroxyvitamin D fluctuations in cardiac surgery are related to age and clinical outcome*. Crit Care Med. 2012 Jul;40(7):2073-81. doi: 10.1097/CCM.0b013e31824e8c42.

[7] WHO wnday, March 28, 2016 World's older population grows dramatically NIH-funded Census Bureau report offers details of global aging phenomenon.

[8] Hilger J, Friedel A, Herr R, et al. A systematic review of vitamin D status in populations worldwide. Br J Nutr. 2014; 111: 23-45.

[9] Boucher BJ. The Problems of Vitamin D Insufficiency in Older People. Aging Dis. 2012; 3: 313-329.

[10] Watson J, Lee M, Garcia-Casal M. Consequences of inadequate intakes of Vitamin A, Vitamin B12, Vitamin D, Calcium, Iron and folate in Older persons. Current geriatric reports. 2018; 7: 103-113.

[11] Morley JE. A brief history of geriatrics. J Gerontol A Biol Sci Med Sci. 2004; 59: 1132-1152.

[12] Morley JE. The new geriatric giants. Clin Geriatr Med. 2017; 33(3): 11-12.

[13] Puvill T, Lindenberg J, Gussekloo J, et al. Associations of various health-ratings with geriatric giants, mortality and life satisfaction in older people. PLOS One. 2016; 11: 1-13.

[14] Cruz-Jentoft AJ, Bahat G, Bauer J, et al. Writing Group for the European Working Group on Sarcopenia in Older People 2 (EWGSOP2), and the Extended Group for EWGSOP2. Sarcopenia: revised European consensus on definition and diagnosis. Age Ageing. 2019 Jan 1;48(1):16-31.

[15] Harris, R., Strtmayer, E., Boudreau, R., et al. The risk of fracture among men with sarcopenia, obesity, their combination sarcopenic obesity, and men with neither condition: the MrOs Study. 2017 Abstract 1156. ASBMR Annual Meeting.

[16] Tanner SB, Harwell SA. More than healthy bones: a review of vitamin D in muscle health. Ther Adv Musculoskelet Dis. 2015 Aug;7(4):152-9. doi: 10.1177/1759720X15588521.

[17] Wagatsuma, A., Sakuma, K. (2014). Vitamin D signaling in myogenesis: potential for treatment for sarcopenia. Bio. Med. Research. International doi: 10.1155/2014/121254

[18] Bo, Y., Liu, C., Ji, Z., Yang, R., An, Q., Zhang, X. et al. (2018). A high whey protein, vitamin D and E supplement preserves muscle mass, strength, and quality of life in sarcopenic older adults: A double-blind randomized controlled trial. Clin Nutr. doi: 10.1016/j.clnu.2017.12.020

[19] Bolzetta, F., Stubbs, B., Noale, M., et al. Low dose vitamin d supplementation and incident frailty in older people: an eight year longitudal study. Exp Gerontol.2018. 101:1-6. doi: 10.1016/j

[20] Granic, A., Hill, T.R, Davis, K., et al. Vitamin D status, Muscle strength and physical performace decline in very old adults: a prospecticve study . Nutrients. 2017. 13;9(4). doi: 10.3390/nu9040379.

[21] Olive Tang, Stephen P. Juraschek, Lawrence J. Appel. Design Features of Randomized Clinical Trials of Vitamin D and Falls: A Systematic Review. Nutrients. 2018 Aug; 10(8): 964. Published online 2018 Jul 26. doi: 10.3390/nu10080964

[22] Pike JW, Meyer MB. The vitamin D receptor: new paradigms for the regulation of gene expression by 1,25-dihydroxyvitamin D(3). *Endocrinol Metab Clin North Am*. 2010;39(2):255-269. doi:10.1016/j.ecl.2010.02.007

[23] Grønli O, Kvamme JM, Jorde R, Wynn R. Vitamin D deficiency is common in psychogeriatric patients, independent of diagnosis. BMC Psychiatry. 2014 May 8; 14(1): 134. doi: 10.1186/1471-244X-14-134.

[24] Lapid MI, Drake MT, Geske JR, Mundis CB, Hegard TL, Kung S, Frye MA. Hypovitaminosis D in psychogeriatric inpatients. J Nutr Health Aging. 2013 Mar; 17(3): 231-4. doi: 10.1007/s12603-012-0383-7.

[25] Licher, S., de Bruijn, R. F., Wolters, F. J., Zillikens, M. C., Ikram, M. A., & Ikram, M. K. (2017). Vitamin D and the risk of dementia: the Rotterdam study. Journal of Alzheimer's Disease, 60(3), 989-997.

[26] Jayedi, A., Rashidy-Pour, A., & Shab-Bidar, S. (2018). Vitamin d status and risk of dementia and alzheimer's disease: A meta-analysis of dose-response. Nutritional neuroscience, 1-10.

[27] Pludowski P, Grant WB, Konstantynowicz J and Holick MF (2019) Editorial: Classic and Pleiotropic Actions of Vitamin D. Front. Endocrinol. 10:341. doi: 10.3389/fendo.2019.00341.

[28] Rusińska A, Płudowski P, Walczak M, Borszewska-Kornacka MK, et al. Vitamin D Supplementation Guidelines for General Population and Groups at Risk of Vitamin D Deficiency in Poland-Recommendations of the Polish Society of Pediatric Endocrino logy and Diabetes and the Expert Panel With Participation of National Specialist Consultants and Representatives of Scientific Societies-2018 Update. Front Endocrinol (Lausanne). 2018 May 31;9:246. doi: 10.3389/fendo.2018.00246.

[29] Holick MF.The vitamin D deficiency pandemic: Approaches for diagnosis, treatment and prevention. Rev Endocr Metab Disord. 2017 Jun;18(2):153-165. doi: 10.1007/s11154-017-9424-1.

[30] Marcinowska-Suchowierska E, Płudowski P. Manegement of osteoporosis in Poland.Calcium and vitamin D, WCO, IFO-ESCEO Congrss, Kraków 19-2204.2018, Lecture, Osteopor.Int. 2018,29. supl.1, Abs. NS74.

[31] Robien K., Oppeneer S.J., Kelly J.A., Hamilton-Reeves J.M.. Drug–Vitamin D Interactions: A Systematic Review of the Literature. Nutr. Clin. Pract. 2013 28, 194-208.

[32] Mazidi M., Rezaie P., Vatanparast H. and Kengne A.P. Effect of statins on serum vitamin D concentrations: a systematic review and meta-analysis. Eur. J. Clin. Invest. 2017;47, 93-101.

[33] Wang Z., Schuetz E.G., Xu Y., and Thummel K.E. Interplay between Vitamin D and the Drug Metabolizing Enzyme CYP3A4. J. Steroid Biochem. Mol. Biol.2013; 136, 54-58

[34] Bischoff-Ferrari H. A ., Fischer K., Orav E.J., Dawson-Hughes B ., et al. . Statin Use and 25-Hydroxyvitamin D Blood Level Response to Vitamin D Treatment of Older Adults. J Am Geriatr Soc. 2017; 65, 1267-1273.

[35] Arora E., Singh H., Gupta Y.K. Impact of antiepileptic drugs on bone health: Need for monitoring, treatment, and prevention strategies. J. Family Med. Prim. Care. 2016; 5, 248-253.

[36] Jette´N., Lix L.M., Metge C.J., et al. Association of Antiepileptic Drugs With Nontraumatic Fractures A Population-Based Analysis. Arch. Neurol.2011. 68, 107-112.

[37] Rice B.J., White A.G., Scarpati L.M., Wan G., and Nelson W.W. Long-term Systemic Corticosteroid Exposure: A Systematic Literature Review. Clin. Ther. 2017; 39, 2216-2229

[38] Kweder H, Housam E.. Vitamin D deficiency in elderly: Risk factors and drugs impact on vitamin D status. Avicenna J Med. 2018 Oct-Dec; 8(4): 139-146.

[39] Robien K, Oppeneer SJ, Kelly JA, et al. Drug-vitamin D interactions: a systematic review of the literature. Nutr Clin Pract. 2013 Apr;28(2):194-208. doi: 10.1177/0884533612467824.

[40] Tebben PJ, Singh RJ, Kumar R. Vitamin D–Mediated Hypercalcemia: Mechanisms, Diagnosis, and Treatment. Endocr Rev. 2016;37(5):521-547.

[41] Gupta AK, Jamwal V, Sakul et al. Hypervitaminosis D and systemic manifestations: a comprehensive review. JIMSA. 2014;27(4):236-237.

[42] Mudde AH, van den Berg H, Boshuis PG, et al. Ectopic production of 1,25-dihydroxyvitamin D by B-cell lymphoma as a cause of hypercalcemia. Cancer. 1987;59:1543-1546.

[43] Bell NH, Stern PH, Pantzer E, Sinha TK, DeLuca HF. Evidence that increased circulating 1α, 25-dihydroxyvitamin D is the probable cause for abnormal calcium metabolism in sarcoidosis. J Clin Invest. 1979;64:218-225.

[44] Dudenkov DV, Yawn BP, Oberhelman SS, et al. Changing incidence of serum 25-hydroxyvitamin D values above 50 ng/ml: a 10-year population-based study.Mayo Clin Proc. 2015;90:577-586.

[45] Holick MF. Vitamin D is not as toxic as was once thought: a historical and up-to-date perspective. Mayo Clin Proc.2015;90(5):561-564.

[46] Ekwaru JP, Zwicker JD, Holick MF, Giovannucci E, Veugelers PJ. The importance of body weight for the dose response relationship of oral vitamin D supplementation and serum 25-hydroxyvitamin D in healthy volunteers. PLoS One. 2014;9(11):e111265.

[47] Marcinowska – Suchowierska, Kupisz – Urbańska M, Łukaszkiewicz J, Płudowski P, Glenville J.. Vitamin D toxicity – a clinical perspective. Frontiers in Endocrinology, 2018. doi:10.3389/fendo.2018.00550.

Section 2

Vitamin D, Immune System and Infections

Chapter 4

Vitamin D and the Immune System

Vikram Singh Chauhan

Abstract

In the past few decades, various novel actions of vitamin D have been discovered. The mechanism of action of calcitriol or vitamin D is mediated by the Vitamin D receptor (VDR), a subfamily of nuclear receptors, which acts as a transcription factor in the target cells after formation of a heterodimer with the retinoid X receptor (RXR). As the VDR has been found in virtually all cell types, vitamin D exerts multiple actions on different tissues. Vitamin D has important immunomodulatory actions, which includes enhancement of the innate immune system and inhibition of the adaptative immune responses. These actions are associated with an increase in production of interleukin (IL)-4 by T helper (Th)-2 lymphocytes and the up-regulation of regulatory T lymphocytes. Vitamin D can regulate the immune responses in secondary lymphoid organs as well as in target organs through a number of mechanisms. Vitamin D inhibits the expression of APC cytokines, such as interleukin-1 (IL-1), IL-6, IL-12, and tissue necrosis factor- α (TNF-α) and decreases the expression of a set of major histocompatibility complex (MCH) class II cell surface proteins in macrophages. Vitamin D also inhibits B cell differentiation and antibody production. These actions reflect an important role of Vitamin D in balancing the immune system.

Keywords: Vitamin D, Immunity, Vitamin D receptor

1. Introduction

Vitamin D is now recognized as a vitamin as well as a pro hormone. It exists in two major forms: vitamin D2 (ergocalciferol) and vitamin D3 (cholecalciferol). Vitamin D3 is formed in the human skin and is obtained in the diet through the intake of animal-based foods such as fish oils, whereas vitamin D2 is present in plant sources [1]. Vitamin D is traditionally known to be involved in the regulation of calcium and phosphate metabolism. Apart from its role in maintaining bone mineralization, vitamin D also has a well described function as an immunomodulatory hormone [2]. The Vitamin D receptor (VDR) and metabolizing enzymes are expressed by numerous types of immune cells such as lymphocytes, macrophages, monocytes and dendritic cells [3, 4]. Preliminary studies have revealed that vitamin D has noteworthy biologic activities on the innate and adaptive immune systems. Some preclinical studies have demonstrated that administration of vitamin D leads to changes in the occurrence and progression of many immune-related diseases [2, 5]. This is supported by clinical data that explains the possible association of vitamin D with the incidence of many disorders such as type 1 diabetes, psoriasis, rheumatoid arthritis, multiple sclerosis and infectious diseases. The purpose of the present chapter is to provide a summary of the effects of vitamin D on the immune system and the link between vitamin D and numerous types of immune-related diseases and conditions.

2. Vitamin D and the immune system

A significant role of vitamin D in the regulation of the immune system has been discovered in the last few decades. In 1983, the contribution of macrophages in producing vitamin D was documented by separation of VDR in activated human inflammatory cells [6, 7]. The role of vitamin D in the inhibition of T cell proliferation was discovered by Rigby, *et al* in 1984 [8]. Further evidences were found for elaborating the role of vitamin D in the regulation of the immune system [8].

T cells and B cells respond to 1, 25$(OH)_2$D in a paracrine or autocrine manner in an immune environment. The action of 1,25$(OH)_2$D on the inhibition of T helper cells was documented in preclinical studies. These effects include directly lowering the dendritic cell capability to activate T helper 17, inhibition of T helper 17-related IL-17 and hampering the ability to support T helper 17 polarization of naïve CD4+ T cells production [9]. In an autoimmune uveitis preclinical model, oral administration of 1,25$(OH)_2$D prevented and inhibited immunological responses, as shown by reduction of both ROR-gamma-t (Retinoic acid Receptor-related Orphan Receptor gamma t) and IL-17 in CD4+ T cells, which are two indicators of T helper 17 cell function. Moreover, 1, 25$(OH)_2$D inhibited bone marrow-derived dendritic cell ability to influence T helper 17 polarization of naive CD4+ T cells [9].

1, 25$(OH)_2$D has also been involved in the inhibition of immunoglobulin production and B cell proliferation and differentiation [10]. Low 1, 25(OH) [2] D level had been found in patients with systemic lupus erythematosus (SLE), suggesting that vitamin D could be involved in the regulation of autoantibody expression. Chen, *et al* showed that 1, 25$(OH)_2$D has a direct effect on B cells, including inhibition of proliferation, on generation of class-switched memory B cells and on immunoglobulin production in patients with SLE [10].

Vitamin D is also involved macrophage regulation and affects their cytokine expression. It increases prostaglandin E2 production from macrophages, which has a role in the inflammatory process and inhibits the expression of granulocyte-macrophage colony-stimulating factor. Moreover, 1, 25$(OH)_2$D induces macrophages and epithelial cells to produce cathelicidin, a peptide involved in antimicrobial action [11, 12]. Cathelicidin is responsible for activating the innate immune response by binding to its transmembrane receptor and is correlated to higher levels of the enzyme 1-alpha-hydroxylase in macrophages and keratinocytes [13]. The enzyme 1-alpha-hydroxylase further increases the production of cathelicidin through the production of 1,25$(OH)_2$D.

Vitamin D is also involved in the activation of dendritic cells which enhance expression of CD4+/CD25+ regulatory T cells (T reg). In preclinical study by Gregori *et al*, 1, 25$(OH)_2$D activated dendritic cells with a tolerogenic phenotype and caused an increased percentage of CD4+/CD25+ T reg in the spleen and lymph nodes. These regulatory T cells have a role in the transfer of transplantation tolerance [14].

3. Vitamin D and the innate immune system

Innate antigen presenting cells (APC), specifically dendritic cells (DC) are principal targets for the immune modulatory effects of vitamin D. APCs have a crucial role in the initiation of the adaptive immune response as they present antigens to B cells and T cells and are able to modulate them by immunogenic signals such as the expression of cytokines. Vitamin D and its analogs modify the function of DCs to induce a more tolerogenic and immature state. Immature DCs result in decreased levels of MHC class II and co-stimulatory molecule expression (CD40, CD80, CD86), which negatively affects antigen presentation accompanied by a lower IL-12 secretion, but an increased production of the tolerogenic interleukin IL-10. High-dose vitamin D supplementation in healthy humans (1 µg twice daily for 7 days) results in significant reduction in the proinflammatory cytokine IL-6 produced by peripheral mononuclear cells. A combination of all these effects results in the induction of potential regulatory T cells which are crucial for controlling immune responses and the development of autoreactivity [15]. A clinical study in 95 patients treated with adjunctive vitamin D therapy, added on to standard tuberculosis therapy demonstrated augmented resolution of inflammatory responses [16].

4. Vitamin D and the adaptive immune system

The expression of the nuclear VDR and vitamin D-activating enzymes in both T- and B types of human adaptive immune cells have been reported in studies. The activation and proliferation of T and B cells results in up-regulation of VDR expression, which ultimately regulates more than 500 vitamin D responsive genes [15].

Following are the proposed mechanisms for influence of vitamin D on T cell function [15]:

1. Direct, endocrine effects on T cells mediated via systemic vitamin D.

2. Direct, intracrine conversion of 25(OH) D to calcitriol by T cells.

3. Direct, paracrine effects of calcitriol on T cells following monocytes or dendritic cells induced conversion of 25(OH) D to calcitriol.

4. Indirect effects on antigen presentation to T cells mediated via localized APCs by calcitriol.

All these effects of vitamin D result in shifting from a proinflammatory status to a more tolerogenic immune status, including very diverse effects on T cell subtypes: Vitamin D suppresses T helper cell proliferation, differentiation and modulates synthesis of cytokines [15].

5. Vitamin D and autoimmune diseases

Clinical studies investigated the association of vitamin D levels with the risk of developing autoimmunity and effect of vitamin D administration on autoimmune diseases. A systematic review of 219 studies demonstrated that vitamin D levels of<30 ng/mL are significantly associated with autoimmune disease. In patients with type-1 diabetes, the risks are significantly reduced in infants treated with vitamin D after the seventh month [17].

6. Vitamin D and Type 1 Diabetes Mellitus

Type 1 Diabetes Mellitus (T1DM) is an autoimmune disease with T cell mediated destruction of pancreatic β-cells. It is hypothesized that Vitamin D supplementation early in life could be protective therapy against the development of T1DM [18]. Vitamin D supplementation in the first year of life in children produced a 33% risk reduction of developing T1D in a subgroup analysis of the EURODIAB study [19]. A meta-analysis of four clinical studies also revealed a significantly reduced risk of development of T1D among infants receiving vitamin D supplementation [20]. Many trials on vitamin D and T1D are currently ongoing which will hopefully expand our understanding of this topic.

7. Vitamin D and multiple sclerosis

Hypovitaminosis D is one of the important risk factors for the increased risk of development of multiple sclerosis (MS). In a cohort of the Nurses' Health Study (92953 women) and Nurses' Health Study II (95310 women), the intake of Vitamin D $\geq$ 400 IU/day was associated with the reduced risk of developing MS. [21] In a study by Merja et al., vitamin D3 add on treatment to interferon β-1b reduces MRI disease activity in MS [22]. Currently ongoing studies such as *SOLAR* and the *EVIDIMS* study will explore many aspects of the role of vitamin D in the management of MS in the coming years.

8. Vitamin D and psoriasis

Vitamin D is involved in the proliferation and maturation of keratinocytes. This action of vitamin D created interest as a topical therapeutic option in the treatment of psoriasis. A significant association between low vitamin D levels and psoriasis has been reported. Although the exact role of vitamin D in the pathogenesis of psoriasis is unclear, possible mechanisms include the regulation of the cutaneous immune system (inhibition of T cell proliferation, T reg induction) and down-regulation of pro-inflammatory cytokines. However robust clinical data regarding a role of vitamin D in psoriasis is still awaited [23].

9. Vitamin D and rheumatoid arthritis

In addition to inhibiting inflammatory cytokines such as IL-6, TNFα, IL-17 in synovial fluid, vitamin D also reduces fibroblast erosion [24]. Vitamin D supplementation was found to be associated with lower risk of RA in a prospective cohort of 29,368 women over a follow up period of 11 years [25]. A randomized controlled trial (RCT) by Buondonno et al. [26] evaluated the effect of administration of cholecalciferol on T helper cell sub-types and osteoclast precursors. Single dose of cholecalciferol (300,000 IU) along with standard treatment showed improvements in inflammatory cytokines in this study [26]. Further studies are required to estimate the dose of Vitamin D in the treatment of RA.

10. Conclusion and future perspectives

The role of Vitamin D in autoimmune disease is a major area of research. Addressing questions as to whether vitamin D levels are related to the risk of developing autoimmunity and whether vitamin D supplementation can modify the course of autoimmune diseases, several studies performed over the last four decades support the role of vitamin D in the prevention of autoimmune diseases. However there is still a need of randomized controlled clinical trials in this field. Upcoming clinical trials will find out the optimal mode and dosage of supplementation of vitamin D. However, with available data, vitamin D emerges as a promising nutrient in the prevention and adjunctive treatment of diseases caused by impaired immune-homeostasis.

Author details

Vikram Singh Chauhan
Dr. Chauhan's Clinic and Jabalpur Hospital and Research Center, Jabalpur, India

*Address all correspondence to: vikramsinghchauhan@gmail.com

References

[1] Valero-Zanuya M, Hawkins-Carranza F: Metabolism, endogenous and exogenous sources of vitamin D. Rev Esp Enferm Metab Oseas. 2007; 16: 63-70.

[2] Prietl, B.; Treiber, G.; Pieber, T.R.; Amrein, K. Vitamin D and immune function. Nutrients 2013, 5, 2502-2521.

[3] Battault, S.; Whiting, S.J.; Peltier, S.L.; Sadrin, S.; Gerber, G.; Maixent, J.M. Vitamin D metabolism, functions and needs: From science to health claims. Eur. J. Nutr. 2013, 52, 429-441

[4] Adams, J.S.; Rafison, B.; Witzel, S.; Reyes, R.E.; Shieh, A.; Chun, R.; Zavala, K.; Hewison, M.; Liu, P.T. Regulation of the extrarenal CYP27B1-hydroxylase. J. Steroid Biochem. Mol. Biol. 2014, 144, 22-27

[5] Aranow, C. Vitamin D and the immune system. J. Investig. Med. 2011, 59, 881-886

[6] Adams JS, Sharma OP, Gacad MA, Singer FR. Metabolism of 25-hydroxyvitamin D3 by cultured pulmonary alveolar macrophages in sarcoidosis. J Clin Invest 1983; 72:1856-60.

[7] Provvedini DM, Tsoukas CD, Deftos LJ, Manolagas SC. 1,25-dihydroxyvitamin D3 receptors in human leukocytes. Science 1983; 221: 1181-3.

[8] Rigby WF, Stacy T, Fanger MW. Inhibition of T lymphocyte mitogenesis by 1, 25-dihydroxyvitamin D3 (calcitriol). J Clin Invest 1984; 74:1451-5.

[9] Tang J, Zhou R, Luger D, Zhu W, Silver PB, Grajewski RS, et al. Calcitriol suppresses antiretinal autoimmunity through inhibitory effects on the Th17 effector response. J Immunol 2009;182:4624-32.

[10] Chen S, Sims GP, Chen XX, Gu YY, Chen S, Lipsky PE. Modulatory effects of 1, 25-dihydroxyvitamin D3 on human B cell differentiation. J Immunol 2007; 179:1634-47.

[11] Cantorna MT, Mahon BD. Mounting evidence for vitamin D as an environmental factor affecting autoimmune disease prevalence. Exp Biol Med 2004; 229:1136-42.

[12] Wang TT, Nestel FP, Bourdeau V, Nagai Y, Wang Q, Liao J, et al. Cutting edge: 1, 25-dihydroxyvitamin D3 is a direct inducer of antimicrobial peptide gene expression. J Immunol 2004; 173:2909-12.

[13] Liu PT, Stenger S, Li H, Wenzel L, Tan BH, Krutzik SR, et al. Toll-like receptor triggering of a vitamin D-mediated human antimicrobial response. Science 2006; 311:1770-3.

[14] Gregori S, Casorati M, Amuchastegui S, Smiroldo S, Davalli AM, Adorini L. Regulatory T cells induced by 1 alpha, 25-dihydroxyvitamin D3 and mycophenolate mofetil treatment mediate transplantation tolerance. J Immunol 2001; 167:1945-53.

[15] Prietl B, Treiber G, Pieber TR, Amrein K. Vitamin D and immune function. Nutrients. 2013 Jul;5(7):2502-21.

[16] Coussens, A.K.; Wilkinson, R.J.; Hanifa, Y.; Nikolayevskyy, V.; Elkington, P.T.; Islam, K.; Timms, P.M.; Venton, T.R.; Bothamley, G.H.; Packe, G.E.; *et al.* Vitamin D accelerates resolution of inflammatory responses during tuberculosis treatment. *Proc. Natl. Acad. Sci. USA* 2012, *109*, 15449-15454.

[17] Antico, A.; Tampoia, M.; Tozzoli, R.; Bizzaro, N. Can supplementation with vitamin D reduce the risk or

modify the course of autoimmune diseases? A systematic review of the literature. *Autoimmun. Rev.* 2012, *12*, 127-136.

[18] Zipitis, C.S.; Akobeng, A.K. Vitamin D supplementation in early childhood and risk of type 1 diabetes: A systematic review and meta-analysis. *Arch. Dis. Child.* 2008, *93*, 512-517.

[19] Vitamin D supplement in early childhood and risk for Type I (insulin-dependent) diabetes mellitus. The EURODIAB Substudy 2 Study Group. Diabetologia 1999, 42, 51-54

[20] Zipitis, C.S.; Akobeng, A.K. Vitamin D supplementation in early childhood and risk of type 1 diabetes: A systematic review and meta-analysis. *Arch. Dis. Child.* 2008, *93*, 512-517

[21] Munger, K.L.; Zhang, S.M.; O'Reilly, E.; Hernán, M.A.; Olek, M.J.; Willett, W.C.; Ascherio, A. Vitamin D intake and incidence of multiple sclerosis. *Neurology* 2004, *62*, 60-65].

[22] Soilu-Hänninen, M.; Aivo, J.; Lindström, B.-M.; Elovaara, I.; Sumelahti, M.-L.; Färkkilä, M.; Tienari, P.; Atula, S.; Sarasoja, T.; Herrala, L.; *et al.* A randomised, double blind, placebo controlled trial with vitamin D3 as add on treatment to interferon β-1b in patients with multiple sclerosis. *J. Neurol. Neurosurg. Psychiatr.* 2012, *83*, 565-571

[23] Barrea L, Savanelli MC, Di Somma C, Napolitano M, Megna M, Colao A, Savastano S. Vitamin D and its role in psoriasis: An overview of the dermatologist and nutritionist. Reviews in Endocrine and Metabolic Disorders. 2017 Jun;18(2):195-205.

[24] Bellan M, Sainaghi PP, Pirisi M. Role of vitamin D in rheumatoid arthritis. Ultraviolet Light in Human Health, Diseases and Environment. 2017:155-68.

[25] Merlino LA, Curtis J, Mikuls TR, Cerhan JR, Criswell LA, Saag KG. Vitamin D intake is inversely associated with rheumatoid arthritis: results from the Iowa Women's Health Study. Arthritis & Rheumatism: Official Journal of the American College of Rheumatology. 2004 Jan;50(1):72-7.

[26] Buondonno I, Rovera G, Sassi F, Rigoni MM, Lomater C, Parisi S, Pellerito R, Isaia GC, D'Amelio P. Vitamin D and immunomodulation in early rheumatoid arthritis: A randomized double-blind placebo-controlled study. PLoS One. 2017 Jun 5;12(6):e0178463.

Chapter 5

Viral Infections, Including Influenza and Corona Virus Disease 2019, and Vitamin D: A Mini-Review

Srđana Čulić

Abstract

Recent research about the influence of vitamin D (VD) deficiency on the occurrence of viral infections suggests that children with VD deficiency have attenuated immune response. This, in turn, increases the severity of viral infections, especially those of the respiratory tract, that show a typical seasonality pattern during the winter months. Despite the immunization of children at the global level, outbreaks of influenza do frequently occur. Over the past months, we have witnessed that the explosive pandemic of the corona virus disease 2019 (COVID-19) has caused significant mortality in some countries. Numerous studies have shown that VD deficiency is increasingly prevalent worldwide, and that it is potentially associated with the onset of viral infections. Persons with hypovitaminosis D and subsequent secondary immunodeficiencies ought to be identified and treated, while preventive supplementation of VD should be recommended to the general population to avoid VD deficiency during the winter. In this way, the burden of viral infections on population health and economy could be reduced. This paper also reviews the influence of VD on infections caused by hepatitis B and C viruses, human papillomavirus, Epstein–Barr virus, Human herpes virus 6, herpes simplex virus, and human immunodeficiency virus.

Keywords: viral infections, vitamin D, hypovitaminosis, influence

1. Introduction

The non-skeletal effect of vitamin D (VD) has been a hot topic of research for almost 20 years, and benefits have been found for many health conditions, including cancer, diabetes, autoimmune diseases, cardiovascular diseases [1, 2]. The increase in global VD deficiency is most likely due to poor sun exposure and poor diet [3].

The dietary sources of VD cannot fulfill the body's requirements [4]. Sun exposure accounts for >90% of VD production in humans. Most people are now spending more time indoors, therefore, their exposure to sunlight is often limited. In the summer, due to fear of malignant skin diseases, use of creams with high ultraviolet (UV) protection is common, which further contributes to VD deficiency [5]. Air pollution in large urban industrial agglomerations with insufficient insolation also predisposes

IntechOpen

to VD deficiency [6, 7]. Taken together, hypovitaminosis D has become a pandemic in itself, identified across ethnicities and age groups worldwide [8–10]. Diekmann investigated the VD status of residents in a German nursing home in Nurnberg, and found VD deficiency (<50 nmol/L) in 93.9% of the residents [11]. Hypovitaminosis D is common in elderly people [12].

VD was classified as a vitamin for historical reasons, although it is actually a hormone in the group of secosteroids (steroids with an open B ring). Until recently, scientists focused on how VD affects the maintenance of plasma calcium and phosphate regulation, particularly in children who have rickets, and in adults, and older people with osteopenia and osteoporosis [13]. New research indicates that this vitamin/hormone plays a significant role in the functioning of the immune system, in fact, it is essential for its optimal functioning [14].

Why is VD so important? Firstly, VD functions as a natural steroid. It is the secosteroid vitamin/hormone, which regulates the immune system function as an immunomodulator. This means that their end-targets are lymphocyte activation and proliferation, and differentiation of promyelocytes and monocytes. Secondly, the VD receptor (VDR) has been identified in most tissues. VD influences the innate and adaptive immune responses. This immunomodulator also targets dendritic cells (DCs), as well as B-lymphocytes, modulating both innate and adaptive immune responses [15].

Thirdly, VD influences the cytokine network through inhibition of secretion of several cytokines by T cells. This immunomodulatory effect may be very important in treatment of viral infections and autoimmune diseases. Different reports have demonstrated the ability of VD to reduce the synthesis of interferon-γ (IFN-γ) and interleukin-2 (IL-2) in peripheral blood lymphocytes (PBL) and T-cell lines [16–18]. VD inhibits IFN-γ production and increased IL-10 production by peripheral blood mononuclear cells (PBMCs) [19]. Initial plasma IFN-γ and IL-10 are higher in COVID-19 Intensive Care Unit (ICU) patients and cytokine storm can occur [20–22].

Furthermore, VD can suppress cytokine storm by reducing the severity of influenza A. It significantly decreases the levels of tumor necrosis factor-alpha (TNF-α), interferon-beta (IFN-β), and IFN-stimulated gene-15 [23]. This is very important in case of severe clinical presentations of viral infection, especially those of the respiratory system [6]. VD also influences the acquired immunity and regenerate endothelial function and lining [24]. This effect is also important in order to minimize the alveolar damage in acute respiratory distress syndrome (ARDS) which can appear after viral acute respiratory infections (ARI) [25].

The condition of the average person's immune system worsens in winter. To explain this, one hypothesis has focused on VD levels, which depend in part on UV light exposure (higher in summer) that positively modulates the immune system. The best evidence is that VD supplementation reduces the incidence of ARI, according to a meta-analysis of randomized trials. VD supplementation is safe protecting against ARI and very deficient patients experience the most benefit [26]. This effect can explain the variation in influenza incidence in summer and in winter. Epidemiologic evidence links poor VD status to high susceptibility to viral infections and autoimmune diseases. Generally, hypovitaminosis D has been linked to the increased susceptibility to viral infections. It is an area of growing interest in scientific community [27–30].

The latest research indicates an interesting interaction between VD and the viruses, focusing on its antiviral and immunoregulatory activity such as the induction of autophagy and apoptosis [31]. This mini review is focused on the influence of VD on morbidity from viral infections including influenza and corona virus disease 2019 (COVID-19), which have been of special interest in the recent months.

The optimal level of VD in serum is recommended at >75 nmol/L [32, 33]. The reference ranges of VD are inconsistent according to different recommendation [34]. The simplest and most acceptable differentiation is that VD insufficiency is considered when VD levels are between 50 and 75 nmol/L, while levels ≤50 nmol/L are considered inadequate and suggest VD deficiency [8]. Deficiency can be strong (30 – 49.9 nmol/L), significant (20 – 29.9 nmol/L) or extreme (< 20 nmol/L) [32].

1.1 Epstein–Barr virus, human herpes virus-6

Alvarez-Lafuente revealed that low levels of VD have been described as one of the possible factors involved in the etiopathogenesis of multiple sclerosis (MS) [35]. Epstein–Barr virus (EBV) and human herpes virus 6 (HHV-6) infections have also been proposed as MS triggers [36, 37]. Possible effect of VD levels on viral load have been suggested [35]. VD levels could be involved in the regulation of the replication/reactivation of EBV in peripheral blood cells of MS patients; moreover, viral load seems to be higher when VD levels in serum are low [35]. Maghzi revealed that levels of VD in patients with infectious mononucleosis were significantly lower at the time of infection than in the control group and concluded that it could be a risk factor for the onset of autoimmune disease in general [38].

Hypovitaminosis D, Epstein–Barr virus (EBV) and human herpes virus 6 (HHV-6) infections have been described as possible MS triggers, but the pathogenesis of MS associated with HHV-6 infection remains unknown [39]. The presence of EBV in the CNS and demonstration of the underlying mechanism (s) linking EBV to the pathogenesis of MS remain to be elucidated. Astrocytes and microglia, in addition to B-cells can also be infected [40]. EBV is present and transcriptionally active in the brain of most cases of MS and supports a role for the virus in MS pathogenesis [40].

Pérez-Pérez analyzes the association between VD and viruses EBV and HHV-6 in 482 patients with multiple sclerosis [41]. The VD levels were significantly higher in the first school semester of the year than in the second and EBV viral load was significantly higher when VD levels were low [41]. Elevated EBV antibody levels and hypovitaminosis D may have impact on the relapsing–remitting form of MS [42]. High-dose oral VD supplementation can help the humoral immune responses against the latent EBV antigen, Ebstein-Barr nuclear antigen (EBNA)1 by decreasing the antibody levels from baseline to week 48 [42].

1.2 Human papillomavirus

There are a few clinical studies about the influence of VD deficiency on occurrence of human papillomavirus (HPV) infection, but two authors are particularly worth mentioning because they revealed that VD deficiency enhance severity of HPV cervical infection. Özgü E et al. investigated whether VD deficiency could be a reason for the HPV infection persistence in cervical premalignant lesions [43]. They concluded that, the deficiency of VD and its metabolites could be a possible reason for HPV DNA persistence and related cervical intraepithelial neoplasia [43].

Another group of authors headed by Shim studied the association of sufficient level of VD with cervical-vaginal HPV infection due to high-risk HPV (cancer-causing) or vaccine-type HPV and revealed that infections were increased in women with VD levels that were severely deficient [44].

These studies are a good guide to some new research into finding evidence of the benefits of VD in the fight against HPV. It is particularly important that supplementation of VD could possibly be considered in therapy of infections caused by HPV.

1.3 Herpes simplex virus

Investigations of VD potential to prevent herpes virus infection or reactivation are limited. Kumar has investigated the herpes labialis cells supplementation with VD before herpes simplex virus (HSV)-1 infection and studied the effect after 6, 12, and 24 h post-infections [45]. The supplementation of VD downregulate the viral load and Toll-like receptors (TLR) 2 mRNA during the initial phase of the infection [45]. The influence of VD was examined by Choi in vivo mouse model and observed that VD improved herpes simplex virus-induced Behçet's disease-like inflammation by down-regulating the expression of TLR and pro-inflammatory cytokines [46].

Öztekin A and authors have studied the association between VD and recurrent herpes labialis (RHL) in a population with RHL. They compared VD levels in healthy volunteers with and without RHL [47]. The individuals with RHL had significant VD deficiency, with VD levels below the recommended levels in more than 96% of the population. Most importantly, the study established a significant association between low serum VD levels and presence of RHL [47].

1.4 Human immunodeficiency virus

VD deficiency is also prevalent among patients with human immunodeficiency virus (HIV) infection. High levels of VD and VDR expression are also associated with natural resistance to HIV-1 infection [48]. VD deficiency is linked to a stronger inflammatory response and immune activation, low peripheral blood CD4+ T-cells, faster progression of HIV disease, and shorter survival time in HIV-infected patients [48]. VD supplementation and restoration of VD level to the recommended serum values in HIV-infected patients may improve immunologic recovery in combination with the antiretroviral therapy by reducing the level of inflammation and immune activation, and by increasing the immune response to viral pathogens [48]. Jiménez-Sousa suggests that VD deficiency may contribute to the pathogenesis of HIV infection and VD supplementation can reverse alterations of the immune system. Author supports VD supplementation as prophylaxis, especially in individuals with more severe VD deficiency [48].

People diagnosed with HIV are vulnerable to VD insufficiency and deficiency. The supplementation acts against HIV disease progression by boosting the immune response [49]. In vitro findings suggest that the VD treatment may reduce HIV-1 transmission modulating levels and function of T cells, and the production of antiviral factors [50].

1.5 Hepatitis B and C virus

VD deficiency is involved in the pathogenesis of chronic liver diseases caused by hepatitis B (HBV), and C viruses (HCV). High prevalence of VD deficiency with serum levels below 20 mg/mL in patients with HBV and HCV infections has been reported. Current literature was reviewed in order to understand the effects of VD supplementation in combination with IFN-based therapy on the virologic response in HBV and HCV infected patients. Hoan revealed that is important to know the significance of VD hypovitaminosis in the outcome of HBV- and HCV-related chronic liver diseases [51].

VD signaling is involved in infectious and non-infectious liver diseases. It is very important to understand the risk factors for the development of HBV. Probably there is relationship between VDR polymorphisms and the risk of HBV infection. Another group of authors headed by He Q in meta-analysis indicates that VDR polymorphisms FokI genotype FF, Ff and allele F increase the risk of HBV infection and possibly has a role in the HBV susceptibility [52].

Low serum levels of VD are associated with increased HBV replication. HBV-transfected cells, inhibit VD impact [53]. The analysis of the immunological response of VD supplementation in chronic HCV patients by Kondo revealed that VD could improve the sensitivity of Peg-IFN/RBV therapy on HCV-infected hepatocytes by reducing the cytokine IP-10 production from PBMCs and expression of IFN-stimulated genes expression in the liver. Th1 responses in subjects treated with VD3/Peg-IFN/RBV were significantly higher than in those treated with Peg-IFN/RBV at 12 weeks after Peg-IFN/RBV therapy ($p < 0.05$) [54].

A recent study shows that supplementation of VD significantly improves sustained viral response via IFN-based therapy. VD reduces the extra- and intracellular levels of HCV core antigen in a concentration-dependent manner. This finding confirmed the improved efficacy of anti-HCV treatment via the combination of VD and IFN [55]. Calcitriol and VD_3, both remarkably inhibit HCV production in a VDR-independent mechanism [56]. A group of authors led by Murayama using an HCV cell culture system identified several compounds with anti-HCV activity by screening VD derivatives, which reduce HCV production by suppressing the expression of apolipoprotein in host cells [57].

2. Respiratory viruses

Acute respiratory viral infections (ARVI) remain the leading cause of morbidity and mortality worldwide, and a major global health problem because the availability of the effective antiviral drugs is limited. Such epidemics have significant negative economic consequences worldwide because of the increased absence from work and school resulting in long lasting economic crises. This can also lead to an overall collapse of the health care system. A number of observational studies revealed that VD deficiency is associated with increased risk of ARVI. Meta-analysis of trials revealed that there is protective effect of VD supplementations on the prevention on ARVI [58]. VD and its metabolites have immunomodulatory effect on respiratory epithelial cells surface markers infected with respiratory viruses (RV) modulating secretion of interferon 1, TNF and IL-6 [58]. VD mediates viral entry in epithelial cells and stimulates the expression of potent antimicrobial peptides in the respiratory tract epithelial cells protecting the lung from infection [58, 59].

Esposito and colleagues reviewed all of the studies published in PubMed over 15 years concerning VD deficiency and supplementations in children with respiratory tract infections. They concluded that VD seems to be very important because of its part of immune system. However, further studies are needed to evaluate the impact of VD deficiency in terms of the epidemiology and the outcome of pediatric respiratory tract infections [25, 60].

Brockman-Schneider and colleagues hypothesized that VD could directly reduce rhinovirus (RV) replication in airway epithelium but they found that VD does not directly affect RV replication in airway epithelial cells, but can instead influence chemokine synthesis and alters the growth and differentiation of airway epithelial cells [61].

2.1 Influenza virus

Influenza appears in a seasonal cycles [62, 63]. Seasonality to influenza correlates with a seasonal drop in VD serum levels and is associated with solar radiation, which triggers seasonal VD skin production. Common winter VD deficiency has negative effects on innate and acquired immunity. UV radiation from artificial sources or from sunlight reduces the incidence of viral respiratory infections [64].

VD supplementation is associated with reduced incidence and severity during influenza A virus (IAV) infection restoring the autophagic flux inhibited by IAV by upregulating the expression of Syntax in-17 (STX17) and V-type proton ATPase subunit (ATP6V0A2). It causes a concomitant decrease in cellular apoptosis via a VDR. VD is useful for limiting IAV-induced cellular injury via its pro-autophagic action [65].

Zhou and colleagues studied the clinical efficacy of VD for preventing influenza A in 400 infants. They revealed that a high-dose VD (1200 IU) is suitable and safe for the prevention of seasonal influenza because of rapid relief from symptoms, rapid decrease in viral loads and quick recovery [66]. This study suggests that VD supplementation during the winter may reduce the incidence of influenza A in infants [66]. Urashima investigated the effect of VD supplementation (1200 IU/d) during the winter on the incidence of seasonal influenza A in schoolchildren and proved that it can reduce it [67].

Very cheap prophylaxis with use of VD as a prophylactic therapy for influenza starting at the end of October till the end of April is very useful; Would be crucial to prove it from a potential easy and cheap prophylaxis or therapy support perspective as far as influenza infections are concerned. Gruber-Bzura explore the preventive effect of VD supplementation on viral influenza infections also [68].

In people diagnosed with hypovitaminosis D at the beginning of the autumn supplementation with 2000 IU of VD helps to bring levels to normal, but if extremely low serum VD values are proven, the reimbursement doses may be even higher.

2.2 Novel beta-coronavirus SARS-CoV-2

Coronaviruses are seasonal, with little transmission in the summer. Coronavirus disease (COVID-19) is caused by a novel beta-corona virus, renamed by the WHO to severe acute respiratory syndrome coronavirus 2 (SARS-CoV-2) to destigmatize the association of the virus with any geographic location or nationality. COVID-19 is a potentially fatal disease and has been declared as a global pandemic nowadays.

A number of additional preprints and publications regarding VD on COVID-19 have appeared. Some reviews tried to explain the involvement of micronutrient VD in COVID19 treatment and prophylaxis. Vitamin D supplementation could possibly improve clinical outcomes of patients infected with COVID-19 [69].

Lau revealed that VD insufficiency prevalence in ICU patients was 84.6%, vs. 57.1% in floor patients and concluded that may be an underlying driver of COVID-19 severity [70]. Rharusun in his retrospective Indonesian cohort study revealed that majority of the death cases were older male with pre-existing condition and hypovitaminosis D. Majority of the COVID-19 cases with insufficient and deficient VD status died [71]. Bloukh conclude that adequate serum vitamin D levels are needed for the prevention of severe cases of COVID-19 [72, 73]. The elderly have lower levels of vitamin D due to a variety of biological and behavioral factors [74, 75].

VD deficiency has been found to contribute to ARDS and case-fatality rates increase with age and with chronic disease comorbidity, both of which are associated with hypovitaminosis D. This supports the view that VD deficiency may also favor the emergence of more severe forms of the disease. It is also well known that older people, especially those housed in homes, have a high percentage of VD deficiency. Unfortunately, today we are witnessing an explosive rate of infections in nursing homes with poor outcomes. VD prevention and treatment for deficiency worldwide would greatly help to overcome this pandemic. VD is known to regenerate endothelial lining, which may be beneficial in minimizing the alveolar damage caused in ARDS. In animal model VD reduce lung permeability by modulation of renin-angiotensin system activity and ACE2 expression [76]. Grant recommends that raising serum VD concentrations to 100 – 150 nmol/l should be able to reduce the risk of COVID-19 infection and death [77].

McCullough recommends reaching those concentrations rapidly by taking large doses of VD for a few weeks, followed by several thousand IU/d VD for the duration of the COVID-19 pandemic. Such doses have been found not to have adverse health effects. Randomized controlled trials and large population studies should be conducted to evaluate these recommendations [78].

There have been a few investigations of VD effect on interstitial pneumonia. Tsujino and his colleagues used human pulmonary fibroblast cell lines (HPFCs) and a mouse model of Bleomycin-induced pulmonary fibrosis. They evaluated whether VD was activated in the lungs and had a preventive effect against interstitial pneumonia [79]. Expression of the VDR gene and genes for enzymes metabolizing VD were evaluated in two HPFCs, as well as the suppressive effect of VD on induction of inflammatory cytokines [79]. Symptoms of Bleomycin-induced pulmonary fibrosis were improved and expression of fibrosis markers/fibrosis inducers was decreased by a high VD diet, so they concluded that VD is activated locally in lung tissues and high dietary intake may have a preventive effect against interstitial pneumonia [79]. Martineau concluded that VD supplementation is safe and protects against acute respiratory tract infection overall. Patients who were very VD deficient experienced the most benefit [80].

Daneshkhah investigates if there is a link between severe cases of COVID-19 expressing cytokine storm and VD deficiency [81]. Age-specific case fatality (CFR) was investigated for the elderly (age $\geq$ 70 yr), Italy and Spain present the highest CFR (>1.7 times that of other countries). A more severe deficiency of VD lower than 25 nmol/L is reported in Italy and Spain compared to other countries. His investigation suggests that elimination of severe VD deficiency reduces the risk of high CRP levels, which may be used as a surrogate marker of cytokine storm expected to reduce in severe COVID-19 cases of up to 15% [81].

Kakodkar in his review points out that VD regenerates endothelial lining and is beneficial in lowering the alveolar damage and ARDS [82]. This protective effect is 19% better on those on a daily bolus compared to those on a monthly one while in those with deficiency protective effect is 70% better. The author and his colleagues consider this vitamin very important in the prevention and treatment of COVID-19 [82].

Recent study of COVID-19 and VD indicate that the severity of the clinical picture of COVID-19 depends of VD deficiency that is more prevalent in patients with severe COVID-19 disease. The inflammatory response is higher with increased chances of mortality [83]. Antiviral and anti-inflammatory action of VD is high and supplementation can have preventive effect on the development of severe COVID-19 forms [84].

A clinical trial on the severity of COVID-19 clinical imaging and VD deficiency should be performed and useful. Caccialanza R. and other authors propose a pragmatic protocol for early nutritional supplementation of non-critically ill patients hospitalized for COVID-19, explaining that most patients present at admission have severe inflammation and anorexia leading to a drastic reduction of food intake [85]. Many published data revealed that VD has immunomodulatory effect. Prevention by supplementation is recommended [86]. There is a link between immunodeficiency in individuals with obesity and greater viral pathogenicity because of VD deficiency/insufficiency in this population [87]. Among patients with COVID-19 in intensive care units (ICU) the prevalence of obesity was 47.5% (49/103). In a multivariate analysis, severe obesity (BMI ≥35 kg/m2) was associated with ICU admission [88].

The first preliminary data collected by Giancarlo Isaia in Turin indicate that patients hospitalized for COVID-19 have a very high prevalence of hypovitaminosis D. Italy is currently the country with the third highest number of Coronavirus cases after the United States and Spain. If we compare the data of southern and northern Italy, published on-line by Statista Research Department, we can see that in southern Italy, which is also poorer, there are significantly fewer infected with SARS-Cov-2 [89].

Vitamin D levels are severely low in the aging population especially in Spain, Italy, and Switzerland. This is also the most vulnerable group of the population in relation to COVID-19 [90–92]. There is a variation in mortality of COVID-19 between different countries and countries in southern hemisphere have a relatively low mortality. For instance, there is a big difference between Australia's 2 per million in 10th the UK's 68 per million by April 3rd 2020., which may support the hypothesis that VD is a factor that determines the severity of the disease [93].

3. Discussion

The viruses that have already been circulating among the population earlier are less severe than the new ones, which have an advantage because the population was not previously immunized to them. Many respiratory viruses are winter-seasonal in temperate regions. For influenza, it has been shown in the lab that absolute humidity strongly affects flu transmission, where drier conditions are more favorable.

There is a significant correlation between VD deficiency in children and the incidence and severity of lower respiratory tract infection (LTRI). Children with LRTI have significantly lower mean VD levels as compared to controls and their disease manifestation was severe [94].

The hypothesis that hypovitaminosis D can influence severity of influenza or COVID-19 has to be confirmed by future research.

Analyzing the immune mechanisms might help us to understand why some people show severe complications while others can be asymptomatic. We have to discover the influence of VD on specific targets in immune system immunomodulating the response on virus influenzas and SARS-CoV-2.

This knowledge can be useful for preventive therapeutic purposes when VD can be used as an immune-protector and antiviral factor. Increasingly, there is a growing awareness that this secosteroid hormone/vitamin is a very important factor in the proper functioning of the immune system in response to various viral infections and consequent complications such as autoimmune or malignant diseases.

In recent years, we have witnessed explosive flu epidemics, generally respiratory infections including this year pandemic of COVID-19 that we can associate with the worldwide epidemic of hypovitaminosis D. It would be necessary that organizations, societies, and country government institutional bodies be lobbied to recommend VD in winter time and adopt guidelines for the prevention of hypovitaminosis D, in order to prevent or at least minimize the outcome of this pandemic with is causing grave and tragic consequences on the health of mankind and of course the economy.

Interventional and observational epidemiological studies provide evidence that VD deficiency may confer increased risk of influenza and respiratory tract infection. Cell culture experiments support the thesis that VD has direct anti-viral effects particularly against enveloped viruses [95].

3.1 Recommendations

For optimal functioning of the immune system and protection against infections caused by viruses, serum VD concentration has to be between 75 and 150 nmol/L. Preventive doses for adults in risk of hypovitaminosis D have to be from 1200-2000 IU and for children at risk for hypovitaminosis D have to be from 800-1200 IU.

For proven VD deficiency for adults, 4000 IU have to be prescribed for the first 8 weeks and then maintained at 1200-2000 IU and for children 2000 IU 8 weeks and maintained 1200-1400 IU depending on the severity of the deficit.

Considering the recommendations presented in **Table 1**, a personalized approach to the treatment and prevention of VD deficiency is extremely important. It is important to identify in the population individuals with secondary immune deficiency caused by hypovitaminosis VD. Such persons have to be treated with higher doses.

In children and adults, we have to bring serum VD levels to >75 nmol/L and maintain them between 90 and 120 nmol / L especially in epidemic conditions to 150 nmol/L After VD replacement therapy, a rechecking of the serum VD concentration is recommended after two months. In period of maintenance therapy rechecking has to be every two months. As can be seen in the preprints and publications on severity of COVID-19 infections those with concentrations >75 nmol/L still have symptomatic infections. Thus, going to 100 to 150 nmol/L would result in reduced risk of symptoms better than just >75 nmol/L.

It is known that VD concentrations decrease with age because the skin is old and has reduced capacity to produce VD and the intestines absorb VD more slowly from food. Elderly Europeans, are thus at risk of hypovitaminosis D during winter [96, 97].

The same is happening worldwide, especially among the older population living in the northern hemisphere. They have to be tested for levels of VD in serum at the beginning of November and at the end of February. The elderly population is the most susceptible to influenza and COVID-19 and has the most frequently fatal complications. It is the same population that is most likely to suffer from hypovitaminosis D, which significantly worsens the condition of the aging immune system [98].

A serum VD lower than 25 nmol/L was found in 2 to 30% of adults, while this percentage may increase to 75% or more in older persons in institutions [90, 91].

The Institute of Medicine (IOM) finds doses <4000 IU/day are safe for old people. Boucher suggest that ≥1000–2000 IU of VD daily is necessary in this

	Therapy for hipovitaminosis D	Prevention of hipovitaminosis D
Children	1. 2000 IU 8 weeks, then VD serum levels control 2. Maintenance 1200-1400 IU, VD serum levels control every two months	1. 800 IU – 1200 IU VD serum levels control every two months
Adults	1. 4000 IU 8 weeks, then VD serum levels control 2. Maintenance 1200-2000 IU, VD serum levels control every two months	1. 1200 IU – 2000 IU VD serum levels control every two months
Elderly	1. 5000 IU 8 weeks, then VD serum levels control 2. Maintenance 2000 - 3000 IU VD serum levels control every two months	1. 2000 - 3000 IU VD serum levels control every two months

Table 1.
Recomandations for daily VD administration.

population with numerous clinical problems related to the indicated age, especially when independence is lost, when hypovitaminosis D is also present worsening the patient's clinical condition. Much higher doses than these are needed for the treatment of the established deficiency [99].

A preventative strategy should be established and endorsed by the organizations, societies, and country governments be lobbied to recommend VD in winter, which is extremely important for maintaining the good health of the world's population. Preventive administration of VD or replacement therapy in the early winter months to early spring could reduce the severity of clinical symptoms in patients with COVID-19 infection. It is necessary to optimize VD status to enhance every one's immunity for protection against SARS-CoV-2 infection. Prevention of influenza outbreaks and COVID-19 must begin as early as the first days of November so that the population enters a season of respiratory infections with a prepared and strengthened immune system. Jakovac in his letter to the editor recommends intensive supplementation as possible prophylaxis with VD with even higher doses [100]. Maintenance of adequate VD status may be an effective and inexpensive prophylactic method against viral infections, but the optimal supplementation regimen has to be defined.

The latest literature by Paul Marik and East Virginia Medical School (EVMS) medical group published on line a protocol explaining prevention and treatment COVID-19 with instructions for applying VD 1000-4000 IU (unknown optimal dose) in prevention and therapy in mildly symptomatic patients [101].

4. Conclusion

Persons with VD deficiency have attenuated immune responses with secondary immunodeficiency. This condition increases the severity of viral infections especially those of respiratory tract that show typical seasonality pattern during the winter months. Children, adults, especially older population have to take supplementation of VD for reason to cure and deficiency prevention. By the general acceptance of the fact that VD supplementation has a positive effect on immunity we can reduce the risk and severity of viral infections with important public health benefits.

Author details

Srđana Čulić
Medical School University of Split, Split, Croatia

*Address all correspondence to: srdjana.culic.sc@gmail.com

References

[1] Pittas AG, Dawson-Hughes B, Sheehan P, Ware JH, Knowler WC, Aroda VR, et al. Vitamin D Supplementation and Prevention of Type 2 Diabetes. N Engl J Med. 2019; 381(6):520-530.

[2] Manson JE, Cook NR, Lee IM, Christen W, Bassuk SS, Mora S, et al. Vitamin D Supplements and Prevention of Cancer and Cardiovascular Disease. N Engl J Med. 2019;380(1):33-44.

[3] Crowe FL, Steur M, Allen NE, Appleby PN, Travis RC, Key TJ. Plasma Concentrations of 25-hydroxyvitamin D in Meat Eaters, Fish Eaters, Vegetarians and Vegans: Results From the EPIC-Oxford Study Public Health Nutr. 2011;14(2):340-346.

[4] Saternus R, Vogt T, Reichrath J. A Critical Appraisal of Strategies to Optimize Vitamin D Status in Germany, a Population With a Western Diet. Nutrients. 2019;11(11):2682.

[5] Engelsen O. The relationship between ultraviolet radiation exposure and vitamin D status. Nutrients. 2010;2(5):482-495.

[6] Hoseinzadeh E, Taha P, Wei C, Godini H, Ashraf GM, Taghavi M, et al. The impact of air pollutants, UV exposure and geographic location on vitamin D deficiency. Food Chem Toxicol. 2018;113:241-254.

[7] Mousavi SE, Amini H, Heydarpour P, Amini Chermahini F, Godderis L.Air pollution, environmental chemicals, and smoking may trigger vitamin D deficiency: Evidence and potential mechanisms. Environ Int. 2019;122:67-90.

[8] Caccamo D, Ricca S, Currò M, Ientile R. Health Risks of Hypovitaminosis D: A Review of New Molecular Insights. Int J Mol Sci. 2018;19(3):892.

[9] Ritterhouse LL, Lu R, Shah HB, Robertson JM, Fife DA, Maecker HT, et al. Vitamin D deficiency in a multiethnic healthy control cohort and altered immune response in vitamin D deficient European-american healthy controls. PLoS One 2014;9(4):e94500.

[10] Yoshimura N, Muraki S, Oka H, Morita M, Yamada H, Tanaka S, et al. Profiles of Vitamin D Insufficiency and Deficiency in Japanese Men and Women: Association With Biological, Environmental, and Nutritional Factors and Coexisting Disorders: The ROAD Study. Osteoporos Int. 2013;24(11):2775-2787.

[11] Diekmann R, Winning K, Bauer JM, Uter W, Stehle P, Lesser S, et al. Vitamin D status and physical function in nursing home residents: A 1-year observational study. Zeitschrift für Gerontologie und Geriatrie. 2013;46:403-409.

[12] Samefors M, Östgren CJ, Mölstad S, Lannering C, Midlöv P, Tengblad A. Vitamin D deficiency in elderly people in Swedish nursing homes is associated with increased mortality. Eur J Endocrinol. 2014;170(5):667-75.

[13] Uday S, Högler W.Spot the silent sufferers: A call for clinical diagnostic criteria for solar and nutritional osteomalacia. J Steroid Biochem Mol Biol. 2019;188:141-146.

[14] Dimitrov V, White JH. Vitamin D signaling in intestinal innate immunity and homeostasis. Mol Cell Endocrinol. 2017;453:68-78.

[15] Baeke F, Takiishi T, Korf H, Gysemans C, Mathieu C. Vitamin D: modulator of the immune system. Curr Opin Pharmacol. 2010;10(4):482-496.

[16] Borges MC, Martini LA, Rogero MM. Current perspectives on

vitamin D, immune system, and chronic diseases. Nutrition. 2011;27(4):399-404.

[17] Ikemoto Y, Kuroda K, Nakagawa K, Ochiai A, Ozaki R, Murakami K, et al. Vitamin D Regulates Maternal T-Helper Cytokine Production in Infertile Women. Nutrients. 2018 13;10(7):902.

[18] Zhang Z, Chen F, Li J, Luo F, Hou T, Xu J, et al. 1,25$(OH)_2D_3$ suppresses proinflammatory responses by inhibiting Th1 cell differentiation and cytokine production through the JAK/STAT pathway.Am J Transl Res. 2018;10(8):2737-2746.

[19] Ragab D, Soliman D, Samaha D, Yassin A. Vitamin D status and its modulatory effect on interferon gamma and interleukin-10 production by peripheral blood mononuclear cells in culture. Cytokine. 2016;85:5-10.

[20] Sun X, Wang T, Cai D, Hu Z, Chen J, Liao H, et al. Cytokine Storm Intervention in the Early Stages of COVID-19 Pneumonia Cytokine Growth Factor Rev. 2020;S1359-6101(20)30048-4.

[21] Huang C, Wang Y, Li X, Ren L, Zhao J, Hu Y, et al. Clinical features of patients infected with 2019 novel coronavirus in Wuhan, China.Lancet. 2020;395(10223):497-506.

[22] Nile SH, Nile A, Qiu J, Li L, Jia X, Kai G. COVID-19: Pathogenesis, cytokine storm and therapeutic potential of interferons. Cytokine Growth Factor Rev. 2020: doi: 10.1016/j.cytogfr.2020.05.002

[23] Khare D, Godbole NM, Pawar SD, Mohan V, Pandey G, Gupta S, et al. Calcitriol [1, 25[OH]2 D3] Pre- And Post-Treatment Suppresses Inflammatory Response to Influenza A (H1N1) Infection in Human Lung A549 Epithelial Cells. Eur J Nutr. 2013;52(4):1405-1415.

[24] Kim DH, Meza CA, Clarke H, Kim JS, Hickner RC. Vitamin D and Endothelial Function. Nutrients. 2020; 12(2): 575.

[25] Dancer RC, Parekh D, Lax S, D'Souza V, Zheng S, Bassford CR, et al. Vitamin D deficiency contributes directly to the acute respiratory distress syndrome (ARDS). Thorax. 2015;70(7):617-624.

[26] Adrian R Martineau AR, David A Jolliffe DA, Hooper RL, Greenberg L, Aloia JF, Bergman P, et al. Vitamin D supplementation to prevent acute respiratory tract infections: systematic review and meta-analysis of individual participant data. BMJ 2017;356:i6583

[27] Zdrenghea MT, Makrinioti H, Bagacean C, Bush A, Johnston SL, Stanciu LA. Vitamin D modulation of innate immune responses to respiratory viral infections. Rev Med Virol. 2017;27(1). doi: 10.1002/rmv.

[28] Cepeda S J, Zenteno A D, Fuentes S C, Bustos B R. Vitamin D and pediatrics respiratory diseases]. Rev Chil Pediatr. 2019;90(1):94-101.

[29] Bryson KJ, Nash AA, Norval M. Does vitamin D protect against respiratory viral infections? Epidemiol Infect. 2014;142(9):1789-801.

[30] Aygun · H. Vitamin D Can Prevent COVID-19 Infection-Induced Multiple Organ Damage. Naunyn Schmiedebergs Arch Pharmacol. 2020;1-4.doi: 10.1007/s00210-020-01911-4

[31] Teymoori-Rad M, Shokri F, Salimi V, Marashi SM. The interplay between vitamin D and viral infections. Rev Med Virol. 2019;29(2):e2032.

[32] Čulić S, Markić J, Petrović D, Armanda V, Konjevoda P, Pavelić J. Vitamin D Status in Pediatric Patients with Newly Diagnosed Malignant

Disease: Preliminary Results. Central Eur J Paed. 2018:14(2):160-166.

[33] Qamar S, Akbani S, Shamim S, Khan G. Vitamin D Levels in Children With Growing Pains. J Coll Physicians Surg Pak. 2011;21(5):284-287.

[34] Ghanaati S, Choukroun J, Volz U, Hueber R, Mourão CF, Sader R, et al. One hundred years after Vitamin D discovery: Is there clinical evidence for supplementation doses? Int J Growth Factors Stem Cells Dent. 2020;3:3-11

[35] Alvarez-Lafuente R. Vitamin D serum levels and viral load of human herpesvirus 6 and Epstein-Barr virus in patients with multiple sclerosis after one year of follow-up. ECTRIMS Online Library. Oct 27, 2017; 200662; P1007.

[36] Christensen T . Human Herpesviruses in MS. Int MS J. 2007;14(2):41-47.

[37] Christensen T.The role of EBV in MS pathogenesis.Int MS J. 2006;13(2):52-57.

[38] Maghzi H, Ataei B, Khorvash F, Yaran M, Maghzi AH. Association Between Acute Infectious Mononucleosis and Vitamin D Deficiency.Viral Immunol. 2016;29(7):397-400

[39] Amini R, Karampoor S, Zahednasab H, Keyvani H, Gheiasian M, Jalilian FA. Serum levels of matrix metalloproteinase-2, −9, and vitamin D in patients with multiple sclerosis with or without herpesvirus-6 seropositivity. Braz J Infect Dis. 2020. pii: S1413-8670(20)30020-9.

[40] Hassani A, Corboy JR, Al-Salam S, Khan G. Epstein-Barr Virus Is Present in the Brain of Most Cases of Multiple Sclerosis and May Engage More Than Just B Cells. PLoS One. 2018;13(2):e0192109.

[41] Pérez-Pérez S, Domínguez-Mozo MI, García-Martínez MÁ, Aladro Y, Martínez-GinésM,García-DomínguezJM, et al. Study of the possible link of 25-hydroxyvitamin D with Epstein-Barr virus and human herpesvirus 6 in patients with multiple sclerosis. Eur J Neurol. 2018;25(12):1446-1453.

[42] Røsjø E, Lossius A, Abdelmagid N, Lindstrøm JC, Kampman MT, Jørgensen L, et al. Effect of high-dose vitamin D_3 supplementation on antibody responses against Epstein-Barr virus in relapsing-remitting multiple sclerosis. Mult Scler. 2017;23(3):395-402.

[43] Özgü E, Yılmaz N, Başer E, Güngör T, Erkaya S, Yakut Hİ. Could 25-OH vitamin D deficiency be a reason for HPV infection persistence in cervical premalignant lesions? J Exp Ther Oncol. 2016;11(3):177-180.

[44] Shim J, Pérez A, Symanski E, Nyitray AG. Association Between Serum 25-Hydroxyvitamin D Level and Human Papillomavirus Cervicovaginal Infection in Women in the United States. J Infect Dis. 2016;213(12):1886-1892.

[45] Kumar A, Singh MP, Kumar RS, Ratho RK. 25-Hydroxyvitamin D3 and 1,25 Dihydroxyvitamin D3 as an Antiviral and Immunomodulator Against Herpes Simplex Virus-1 Infection in HeLa Cells. Viral Immunol. 2018;31(8):589-593.

[46] Choi B, Lee ES, Sohn S. Vitamin D3 ameliorates herpes simplex virus-induced Behçet's disease-like inflammation in a mouse model through down-regulation of Toll-like receptors. Clin Exp Rheumatol. 2011;29(4 Suppl 67):S13-S19.

[47] Öztekin A, Öztekin C. Vitamin D Levels in Patients with Recurrent Herpes Labialis. Viral Immunol. 2019;32(6):258-262.

[48] Jiménez-Sousa MÁ, Martínez I, Medrano LM, Fernández-Rodríguez A,

Resino S. Vitamin D in human immunodeficiency virus infection: influence on immunity and disease. Front Immunol. 2018;9:458.

[49] Akimbekov NS, Ortoski RA, Razzaque MS. Effects of sunlight exposure and vitamin D supplementation on HIV patients. J Steroid Biochem Mol Biol. 2020;200:105664.

[50] González SM, Aguilar-Jiménez W, Trujillo-Gil E, Zapata W, Su RC, Ball TB, et al. Vitamin D treatment of peripheral blood mononuclear cells modulated immune activation and reduced susceptibility to HIV-1 infection of CD4+ T lymphocytes. PLoS One. 2019;14(9):e0222878.

[51] Hoan NX, Tong HV, Song LH, Meyer CG, Velavan TP.Vitamin D deficiency and hepatitis viruses associated liver diseases: A literature review. World J Gastroenterol. 2018;24(4):445-460.

[52] He Q, Huang Y, Zhang L, Yan Y, Liu J, Song X, et al. Association between vitamin D receptor polymorphisms and hepatitis B virus infection susceptibility: A meta-analysis study. Gene. 2018;645:105-112.

[53] Gotlieb N, Tachlytski I, Lapidot Y, Sultan M, Safran M, Ben-Ari Z. Hepatitis B virus downregulates vitamin D receptor levels in hepatoma cell lines, thereby preventing vitamin D-dependent inhibition of viral transcription and production. Mol Med. 2018;24(1):53..

[54] Kondo Y, Kato T, Kimura O, Iwata T, Ninomiya M, Kakazu E, et al. 1(OH) Vitamin D3 Supplementation Improves the Sensitivity of the Immune-Response During Peg-IFN/RBV Therapy in Chronic Hepatitis C Patients-Case Controlled Trial. PLoS On. 2013;8(5):e63672.

[55] Matsumura T, Kato T, Sugiyama N, Tasaka-Fujita M, Murayama A, Masaki T, et al. 25-Hydroxyvitamin D3 Suppresses Hepatitis C Virus Production. Hepatology. 2012;56(4):1231-1239.

[56] Ravid A, Rapaport N, Issachar A, Erman A, Bachmetov L, Tur-Kaspa R, et al. 25-Hydroxyvitamin D Inhibits Hepatitis C Virus Production in Hepatocellular Carcinoma Cell Line by a Vitamin D Receptor-Independent Mechanism. Int J Mol Sci. 2019;13;20(9):2367.

[57] Murayama A, Saitoh H, Takeuchi A, Yamada N, Matsumura T, Shiina M, et al. Vitamin D derivatives inhibit hepatitis C virus production through the suppression of apolipoprotein. Antiviral Res. 2018;160:55-63

[58] Greiller CL, MartineauAR. Modulation of the Immune Response to Respiratory Viruses by Vitamin D. Nutrients 2015; 7(6): 4240-70.

[59] Jolliffe DA, Greiller CL, Mein CA, Hoti M, Bakhsoliani E, Telcian AG, et al. Vitamin D receptor genotype influences risk of upper respiratory infection. Br J Nutr. 2018;120:891-900.

[60] Esposito S, Baggi E, Bianchini S, Marchisio P, Principi N. Role of vitamin D in children with respiratory tract infection. Int J Immunopathol Pharmacol. 2013;26(1):1-13.

[61] Brockman-Schneider RA, Pickles RJ, Gern JE. Effects of vitamin D on airway epithelial cell morphology and rhinovirus replication. PLoS One. 2014;9(1):e86755.

[62] Martinez ME. The calendar of epidemics: Seasonal cycles of infectious diseases. PLoS Pathog. 2018;14(11):e1007327.

[63] Cohen J. Sick Time. Science. 2020;367(6484):1294-1297.

[64] Cannell JJ, Vieth R, Umhau JC, Holick MF, Grant WB, Madronich S, Garland CF, Giovannucci E. Epidemic influenza and vitamin D. Epidemiol Infect. 2006;134(6):1129-1140.

[65] Godbole NM, Sinha RA, Tiwari S, Pawar SD, Dhole TN. Analysis of influenza virus-induced perturbation in autophagic flux and its modulation during Vitamin D3 mediated anti-apoptotic signaling. Virus Res. 2020;282:197936.

[66] Zhou J, Du J, Huang L, Wang Y, Shi Y, Lin H. Preventive Effects of Vitamin D on Seasonal Influenza A in Infants: A Multicenter, Randomized, Open, Controlled Clinical Trial. Pediatr Infect Dis J. 2018;37(8):749-754.

[67] Urashima M, Segawa T, Okazaki M, Kurihara M, Wada Y, Ida H. Randomized trial of vitamin D supplementation to prevent seasonal influenza A in school children. Am J Clin Nutr. 2010;91(5):1255-1260.

[68] Gruber-Bzura BM. Vitamin D and Influenza-Prevention or Therapy? Int J Mol Sci. 2018;19(8):pii: E2419.

[69] Alipio, Mark, Vitamin D Supplementation Could Possibly Improve Clinical Outcomes of Patients Infected with Coronavirus-2019 (COVID-19) (April 9, 2020). Available at SSRN: https://ssrn.com/abstract=3571484 or http://dx.doi.org/10.2139/ssrn.3571484

[70] Lau FH, Majumder R, Torabi R, Saeg F, Hoffman R, Cirillo JD, Greiffenstein P, et al. Vitamin D Insufficiency is Prevalent in Severe COVID-1. https://www.medrxiv.org/content/101101/2020.04.24.20075838v1

[71] Raharusun, Prabowo and Priambada, Sadiah and Budiarti, Cahni and Agung, Erdie and Budi, Cipta, Patterns of COVID-19 Mortality and Vitamin D: An Indonesian Study (April 26, 2020). Available at SSRN: https://ssrn.com/abstract=3585561 or http://dx.doi.org/10.2139/ssrn.3585561

[72] Bloukh SH. Shaikh AA, Pathan HM, Edis Z. Prevalence of COVID-19: A Look behind the Scenes from the UAE and India. - 2020 – preprints.org file:///C:/UsersDownloads/preprints202004.0179.v2%20(2).pdf

[73] Ghavideldarestani M, Honardoost M, Khamsch ME. Role of Vitamin D in Pathogenesis and Severity of COVID-19 Infection. https://www.preprints.org/manuscript/202004.0355/v1/download

[74] Hribar CA, Cobbold PH, Church FC. Potential Role of Vitamin D in the Elderly to Resist COVID-19 and to Slow Progression of Parkinson's Disease. Brain Sci. 2020;*10*(5):284.

[75] Galicio EJ. Vitamin D Level of Mild and Severe Elderly Cases of COVID-19: A Preliminary Report. https://papers.ssrn.com/sol3/papers.cfm?abstract_id=3593258

[76] Xu J, Yang J, Chen J, Luo Q, Zhang Q, Zhang H. Vitamin D alleviates lipopolysaccharide-induced acute lung injury via regulation of the renin-angiotensin system. Mol Med Rep. 2017;16:7432-7438.

[77] Grant WB, Lahore H, Sharon L McDonnell SL, Baggerly CA, French CB, et al. Evidence That Vitamin D Supplementation Could Reduce Risk of Influenza and COVID-19 Infections and Deaths. Nutrients. 2020;12(4):E988.

[78] McCullough PJ, Lehrer DS, Amend J. Daily oral dosing of vitamin D3 using 5000 TO 50,000 international units a day in long-term hospitalized patients: Insights from a seven year experience. J Steroid Biochem Mol Biol 2019;189:228-239

[79] Tsujino I, Ushikoshi-Nakayama R, Yamazaki T, Matsumoto N, Saito I.

Pulmonary activation of vitamin D_3 and preventive effect against interstitial pneumonia. J Clin Biochem Nutr. 2019;65(3):245-251.

[80] Martineau AR, Jolliffe DA , HooperRL, Greenberg L, Aloia JF, Bergman P. Vitamin D Supplementation to Prevent Acute Respiratory Tract Infections: Systematic Review and Meta-Analysis of Individual Participant Data. BMJ. 2017;356:0.

[81] Daneshkhah A, Eshein A , Subramanian H, Roy HK, Backman V.The Role of Vitamin D in Suppressing Cytokine Storm in COVID-19 Patients and Associated Mortality. doi: https://doi.org/10.1101/2020.04.08.20058578. COVID-19 SARS-CoV-2 preprints from medRxiv and bioRxiv

[82] Kakodkar P, Kaka N, Baig MN.A Comprehensive Literature Review on the Clinical Presentation, and Management of the Pandemic Coronavirus Disease 2019 (COVID-19)Cureus. 2020; 12(4): e7560.

[83] Jain A, Chaurasia R, Sengar NS, Singh M, Mahor S, Narain S. Analysis of vitamin D level among asymptomatic and citically ill COVID-19 patients and its correlation with inflammatory markers. Sci Rep 10, 20191 (2020).

[84] Torehan Aslan M, Aslan IO, Ozdemir O. Is vitamin D One of the Key Elements in COVID-19 Days? J Nutr Health Aging.2020;24(9):1038-1039.

[85] Caccialanza R, Laviano A, Lobascio F, Montagna E, Bruno R, Ludovisi S, et al. Early nutritional supplementation in non-critically ill patients hospitalized for the 2019 novel coronavirus disease (COVID-19): Rationale and feasibility of a shared pragmatic protocol. Nutrition. 2020;3:110835.

[86] McCartney DM, Byrne DG. Optimisation of Vitamin D Status for Enhanced Immuno-protection Against Covid-19. Ir Med J. 2020;113(4):58.

[87] Carter SJ, Baranauskas MN, Fly AD. Considerations for obesity, vitamin D, and physical activity amid the COVID-19 pandemic. Obesity (Silver Spring). 2020. doi: 10.1002/oby.22838.

[88] Kalligeros M, Shehadeh F, Mylona EK, Benitez G, Beckwith CG, Chan PA, et al. Association of Obesity with Disease Severity among Patients with COVID-19. Obesity (Silver Spring). 2020 Apr 30. doi: 10.1002/oby.22859.

[89] https://www.statista.com/statistics/1099375/coronavirus-cases-by-region-in-italy/

[90] Isaia G, Giorgino R, Rini GB, Bevilacqua M, Maugeri D, Adami S. Prevalence of hypovitaminosis D in elderly women in Italy: clinical consequences and risk factors. Osteoporos Int. 2003l;14(7):577-582.

[91] Quesada JM, Jans I, Benito P, J A Jimenez JA, R Bouillon R. Vitamin D status of elderly people in Spain. Age Ageing1989;18(6):392-397.

[92] Ilie PC, Stefanescu S, Smith L. The role of vitamin D in the prevention of coronavirus disease 2019 infection and mortality. Aging Clin Exp Res (2020). https://doi.org/10.1007/s40520-020-01570-8

[93] Rhodes JM, Subramanian S, Laird E, Anne Kenny R.Editorial: low population mortality from COVID-19 in countries south of latitude 35 degrees North - supports vitamin D as a factor determining severity.Aliment Pharmacol Ther. 2020 Apr 20.

[94] Kana Ram Jat. Vitamin D Deficiency and Lower Respiratory Tract Infections in Children: A Systematic Review and Meta-Analysis of Observational Studies. Trop Doct. 2017; 47(1):77-84.

[95] Beard JA, Bearden A, Striker R. Vitamin D and the anti-viral state. J Clin Virol. 2011;50(3):194-200.

[96] van der Wielen RP, Löwik MR, van den Berg H, de Groot LC, Haller J, Moreiras O, et al. Serum vitamin concentrations among elderly people in Europe.Lancet. 1995;346(8969):207-210.

[97] MacLaughlin J, Holick MF. Aging decreases the capacity of human skin to produce vitamin D3. J Clin Invest. 1985;76(4):1536-1538.

[98] Basile M, Ciardi L, Crespi I, Saliva E, Bellomo G, Vidali M. Assessing Serum Concentrations of 25-Hydroxy-Vitamin D in North-Western Italy. J Frailty Aging. 2013;2(4):174-178.

[99] Boucher BJ. The Problems of Vitamin D Insufficiency in Older People. Aging Dis. 2012; 3(4):313-329.

[100] Jakovac H. COVID-19 and vitamin D-Is there a link and an opportunity for intervention?Am J Physiol Endocrinol Metab. 2020;318(5):E589.

[101] Marik P, (EVMS Medical Group). Coronavirus / Covid-19 Vitamin C, D, Zinc And Immune System Building Protocol – PREVENTION / TREATMENT.https://greenbeltoutdoors.com/coronavirus-covid-19-vitamin-c-d-zinc-and-immune-system-building-protocol-prevention-treatment-dr-paul-marik-evms-medical-group/

Chapter 6

Vitamin D and Its Relationship with the Pathways Related to Thrombosis and Various Diseases

Syed Mohd, Swati Sharma, Aastha Mishra and Mohammad Zahid Ashraf

Abstract

Vitamin D known for its vital role in diverse biological function such as calcium and phosphorus homeostasis, also exert an anticoagulant effect emphasizing its essential role in the thrombosis pathogenesis. Thrombosis is the formation and propagation of a blood clot or thrombus either in the arterial or the venous system resulting in several severe complications. Various studies have also reported the association of vitamin D deficiency with the increased incidences of thromboembolism. This may be in part due to its anticoagulant effects through upregulation of thrombomodulin, an anticoagulant glycoprotein, and downregulation of Tissue Factor, a critical coagulation factor. The protective effects of vitamin D and its receptor in endothelial cells may further explain some of the reported beneficial effects of vitamin D in the prevention or treatment of cardiovascular diseases. Additionally, the immunomodulatory role of vitamin D has been observed through its ability to alter the secretion of inflammatory cytokines that can induce a pro-coagulant milieu by multiple pathways. Therefore, it becomes pertinent to discuss the close link between vitamin D and human health and to improve our knowledge of the molecular pathways regulated or influenced by vitamin D and its associated metabolites.

Keywords: vitamin D, vitamin D receptor, thrombosis, coagulation, immune response

1. Introduction

Vitamin D is a lipophilic, steroid hormone, obtained from various food sources as well as majorly synthesized by the body in the skin through exposure to ultra-violet irradiation [1, 2]. In nature, vitamin D exists in two forms, vitamin D2, and vitamin D3. 25-hydroxyvitamin D (25(OH)D) is the major circulatory form and 1,25-dihydroxyvitamin D (1,25(OH)2D) is the active form of vitamin D that exerts its activity by binding to and activating the nuclear vitamin D receptor (VDR), which is a ligand-inducible transcription factor [3]. Upon activation, VDR forms a heterodimer with the retinoid-X receptor (RXR) that interacts with particular DNA sequences in the promoter region of target genes called vitamin response elements (VDREs) [4]. Vitamin D exerts a diverse biological function such as cell proliferation, calcium and phosphorus homeostasis, and cell differentiation. Most of these actions are carried out by regulating the expression of target genes through VDR activation [3].

Vitamin D deficiency is a widespread condition, reportedly occurring in 30 to 60% of the general population worldwide [5–7]. Vitamin D is commonly known for its vital role in calcium homeostasis and bone mineralization. It is also crucial in the prevention of rickets during early age and osteomalacia during adult age [8, 9]. Increasing evidence from clinical reports, cross-sectional studies, and cell culture studies further indicate that vitamin D may exert an anticoagulant effect emphasizing an essential role of vitamin D metabolites in the pathogenesis of thrombosis [10–12]. VDR is expressed throughout the body including various immune cells such as macrophages, dendritic cells, and lymphocytes [13–17]. They are also expressed in the vascular endothelial cells [18], which are relevant to hemostasis.

Thrombosis is the formation of a blood clot within the intact vascular system. It can occur in both arterial and venous systems [19]. Rudolf Virchow, a German scientist, and physician proposed the three main factors that may predispose an individual to the development of thrombosis: stasis, endothelial dysfunction, and hypercoagulability. Apart from these three factors, the innate inflammatory system also has an intrinsic link with coagulation, whereby activation of the inflammatory system promotes thrombosis and vice versa [20, 21]. Interventional studies have shown vitamin D treatment enhances endothelial functions and reduces the production of pro-inflammatory cytokines [22–24]. Apart from this, the anti-thrombotic effect of vitamin D on the pro-thrombotic and anti-thrombotic components of the coagulation system has also been well defined [25–27]. In this chapter, we are defining the effect of vitamin D deficiency in the three most important parameters viz. coagulation, endothelial activation, and immune responses affecting the occurrence of thrombosis. This chapter will also discuss the clinical impact of Vitamin D in various diseases including COVID-19.

2. Vitamin D in coagulation

Vitamin D deficiency is defined based on the plasma levels of 25(OH)D. Individuals with plasma levels under 20 ng/mL are considered vitamin D deficient. Vitamin D deficiency is highly prevalent worldwide with approximately 30–50% incidences [28–30]. Several reports have established the significant association of vitamin D deficiency with the increased risk of various cardiovascular diseases (CVDs) and mortality [31–33]. Various studies have also reported the association of vitamin D deficiency with the increased incidences of thromboembolism [34–36]. As suggested by the studies, the underlying molecular mechanism for the antithrombotic potential of vitamin D includes up-regulation of thrombomodulin and downregulation of tissue factor (TF) [25, 36, 37]. Additionally, vitamin D upregulates and increases the level of anti-inflammatory cytokines like IL-10 [24, 38]. The expression profile of more than 200 genes involved in the regulation of cellular proliferation, differentiation, apoptosis, and angiogenesis is directly or indirectly regulated by vitamin D [39]. The experimental shreds of evidence obtained from cell culture studies depicted that biologically active form of vitamin D_3 i.e., 1,25(OH)2D, and its synthetic analogs exerted the anticoagulant effects [40]. Koyama et al. have demonstrated in their experiments on human peripheral monocytes that 1,25(OH)2D exerted the anticoagulant effects by upregulating the expression of thrombomodulin, an anticoagulant glycoprotein, and downregulating the expression of TF, a critical coagulation factor [13]. 1,25 (OH)2D directly suppresses renin gene expression via a vitamin D-response (VDR) element that is present in the renin gene [41]. Different studies on mouse embryonic fibroblasts from VDR Knockout (VDRKO) mice asserted an increase in pro-fibrotic factors including nuclear factor kappa B, interleukin (IL)- 6, and TNF-α suggesting that 1,25 (OH)2D may have antifibrotic effect and hence modulates multiple signaling pathways, like the transforming growth factor-β/Smad signaling [42]. Experiments with VDRKO mice showed enhanced ADP-induced platelet aggregation, down-regulation of thrombomodulin and anti-thrombin, and upregulation of TF at mRNA level [43]. The VDR system has a physiological role in the maintenance of anti-thrombotic homeostasis as exacerbated multiorgan thrombus formation has been observed in VDRKO mice after lipopolysaccharide injection [43]. Recently, it has been documented that human platelets and megakaryocyte lineage also express VDR [44]. Hyppönen et al. documented that serum 25(OH)D level inversely associated with tPA antigen, fibrinogen, and D-dimer, suggesting a possible role for vitamin D3 status in determining thrombolytic profile [45]. It is well studied that inflammation can cause coagulation with high sensitivity C-reactive protein (hs-CRP) [46, 47]. A study comprising of 206 individuals reported significant inverse associations between 25(OH)D and PAI-1 and tPA antigen levels and between 1,25(OH)2D and tPA and hs-CRP levels [48].

However, because of the small number of clinical trials and heterogeneity, more studies need to be conducted to further define the haemostatic abnormalities seen in individuals with vitamin D3-deficiency, and to precisely define the potential benefits of vitamin D3 supplementation as a preventive measure for various CVDs.

3. Vitamin D in endothelium homeostasis

The pathogenesis of cardiovascular diseases is governed by endothelium homeostasis. The vascular endothelium is of mesodermal origin and is located at the confluence between blood and the underlying vascular tissues. It not only works as a barrier function but also exerts several vasoprotective roles, and is considered as the main regulator of blood vessel homeostasis. Due to its inherent capability to perceive humoral and hemodynamic stimuli [49], the endothelium is instrumental in local regulation of vascular tone and structure, regulation of migration and growth of VSMCs, and controlling the adhesion and extravasation of leukocytes [50, 51]. Destabilization and activation of the endothelium take place as a result of injury, hemodynamic alteration, response to inflammatory cytokines, as well as genetic disorders [52, 53]. Endothelial dysfunction is found in various conditions that adversely affect the cardiovascular system, including hypertension, diabetes mellitus, atherosclerosis, chronic renal failure, and Deep venous thrombosis (DVT) [54]. Endothelial cells (ECs) in a quiescent form exhibit an anti-coagulant, vaso-dilatory, and anti-adhesive property [55]. However, when activated they express pro-coagulant, vasoconstricting, and pro-adhesive properties [56]. Hemostasis is facilitated by an equilibrium of anticoagulant and procoagulant factors [56]. On one side of the hemostatic equilibrium, the ECs express anticoagulant factors such as thrombomodulin TM, tissue factor pathway inhibitor (TFPI), and tissue-type plasminogen activator (t-PA). On the other side, they express thrombin receptors, TF, plasminogen activator, and von Willebrand factor (vWF) [56].

The VDR has been identified in endothelium cells, and hydroxylation of 25(OH)D to 1,25(OH)2D also takes place in the endothelium [18, 57]. The expression of VDR and 1-alfa hydroxylase in the endothelium was found to be decreased with 25(OH)D deficiency [58]. In the vascular system, it has been recognized that vitamin D controls the proliferation of endothelial cells and vascular smooth muscle cells [59, 60]. Vitamin D up-regulates the production of nitric oxide (NO) in ECs [31], by increasing eNOS expression [61], which helps in reducing arterial stiffness [62]. Various randomized control trials (RCTs) have demonstrated an improvement in endothelial dysfunction in healthy individuals [23, 63, 64], as well as in patients [65, 66] and improvement of arterial stiffness with improved flow-mediated dilation (FMD) after vitamin D supplementation [67]. A study by Davide Carrara et al. showed restoration of normal vitamin D levels after prolonged supplementation with a high dose of cholecalciferol (50,000 IU/week orally for 8 weeks) is associated with inhibition of peripheral renin-angiotensin system and with an improvement of FMD in essential hypertensive patients with hypovitaminosis [68]. The 25(OH)D presumed to be an inactive sterol is also found to be a potent mediator of endothelial stability in a non-genomic manner at physiologically relevant levels [69].

1,25(OH)2D3 supplementation reduces oxidation stress, NF-kappa B activation, Intercellular Adhesion Molecule 1 (ICAM-1), and Monocyte chemoattractant protein-1 levels in the endothelium cells [70]. Vitamin D also downregulates platelet-activating factor (PAF) induced ICAM-1 expression in the ECs [71]. Another study observed a greater level of p65 subunit of NF-kB, and IL-6 in vitamin D deficient groups as compared to the vitamin D sufficient group [72]. Vitamin D has also been shown to inhibit activation of proinflammatory TF, NF-kB, and its downstream target, IL-6 [73], which is a pro-inflammatory cytokine in cultured vascular ECs [74] In addition, Vitamin D has been demonstrated to reverse Angiotensin II (Ang II) induced oxidative stress, a key mediator of endothelial dysfunction [75]. Ang II not only induces the production of ROS but also activates TF NF-kB, which further upregulates several cytokines such as TNF-alfa, IL-6, and adhesion molecules ICAM-1, Vascular cell adhesion molecule 1 (VCAM-1), and E-selectin prompting vascular injury [76]. In vivo, VDR knockdown leads to an increase in leukocytes-endothelial interaction associated with endothelial cell activation markers VCAM-1 and ICAM-1 in endothelial cells [77].

Given the recognized significance of endothelial function in the homeostasis of the cardiovascular system, the protective effects of VDR in endothelial cells may explain by some of the reported beneficial effects of vitamin D attributed to the prevention or curing of cardiovascular disease [78, 79]. Vitamin D therapy has been observed to be associated with improvement in endothelial function in ischemic heart disease (IHD) patients with vitamin D deficiency or insufficiency [80]. Further, *in vitro* supplementation of vitamin D improved endothelial progenitor cell ability in the formation of colonies in type 2 diabetes mellitus patients [81]. Cuenca *et al.* demonstrated that paricalcitol, a vitamin D substitute attenuates the endothelium damage induced by the chronic kidney disease in the thoracic aorta and directly mediates stability of endothelium in vitro by enhancing cell–cell interactions resembling a protective mechanism [82].

4. Inflammation and thrombosis

Thrombosis and inflammation are the two intrinsically interlinked processes. Inflammation can induce a procoagulant milieu by multiple pathways such as by causing an imbalance between procoagulant and anticoagulant characteristics of the endothelium that can lead to local stimulation of coagulation cascade. TNF-α, a pro-inflammatory cytokine that is a potent inducer of the immune defense mechanism and the first to be released at the site of infection promotes a pro-coagulant state by eliciting the production of TF on the endothelium [83] and suppressing the synthesis of the anticoagulant protein C [84], thereby stimulating fibrin formation. Inflammatory stimuli change the cellular program of the endothelium by expressing adhesion molecules such as p-selectin and E-selectin facilitating a transition toward a more procoagulant phenotype [85].

Other cells of the circulation are also customized by inflammatory molecules toward a pro-thrombotic state such as neutrophils and monocytes expression of TF [86, 87], which is upregulated upon inflammation. The role of sterile inflammation has also been demonstrated in the thrombosis by a direct association between nucleotide-binding domain, leucine-rich-containing family, pyrin domain containing 3 (NLRP3) inflammasome complex, and hypoxia-inducible factor-1 alpha in hypoxia-induced thrombosis associated with an increase in the relative expression of caspase-1, interleukin-1beta and IL-18 transcripts in the individuals with venous thrombosis [20]. In recent years, the role of vitamin D as a regulator of both innate and adaptive immune responses has become very clear [88]. Local synthesis of 1,25-(OH)2D at the site of inflammation can modulate the immune response in a paracrine manner [89]. 1,25(OH)2D binds to the nuclear VDR which has been found to be expressed in various cells of the immune system such as macrophages, activated T-cells, B-cells, Dendritic cells, and monocytes [90, 91].

The immunomodulatory role of vitamin D has been observed through its ability to alter the secretion of inflammatory cytokines [92, 93]. Additionally, multiple studies are suggesting an inverse association between vitamin D level and inflammatory cytokines such as TNF-α, IL-6, and CRP [16–20], which are correctable by vitamin D supplementation [94–96]. Furthermore, lower vitamin D levels have also been associated with an increase in the levels of cellular adhesion molecules such as VCAM and ICAM [97].

Moreover, an increased incidence of auto-immune disorders in higher latitudes has been reported, which could be attributed to low UV-radiation that reduces the ability to synthesize vitamin D [98, 99]. Elderly peoples usually tend to have Hypovitaminosis D [26], which has been associated with an increased risk for chronic diseases where inflammation plays an integral component [100, 101]. A study by EM Akbas *et al.* revealed an inverse association between Vitamin D levels and inflammation through Neutrophil-to-lymphocyte ratio (NLR) and platelet-to-lymphocyte ratio (PLR) which are novel and inexpensive markers of inflammation. They found a significantly higher NLR and PLR in patients with lower 25(OH)D status [102].

Further, several cross-sectional studies have associated vitamin D levels and inflammation. Amer and Qayyam Studied 15,167 men and women aged 18 years and older [103]. They observed a negative association between vitamin D and inflammatory markers such as CRP and IL-6 in the vitamin D deficient groups (<25 nmol/L). This association was not observed in groups with insufficient and sufficient vitamin D status [104]. Bellia et al. examined the association of vitamin D and inflammatory markers in 137 morbidly obese individuals including both men and women. They also observed a significant inverse association between serum 25(OH)D levels and inflammatory markers like CRP, IL-6, and TNF-α [105]. A clinical trial by SS Bidar et al. observed a significant decrease in the systemic inflammatory markers including hsCRP, serum amyloid A, TNF-α, and IL-6 with the increase in circulating vitamin D after a daily intake of vitamin D fortified yogurt drink in the subjects with type 2 diabetes (T2D) [96]. However, in another clinical trial, Jorde et al. [106] observed no significant effects on hsCRP levels in the subjects randomly assigned to the therapy for 1 year with vitamin D3 40,000 IU per week, 20,000 IU per week, or placebo.

5. Clinical impact of vitamin D in various diseases

There is a close link between vitamin D and human health, vitamin D deficiency is widely associated with several diseased conditions by physicians and patients.

The various diseases affected by vitamin D deficiency can be categorized as cardiovascular disease (hypertension, thrombosis), various cancers, autoimmune diseases like multiple sclerosis, rheumatoid arthritis, and metabolic syndromes like osteomalacia, diabetes, and muscle weakness (**Figure 1**).

Osteomalacia is a classical human manifestation associated with vitamin D deficiency. It is a clinical condition in which bone mineralization is hampered due to low concentrations of phosphorus and calcium in the extracellular fluid [107]. Vitamin D plays a crucial role in maintaining an adequate level of serum phosphorus and calcium. In the absence of vitamin D or its deficiency, only 10 to 15% of dietary calcium and 60% of phosphorus are absorbed in the human body [108–110]. With the advent of technologies, molecular biology has permitted a more detailed characterization of the effects of vitamin D deficiency, via working on the animals lacking the VDR and studying their phenotype. Subtle abnormalities in the immune and cardiovascular system have been defined in the global VDRKO mouse, but their relevance to human disease is still obscure [111]. Greater awareness of the high prevalence of vitamin D inadequacy and its associated abnormalities is required among researchers, clinicians, and patients. There has been a large number of trials concerning the effects of vitamin D on the management and prevention in the last two decades. The most studied diseases in this aspect have been discussed below:

5.1 Osteoporosis

The association between osteoporosis and vitamin D deficiency is well established especially in the elderly. Vitamin D deficiency has been linked with the significant suppression in intestinal Calcium absorption and the impairment of its balance, which causes low bone mineral content and density. Decreased bone mineral density (BMD) raises the risk of bone fractures, which contributes significantly to the hospitalization, morbidity, and mortality of elderlies [112, 113]. Several studies have demonstrated the efficacy of vitamin D as a preventive measure for fractures. Clinical trials recommending the use of 700 to 800 IU/d oral vitamin D with or without Ca supplementation reported a significant 26% decrease in the risk of sustaining a hip fracture and a significant 23% decrease in the risk of sustaining any non-vertebral fracture vs. placebo or Calcium alone [114].

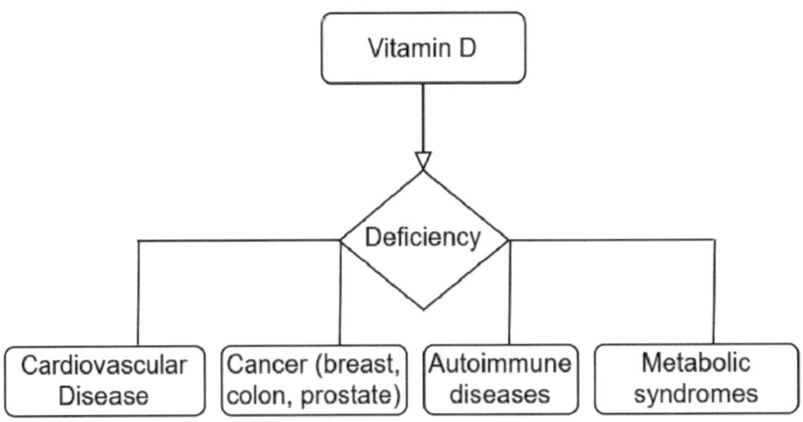

Figure 1.
Reported Association of Vitamin D deficiency with various human disease.

5.2 Muscle weakness

One of the prominent features of vitamin D deficiency is muscle weakness. Several clinical data of patients with nonspecific muscle weakness, muscle aches, and pains have shown vitamin D inadequacy [115, 116]. It has been reported that skeletal muscle tissue contains VDR and needs vitamin D to attain maximum function [117]. Recent studies have associated the increased vitamin D levels with improved muscle performance, and thereby reduced incidences of fall and fracture. A 5-month randomized controlled trial study has exhibited a 72% reduction in the risk of falls as compared with the placebo group in elderly people in a nursing home receiving 800 IU of vitamin D2 plus calcium daily [118].

5.3 Hypertension

Hypertension affects the population globally. Increasing evidence in recent times suggests that vitamin D has a crucial role in regulating blood pressure. Animal studies indicate that 1,25-dihydroxy vitamin D inhibits renin expression in the juxtaglomerular apparatus and blocks the proliferation of vascular smooth muscle cells, which affects systemic blood pressure [119]. People taking oral supplementation of vitamin D were found to have reduced blood pressure. The exposure of skin to UVB rays, a major source of vitamin D formation, has been associated with lower blood pressure [120–122].

5.4 Multiple sclerosis

Multiple sclerosis (MS) is an auto-immune disease characterized by the attack of self- immune system on the myelin sheath which works as a nerve insulator. The transmission of nerve signals gets affected leading to disrupted communication between the body and brain.. There have been several reports claiming the increased frequency of MS in temperate climates than in the tropics [123, 124]. Furthermore, studies also suggest that there is a strong negative correlation between the short annual, winter hours and frequency of occurrence of MS [125, 126]. Hence, these studies could hypothesized that vitamin D synthesized during sun exposure exerted a protective effect [127–129]. In addition, There are few studies that indicated low or insufficient levels of vitamin D in MS patients [130–132].

5.5 Rickets

The re-arrival of worldwide vitamin D deficiency has led to the re-emergence of rickets. Low levels of vitamin D in breastfeeding mothers can, often, lead to deficiencies in their children. The recommended levels of vitamin D supplements are 400 IU/d for infants to avoid diseases such as rickets [8].

5.6 Cancer

Garland and Garland for the first time reported that vitamin D deficiency could be associated with a higher risk of colon cancer mortality. Recent studies have reported an increased risk of several cancers with vitamin D deficiency, suggesting that vitamin D deficiency may account for premature mortality from colon, breast, ovarian, and prostate cancer [133–135]. Vitamin D is a potent hormone and regulates cell growth. VDRs are expressed by various cells and get activated by 1,25(OH)2 D, inducing differentiation into normally functioning cells, and inhibiting proliferation, angiogenesis, invasiveness, and metastatic potential.

Studies reveal that tumor models of lung, colon, kidney, breast, and prostate cancer, vitamin D showed activity against metastasis [136–141]. These studies have also shown the immunomodulatory effect of Vitamin D. It has been reported that when elicited by an inappropriate and overly exuberant immune response, vitamin D acts in a paracrine manner and decreases T cell responsiveness via inhibition of cellular proliferation and reduced lymphokine production. Thus, vitamin D shows a beneficial effect as an immunosuppressant.

5.7 Diabetes

Vitamin D deficiency is known to inhibit pancreatic secretion and turnover of insulin, causing impaired glucose tolerance. An association was found between a low level of vitamin D and a high incidence of type 1 diabetes [142].

5.8 Tuberculosis

Tuberculosis (TB) is one of the global health problems causing 2 million deaths a year. It is estimated that approximately one-third of the global population carries latent TB infection, which poses potential health risks of reactivation in the future. Before the use of antibiotics to treat TB, high doses of vitamin D were widely used [143]. Cross-sectional studies indicated that patients with TB possess a decrease 25(OH)D levels in comparison with the control population.

5.9 Thrombosis

As discussed in previous sections, vitamin D can tackle thrombosis by influencing inflammatory pathways, coagulation factors, and endothelium homeostasis in a pleiotropic manner. **Figure 2** illustrates a possible mechanism through which vitamin D might impart its protective role against the occurrence of thrombosis. Several clinical trials have also highlighted the anti-thrombotic actions of vitamin D. A study by TM Beer *et al.* involving 250 cancer patients for high dose calcitriol supplementation, a total of 13 thrombotic events were observed of which 11 occur placebo-treated and only 2 occur in high dose calcitriol-treated cancer patients [35]. Vitamin D has been found to inhibits *in-vitro* anti beta2GPI antibodies (purified from patients with antiphospholipid syndrome (APS)) induced TF expression indicating the association of vitamin D deficiency and decreased inhibition of TF expression and increased coagulation in APS [34]. M Blondon *et al.* investigated the role of oral supplementation of vitamin D3 in the placebo-controlled RCT in 36,282 postmenopausal women. Subjects were randomized to receive 1000 mg of calcium carbonate and 400 IU of vitamin D3 per day for an average period of 7 years and observed a reduced risk of idiopathic VTE in women randomized to calcium and vitamin D [144]. A 60% lower rate of VTE was observed in 769 renal transplant recipients after combined therapy with calcitriol 0.5ug/day, angiotensin-converting enzyme inhibitor (ACEi), and angiotensin receptor blocker (ARB) [145]. Another prospective study which included a cohort comprising of 40,000 women followed for a mean period of 11 years concluded a 30% lower risk of VTE in women with a habit of more active sun exposure [146]. Moreover, another study determined a 50% increased risk of VTE in winter, during which vitamin D status has been established to be the lowest as compared to another season [147].

5.10 COVID-19

The COVID-19 pandemic has affected all of us globally. The lack of understanding of the mechanism of action of SARS-CoV2 virus has generated an overall

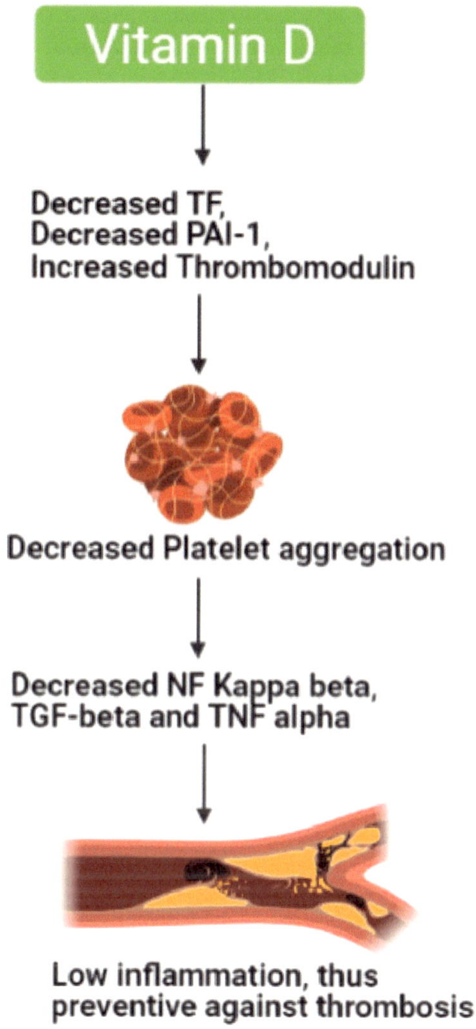

Figure 2.
Possible mechanism of the protective role of vitamin D in the occurrence of thrombosis.

interest in understanding the potential risk factors that may explain the mechanistic basis for disease propagation and control. The role of vitamin D has emerged in COVID-19 as well. The innate immune system forms the first line of defense against invading pathogens including viruses. 1,25(OH)2D enhances innate defense by inducing antimicrobial peptides like cathelicidin that result in the destruction and clearance of viral particles via several molecular mechanisms. It also helps in the recruitment of neutrophils, monocytes/macrophages, and dendritic cells for killing and clearance of viral particles, and initiation of the immune response. Further, the chronic activation of the innate immune system in COVID-19 infection results in a cytokine storm. It has been hypothesized that 1,25(OH)2D helps in curtailing this chronic innate immune response through various biological mechanisms such as downregulation of TLRs and direct inhibition of TNF/NFκB and IFNγ signaling pathways. 1,25(OH)2D, regulates adaptive immune response by limiting maturation of dendritic cells along with their ability to present antigen to T cells, thus limiting shifting of the T cell profile from proinflammatory Th1 and Th17 subsets to Th2 and Treg subsets. Thus, inhibits the pro-inflammatory processes. Although all these findings come from different studies with a variety of pathogens (virus/bacteria) the relevance of these protective actions of vitamin D on SARS-CoV-2 can merit further investigation [148]. In a recent study of hospitalized COVID-19 patients, vitamin D deficiency was reported in 75% of the overall cohort and in 85% of those who required ICU admission [149]. Also, a European study analysis of SARS-CoV-2 severity based on vitamin D status suggested that countries with the highest rate of vitamin D deficiency are associated with the highest rates of COVID-19 infection and mortality [150]. Therefore, vitamin D supplements as a part of standard nutrition in COVID-19 may provide certain clinical benefits though more research related to this subject is solicited [151].

6. Conclusion

Inadequacy or deficiency of vitamin D is a global problem. Though recent studies have established vitamin D as a key regulatory molecule in various physiological processes and have proposed it as a promising predictive/therapeutic tool still the close association of vitamin D with human health, and its deficiency in the body is not widely recognized as a health concern by both common man and physicians. The relation between vitamin D deficiency and the associated risk of various chronic and acute diseases is still obscure and requires intensive research efforts. In recent years, various studies have explored several non-calcemic consequences of vitamin D. There are reports that corelates lower doses of vitamin D with thrombosis and various cardiovascular diseases. Still, there is an impelling need to enhance our knowledge of the molecular pathways regulated/influenced via vitamin D and their effect on various organ systems including the cardiovascular system. This would require conducting large-scale intervention clinical trials to firmly establish the association of vitamin D status to cardiovascular health. Additionally, it is important to state that although deficiency of vitamin D is common and widespread, it can be safely corrected with a variety of supplement types and regimens available and thus should be identified and addressed in the clinical practice of treating diseases associated with it.

Conflict of interest

The authors declare no conflict of interest.

Author details

Syed Mohd[1†], Swati Sharma[1†], Aastha Mishra[2] and Mohammad Zahid Ashraf[1*]

1 Department of Biotechnology, Jamia Millia Islamia, Delhi, India

2 CSIR-Institute of Genomics and Integrative Biology, Delhi, India

*Address all correspondence to: zashraf@jmi.ac.in

† These authors have contributed equally to this work.

References

[1] Black LJ, Seamans KM, Cashman KD, Kiely M. An updated systematic review and meta-analysis of the efficacy of vitamin D food fortification. The Journal of nutrition. 2012 Jun 1;142(6):1102-8.

[2] Visser M, Deeg DJ, Lips P. Low vitamin D and high parathyroid hormone levels as determinants of loss of muscle strength and muscle mass (sarcopenia): the Longitudinal Aging Study Amsterdam. The Journal of Clinical Endocrinology & Metabolism. 2003 Dec 1;88(12):5766-72.

[3] Mangelsdorf DJ, Thummel C, Beato M, Herrlich P, Schütz G, Umesono K, Blumberg B, Kastner P, Mark M, Chambon P, Evans RM. The nuclear receptor superfamily: the second decade. Cell. 1995 Dec 15;83(6):835.

[4] Poon AH, Gong L, Brasch-Andersen C, Litonjua AA, Raby BA, Hamid Q, Laprise C, Weiss ST, Altman RB, Klein TE. Very important pharmacogene summary for VDR. Pharmacogenetics and genomics. 2012 Oct;22(10):758.

[5] Takeyama KI, Masuhiro Y, Fuse H, Endoh H, Murayama A, Kitanaka S, Suzawa M, Yanagisawa J, Kato S. Selective interaction of vitamin D receptor with transcriptional coactivators by a vitamin D analog. Molecular and Cellular Biology. 1999 Feb 1;19(2):1049-55.

[6] Targher G, Pichiri I, Lippi G. Vitamin D, thrombosis, and hemostasis: more than skin deep. InSeminars in thrombosis and hemostasis 2012 Feb (Vol. 38, No. 01, pp. 114-124). Thieme Medical Publishers.

[7] Ross AC, Manson JE, Abrams SA, Aloia JF, Brannon PM, Clinton SK, Durazo-Arvizu RA, Gallagher JC, Gallo RL, Jones G, Kovacs CS. The 2011 report on dietary reference intakes for calcium and vitamin D from the Institute of Medicine: what clinicians need to know. The Journal of Clinical Endocrinology & Metabolism. 2011 Jan 1;96(1):53-8.

[8] Holick MF. Resurrection of vitamin D deficiency and rickets. The Journal of clinical investigation. 2006 Aug 1;116(8):2062-72.

[9] Aaron JE, Stasiak L, Gallagher JC, Longton EB, Nicholson M, Anderson J, Nordin BE. Frequency of osteomalacia and osteoporosis in fractures of the proximal femur. The Lancet. 1974 Feb 16;303(7851):229-33.

[10] Khademvatani K, Seyyed-Mohammadzad MH, Akbari M, Rezaei Y, Eskandari R, Rostamzadeh A. The relationship between vitamin D status and idiopathic lower-extremity deep vein thrombosis. International journal of general medicine. 2014;7:303.

[11] Wu WX, He DR. Low vitamin D levels are associated with the development of deep venous thromboembolic events in patients with ischemic stroke. Clinical and applied thrombosis/hemostasis. 2018 Dec;24(9_suppl):69S–75S.

[12] Koyama T, Hirosawa S. Anticoagulant effects of synthetic retinoids and activated vitamin D3. In Seminars in thrombosis and hemostasis 1998 Jun (Vol. 24, No. 03, pp. 217-226). Copyright© 1998 by Thieme Medical Publishers, Inc..

[13] Koyama T, Shibakura M, Ohsawa M, Kamiyama R, Hirosawa S. Anticoagulant effects of 1α, 25-dihydroxyvitamin D3 on human myelogenous leukemia cells and monocytes. Blood, The Journal of the American Society of Hematology. 1998 Jul 1;92(1):160-7.

[14] Adorini L. Intervention in autoimmunity: the potential of vitamin D receptor agonists. Cellular immunology. 2005 Feb 1;233(2):115-24.

[15] Bhalla AK, Amento EP, Serog B, Glimcher LH. 1, 25-Dihydroxyvitamin D3 inhibits antigen-induced T cell activation. The Journal of Immunology. 1984 Oct 1;133(4):1748-54.

[16] Provvedini DM, Tsoukas CD, Deftos LJ, Manolagas SC. 1, 25-dihydroxyvitamin D3 receptors in human leukocytes. Science. 1983 Sep 16;221(4616):1181-3.

[17] Brennan A, Katz DR, Nunn JD, Barker S, Hewison M, Fraher LJ, O'Riordan JL. Dendritic cells from human tissues express receptors for the immunoregulatory vitamin D3 metabolite, dihydroxycholecalciferol. Immunology. 1987 Aug;61(4):457.

[18] Merke J, Milde P, Lewicka S, Hügel U, Klaus G, Mangelsdorf DJ, Haussler MR, Rauterberg EW, Ritz E. Identification and regulation of 1, 25-dihydroxyvitamin D3 receptor activity and biosynthesis of 1, 25-dihydroxyvitamin D3. Studies in cultured bovine aortic endothelial cells and human dermal capillaries. The Journal of clinical investigation. 1989 Jun 1;83(6):1903-15.

[19] Esmon CT. Basic mechanisms and pathogenesis of venous thrombosis. Blood reviews. 2009 Sep 1;23(5):225-9.

[20] Gupta N, Sahu A, Prabhakar A, Chatterjee T, Tyagi T, Kumari B, Khan N, Nair V, Bajaj N, Sharma M, Ashraf MZ. Activation of NLRP3 inflammasome complex potentiates venous thrombosis in response to hypoxia. Proceedings of the National Academy of Sciences. 2017 May 2;114(18):4763-8.

[21] Engelmann B, Massberg S. Thrombosis as an intravascular effector of innate immunity. Nature Reviews Immunology. 2013 Jan;13(1):34-45.

[22] Ertek S, Akgül E, Cicero AF, Kütük U, Demirtaş S, Çehreli S, Erdoğan G. 25-Hydroxy vitamin D levels and endothelial vasodilator function in normotensive women. Archives of medical science: AMS. 2012 Feb 29;8(1):47.

[23] Harris RA, Pedersen-White J, Guo DH, Stallmann-Jorgensen IS, Keeton D, Huang Y, Shah Y, Zhu H, Dong Y. Vitamin D3 supplementation for 16 weeks improves flow-mediated dilation in overweight African-American adults. American journal of hypertension. 2011 May 1;24(5):557-62.

[24] Schleithoff SS, Zittermann A, Tenderich G, Berthold HK, Stehle P, Koerfer R. Vitamin D supplementation improves cytokine profiles in patients with congestive heart failure: a double-blind, randomized, placebo-controlled trial. The American journal of clinical nutrition. 2006 Apr;83(4):754-9.

[25] Ohsawa M, Koyama T, Yamamoto K, Hirosawa S, Kamei S, Kamiyama R. 1α, 25-dihydroxyvitamin D3 and its potent synthetic analogs downregulate tissue factor and upregulate thrombomodulin expression in monocytic cells, counteracting the effects of tumor necrosis factor and oxidized LDL. Circulation. 2000 Dec 5;102(23):2867-72.

[26] Martinez-Moreno JM, Herencia C, Oca AM, Muñoz-Castañeda JR, Rodríguez-Ortiz ME, Díaz-Tocados JM, Peralbo-Santaella E, Camargo A, Canalejo A, Rodriguez M, Velasco-Gimena F. Vitamin D modulates tissue factor and protease-activated receptor 2 expression in vascular smooth muscle cells. The FASEB Journal. 2016 Mar;30(3):1367-76.

[27] Toderici M, de la Morena-Barrio ME, Padilla J, Miñano A,

Antón AI, Iniesta JA, Herranz MT, Fernández N, Vicente V, Corral J. Identification of regulatory mutations in SERPINC1 affecting vitamin D response elements associated with antithrombin deficiency. Plos one. 2016 Mar 22;11(3):e0152159.

[28] Holick MF. Vitamin D deficiency. New England Journal of Medicine. 2007 Jul 19;357(3):266-81.

[29] Anderson JL, May HT, Horne BD, Bair TL, Hall NL, Carlquist JF, Lappé DL, Muhlestein JB, Group IH. Relation of vitamin D deficiency to cardiovascular risk factors, disease status, and incident events in a general healthcare population. The American journal of cardiology. 2010 Oct 1;106(7):963-8.

[30] Vacek JL, Vanga SR, Good M, Lai SM, Lakkireddy D, Howard PA. Vitamin D deficiency and supplementation and relation to cardiovascular health. The American journal of cardiology. 2012 Feb 1;109(3):359-63.

[31] Kheiri B, Abdalla A, Osman M, Ahmed S, Hassan M, Bachuwa G. Vitamin D deficiency and risk of cardiovascular diseases: a narrative review. Clinical hypertension. 2018 Dec;24(1):1-9.

[32] Lee JH, O'Keefe JH, Bell D, Hensrud DD, Holick MF. Vitamin D deficiency: an important, common, and easily treatable cardiovascular risk factor?. Journal of the American College of Cardiology. 2008 Dec 9;52(24):1949-56.

[33] Pilz S, Tomaschitz A, März W, Drechsler C, Ritz E, Zittermann A, Cavalier E, Pieber TR, Lappe JM, Grant WB, Holick MF. Vitamin D, cardiovascular disease and mortality. Clinical endocrinology. 2011 Nov;75(5):575-84.

[34] Agmon-Levin N, Blank M, Zandman-Goddard G, Orbach H, Meroni PL, Tincani A, Doria A, Cervera R, Miesbach W, Stojanovich L, Barak V. Vitamin D: an instrumental factor in the anti-phospholipid syndrome by inhibition of tissue factor expression. Annals of the Rheumatic Diseases. 2011 Jan 1;70(1):145-50.

[35] Beer TM, Venner PM, Ryan CW, Petrylak DP, Chatta G, Dean Ruether J, Chi KN, Curd JG, DeLoughery TG. High dose calcitriol may reduce thrombosis in cancer patients. British journal of haematology. 2006 Nov;135(3):392-4.

[36] Koyama T, Hirosawa S. Anticoagulant effects of synthetic retinoids and activated vitamin D3. InSeminars in thrombosis and hemostasis 1998 Jun (Vol. 24, No. 03, pp. 217-226). Copyright© 1998 by Thieme Medical Publishers, Inc.

[37] Maillard CH, Berruyer MI, Serre CM, Amiral JE, Dechavanne MA, Delmas PD. Thrombomodulin is synthesized by osteoblasts, stimulated by 1, 25-(OH) 2D3 and activates protein C at their cell membrane. Endocrinology. 1993 Aug 1;133(2):668-74.

[38] Michel G, Gailis A, Jarzebska-Deussen B, Muüschen A, Mirmohammadsadegh A, Ruzicka T. 1, 25-(OH) 2-vitamin D 3 and calcipotriol induce IL-10 receptor gene expression in human epidermal cells. Inflammation Research. 1997 Jan;46(1):32-4.

[39] Nagpal S, Na S, Rathnachalam R. Noncalcemic actions of vitamin D receptor ligands. Endocrine reviews. 2005 Aug 1;26(5):662-87.

[40] Koyama T, Hirosawa S. Anticoagulant effects of synthetic retinoids and activated vitamin D3. InSeminars in thrombosis and hemostasis 1998 Jun (Vol. 24, No. 03,

pp. 217-226). Copyright© 1998 by Thieme Medical Publishers, Inc..

[41] Li YC, Kong J, Wei M, Chen ZF, Liu SQ, Cao LP. 1, 25-Dihydroxyvitamin D 3 is a negative endocrine regulator of the renin-angiotensin system. The Journal of clinical investigation. 2002 Jul 15;110(2):229-38.

[42] Sun J, Kong J, Duan Y, Szeto FL, Liao A, Madara JL, Li YC. Increased NF-κB activity in fibroblasts lacking the vitamin D receptor. American Journal of Physiology-Endocrinology and Metabolism. 2006 Aug;291(2):E315-22.

[43] Aihara KI, Azuma H, Akaike M, Ikeda Y, Yamashita M, Sudo T, Hayashi H, Yamada Y, Endoh F, Fujimura M, Yoshida T. Disruption of nuclear vitamin D receptor gene causes enhanced thrombogenicity in mice. Journal of Biological Chemistry. 2004 Aug 20;279(34):35798-802.

[44] Silvagno F, De Vivo E, Attanasio A, Gallo V, Mazzucco G, Pescarmona G. Mitochondrial localization of vitamin D receptor in human platelets and differentiated megakaryocytes. PLoS One. 2010 Jan 13;5(1):e8670.

[45] Hyppönen E, Berry D, Cortina-Borja M, Power C. 25-Hydroxyvitamin D and pre-clinical alterations in inflammatory and hemostatic markers: a cross sectional analysis in the 1958 British Birth Cohort. PloS one. 2010 May 24;5(5):e10801.

[46] Stewart GJ. Neutrophils and deep venous thrombosis. Pathophysiology of Haemostasis and Thrombosis. 1993;23(Suppl. 1):127-40.

[47] Pabinger I, Ay C. Biomarkers and venous thromboembolism. Arteriosclerosis, thrombosis, and vascular biology. 2009 Mar 1;29(3):332-6.

[48] Jorde R, Haug E, Figenschau Y, Hansen JB. Serum levels of vitamin D and haemostatic factors in healthy subjects: the Tromsø study. Acta haematologica. 2007;117(2):91-7.

[49] Vanhoutte PM. Endothelial dysfunction and atherosclerosis. European heart journal. 1997 Nov 1;18(suppl_E):19-29.

[50] Davignon J, Ganz P. Role of endothelial dysfunction in atherosclerosis. Circulation. 2004 Jun 15;109(23_suppl_1):III-27.

[51] Schuett H, Luchtefeld M, Grothusen C, Grote K, Schieffer B. How much is too much? Interleukin-6 and its signalling in atherosclerosis. Thrombosis and haemostasis. 2009;102(08):215-22.

[52] Pober JS, Sessa WC. Evolving functions of endothelial cells in inflammation. Nature Reviews Immunology. 2007 Oct;7(10):803-15.

[53] Dejana E, Tournier-Lasserve E, Weinstein BM. The control of vascular integrity by endothelial cell junctions: molecular basis and pathological implications. Developmental cell. 2009 Feb 17;16(2):209-21.

[54] Hadi HA, Carr CS, Al Suwaidi J. Endothelial dysfunction: cardiovascular risk factors, therapy, and outcome. Vascular health and risk management. 2005 Sep;1(3):183.

[55] Bombeli T, Mueller M, Haeberli A. Anticoagulant properties of the vascular endothelium. Thrombosis and haemostasis. 1997;77(03):408-23.

[56] Nawroth PP, Handley D, Stern DM. The multiple levels of endothelial cell-coagulation factor interactions. Clinics in haematology. 1986 May 1;15(2):293-321.

[57] Zehnder D, Bland R, Chana RS, Wheeler DC, Howie AJ, Williams MC, Stewart PM, Hewison M. Synthesis of 1, 25-dihydroxyvitamin D3 by human endothelial cells is regulated by inflammatory cytokines: a novel autocrine determinant of vascular cell adhesion. Journal of the American Society of Nephrology. 2002 Mar 1;13(3):621-9.

[58] Jablonski KL, Chonchol M, Pierce GL, Walker AE, Seals DR. 25-Hydroxyvitamin D deficiency is associated with inflammation-linked vascular endothelial dysfunction in middle-aged and older adults. Hypertension. 2011 Jan;57(1):63-9.

[59] Mitsuhashi T, Morris RC, Ives HE. 1, 25-dihydroxyvitamin D3 modulates growth of vascular smooth muscle cells. The Journal of clinical investigation. 1991 Jun 1;87(6):1889-95.

[60] Mantell DJ, Owens PE, Bundred NJ, Mawer EB, Canfield AE. 1α, 25-dihydroxyvitamin D3 inhibits angiogenesis in vitro and in vivo. Circulation research. 2000 Aug 4;87(3):214-20.

[61] Molinari C, Uberti F, Grossini E, Vacca G, Carda S, Invernizzi M, Cisari C. 1α, 25-dihydroxy cholecalciferol induces nitric oxide production in cultured endothelial cells. Cellular Physiology and Biochemistry. 2011;27(6):661-8.

[62] Andrukhova O, Slavic S, Zeitz U, Riesen SC, Heppelmann MS, Ambrisko TD, Markovic M, Kuebler WM, Erben RG. Vitamin D is a regulator of endothelial nitric oxide synthase and arterial stiffness in mice. Molecular Endocrinology. 2014 Jan 1;28(1):53-64.

[63] Tarcin O, Yavuz DG, Ozben B, Telli A, Ogunc AV, Yuksel M, Toprak A, Yazici D, Sancak S, Deyneli O, Akalin S. Effect of vitamin D deficiency and replacement on endothelial function in asymptomatic subjects. The Journal of Clinical endocrinology & metabolism. 2009 Oct 1;94(10):4023-30.

[64] Kamen DL, Oates J. A pilot randomized, controlled trial of vitamin D repletion to determine if endothelial function improves in patients with systemic lupus erythematosus. The American journal of the medical sciences. 2015 Oct;350(4):302.

[65] Carrara D, Bernini M, Bacca A, Rugani I, Duranti E, Virdis A, Ghiadoni L, Taddei S, Bernini G. Cholecalciferol administration blunts the systemic renin–angiotensin system in essential hypertensives with hypovitaminosis D. Journal of the Renin-Angiotensin-Aldosterone System. 2014 Mar;15(1):82-7.

[66] Chitalia N, Ismail T, Tooth L, Boa F, Hampson G, Goldsmith D, Kaski JC, Banerjee D. Impact of vitamin D supplementation on arterial vasomotion, stiffness and endothelial biomarkers in chronic kidney disease patients. PloS one. 2014 Mar 19;9(3):e91363.

[67] Dong Y, Stallmann-Jorgensen IS, Pollock NK, Harris RA, Keeton D, Huang Y, Li K, Bassali R, Guo DH, Thomas J, Pierce GL. A 16-week randomized clinical trial of 2000 international units daily vitamin D3 supplementation in black youth: 25-hydroxyvitamin D, adiposity, and arterial stiffness. The Journal of Clinical Endocrinology & Metabolism. 2010 Oct 1;95(10):4584-91.

[68] Carrara D, Bruno RM, Bacca A, Taddei S, Duranti E, Ghiadoni L, Bernini G. Cholecalciferol treatment downregulates renin–angiotensin system and improves endothelial function in essential hypertensive patients with hypovitaminosid D. Journal of hypertension. 2016 Nov 1;34(11):2199-205.

[69] Gibson CC, Davis CT, Zhu W, Bowman-Kirigin JA, Walker AE, Tai Z, Thomas KR, Donato AJ, Lesniewski LA, Li DY. Dietary vitamin D and its metabolites non-genomically stabilize the endothelium. PloS one. 2015 Oct 15;10(10):e0140370.

[70] Kanikarla-Marie P, Jain SK. 1, 25 (OH) 2D3 inhibits oxidative stress and monocyte adhesion by mediating the upregulation of GCLC and GSH in endothelial cells treated with acetoacetate (ketosis). The Journal of steroid biochemistry and molecular biology. 2016 May 1;159:94-101.

[71] Chen SF. 1 alpha, 25-Dihydroxyvitamin D3 decreased ICAM-1 and ELAM-1 expressions on pulmonary microvascular endothelial cells and neutrophil motivation. The Journal of steroid biochemistry and molecular biology. 1995 Jan 1;52(1):67-70.

[72] Rahman A, Fazal F. Blocking NF-κB: an inflammatory issue. Proceedings of the American Thoracic Society. 2011 Nov 1;8(6):497-503.

[73] Equils O, Naiki Y, Shapiro AM, Michelsen K, Lu D, Adams J, Jordan S. 1, 25-Dihydroxyvitamin D3 inhibits lipopolysaccharide-induced immune activation in human endothelial cells. Clinical & Experimental Immunology. 2006 Jan;143(1):58-64.

[74] Suzuki Y, Ichiyama T, Ohsaki A, Hasegawa S, Shiraishi M, Furukawa S. Anti-inflammatory effect of 1α, 25-dihydroxyvitamin D3 in human coronary arterial endothelial cells: Implication for the treatment of Kawasaki disease. The Journal of steroid biochemistry and molecular biology. 2009 Jan 1;113(1-2):134-8.

[75] Xu W, Hu X, Qi X, Zhu R, Li C, Zhu Y, Yin S, Cheng L, Zhu R. Vitamin D ameliorates angiotensin II-induced human endothelial progenitor cell injury via the PPAR-γ/HO-1 pathway. Journal of vascular research. 2019;56(1):17-27.

[76] Liang B, Wang X, Zhang N, Yang H, Bai R, Liu M, Bian Y, Xiao C, Yang Z. Angiotensin-(1-7) attenuates angiotensin II-induced ICAM-1, VCAM-1, and MCP-1 expression via the MAS receptor through suppression of P38 and NF-κB pathways in HUVECs. Cellular Physiology and Biochemistry. 2015;35(6):2472-82.

[77] Bozic M, Álvarez Á, de Pablo C, Sanchez-Niño MD, Ortiz A, Dolcet X, Encinas M, Fernandez E, Valdivielso JM. Impaired vitamin D signaling in endothelial cell leads to an enhanced leukocyte-endothelium interplay: implications for atherosclerosis development. PLoS One. 2015 Aug 31;10(8):e0136863.

[78] Autier P, Gandini S. Vitamin D supplementation and total mortality: a meta-analysis of randomized controlled trials. Archives of internal medicine. 2007 Sep 10;167(16):1730-7.

[79] Wang L, Manson JE, Song Y, Sesso HD. Systematic review: vitamin D and calcium supplementation in prevention of cardiovascular events. Annals of internal medicine. 2010 Mar 2;152(5):315-23.

[80] Hashemi SM, Mokhtari SM, Sadeghi M, Foroozan R, Safari M. Effect of vitamin D therapy on endothelial function in ischemic heart disease female patients with vitamin D deficiency or insufficiency: A primary report. ARYA atherosclerosis. 2015 Jan;11(1):54.

[81] Hammer Y, Soudry A, Levi A, Talmor-Barkan Y, Leshem-Lev D, Singer J, Kornowski R, Lev EI. Effect of vitamin D on endothelial progenitor cells function. PloS one. 2017 May 17;12(5):e0178057.

[82] Vila Cuenca M, Ferrantelli E, Meinster E, Pouw SM, Kovačević I, de Menezes RX, Niessen HW, Beelen RH, Hordijk PL, Vervloet MG. Vitamin D attenuates endothelial dysfunction in uremic rats and maintains human endothelial stability. Journal of the American Heart Association. 2018 Sep 4;7(17):e008776.

[83] Kirchhofer D, Tschopp TB, Hadvary P, Baumgartner HR. Endothelial cells stimulated with tumor necrosis factor-alpha express varying amounts of tissue factor resulting in inhomogenous fibrin deposition in a native blood flow system. Effects of thrombin inhibitors. The Journal of clinical investigation. 1994 May 1;93(5):2073-83.

[84] Yamamoto K, Shimokawa T, Kojima T, Loskutoff DJ, Saito H. Regulation of murine protein C gene expression in vivo: effects of tumor necrosis factor-α, interleukin-1, and transforming growth factor-β. Thrombosis and haemostasis. 1999;82(10):1297-301.

[85] van Hinsbergh VW. Endothelium—role in regulation of coagulation and inflammation. InSeminars in immunopathology 2012 Jan (Vol. 34, No. 1, pp. 93-106). Springer-Verlag.

[86] Eilertsen KE, Østerud B. Tissue factor:(patho) physiology and cellular biology. Blood coagulation & fibrinolysis. 2004 Oct 1;15(7):521-38.

[87] Darbousset R, Thomas GM, Mezouar S, Frere C, Bonier R, Mackman N, Renné T, Dignat-George F, Dubois C, Panicot-Dubois L. Tissue factor–positive neutrophils bind to injured endothelial wall and initiate thrombus formation. Blood, The Journal of the American Society of Hematology. 2012 Sep 6;120(10):2133-43.

[88] Hewison M. An update on vitamin D and human immunity. Clinical endocrinology. 2012 Mar;76(3):315-25.

[89] Holick MF, Chen TC. Vitamin D deficiency: a worldwide problem with health consequences. The American journal of clinical nutrition. 2008 Apr 1;87(4):1080S–6S.

[90] Veldman CM, Cantorna MT, DeLuca HF. Expression of 1, 25-dihydroxyvitamin D3 receptor in the immune system. Archives of biochemistry and biophysics. 2000 Feb 15;374(2):334-8.

[91] Mahon BD, Wittke A, Weaver V, Cantorna MT. The targets of vitamin D depend on the differentiation and activation status of CD4 positive T cells. Journal of cellular biochemistry. 2003 Aug 1;89(5):922-32.

[92] van Etten E, Mathieu C. Immunoregulation by 1, 25-dihydroxyvitamin D3: basic concepts. The Journal of steroid biochemistry and molecular biology. 2005 Oct 1;97(1-2):93-101.

[93] Adams JS, Hewison M. Unexpected actions of vitamin D: new perspectives on the regulation of innate and adaptive immunity. Nature clinical practice Endocrinology & metabolism. 2008 Feb;4(2):80-90.

[94] Dutta D, Mondal SA, Choudhuri S, Maisnam I, Reza AH, Bhattacharya B, Chowdhury S, Mukhopadhyay S. Vitamin-D supplementation in prediabetes reduced progression to type 2 diabetes and was associated with decreased insulin resistance and systemic inflammation: an open label randomized prospective study from Eastern India. Diabetes research and clinical practice. 2014 Mar 1;103(3):e18-23.

[95] Timms PM, Mannan N, Hitman GA, Noonan K, Mills PG, Syndercombe-Court D, Aganna E, Price CP, Boucher BJ. Circulating MMP9, vitamin D and variation in the TIMP-1 response with VDR genotype:

mechanisms for inflammatory damage in chronic disorders?. Qjm. 2002 Dec 1;95(12):787-96.

[96] Shab-Bidar S, Neyestani TR, Djazayery A, Eshraghian MR, Houshiarrad A, Kalayi A, Shariatzadeh N, Khalaji N, Gharavi AA. Improvement of vitamin D status resulted in amelioration of biomarkers of systemic inflammation in the subjects with type 2 diabetes. Diabetes/ metabolism research and reviews. 2012 Jul;28(5):424-30.

[97] Dobnig H, Pilz S, Scharnagl H, Renner W, Seelhorst U, Wellnitz B, Kinkeldei J, Boehm BO, Weihrauch G, Maerz W. Independent association of low serum 25-hydroxyvitamin D and 1, 25-dihydroxyvitamin D levels with all-cause and cardiovascular mortality. Archives of internal medicine. 2008 Jun 23;168(12):1340-9.

[98] Ponsonby AL, McMichael A, Van Der Mei I. Ultraviolet radiation and autoimmune disease: insights from epidemiological research. Toxicology. 2002 Dec 27;181:71-8.

[99] Staples JA, Ponsonby AL, Lim LL, McMichael AJ. Ecologic analysis of some immune-related disorders, including type 1 diabetes, in Australia: latitude, regional ultraviolet radiation, and disease prevalence. Environmental Health Perspectives. 2003 Apr;111(4):518-23.

[100] Boucher BJ. The problems of vitamin d insufficiency in older people. Aging and disease. 2012 Aug;3(4):313.

[101] Dudani SJ, Kalhan S, Sharma SP. Vitamin D and multiple sclerosis: Potential pathophysiological role and clinical implications. International Journal of Applied and Basic Medical Research. 2011 Jul;1(2):71.

[102] Akbas EM, Gungor A, Ozcicek A, Akbas N, Askin S, Polat M. Vitamin D and inflammation: evaluation with neutrophil-to-lymphocyte ratio and platelet-to-lymphocyte ratio. Archives of medical science: AMS. 2016 Aug 1;12(4):721.

[103] Amer M, Qayyum R. Relation between serum 25-hydroxyvitamin D and C-reactive protein in asymptomatic adults (from the continuous National Health and Nutrition Examination Survey 2001 to 2006). The American journal of cardiology. 2012 Jan 15;109(2):226-30.

[104] Laird E, McNulty H, Ward M, Hoey L, McSorley E, Wallace JM, Carson E, Molloy AM, Healy M, Casey MC, Cunningham C. Vitamin D deficiency is associated with inflammation in older Irish adults. The Journal of Clinical Endocrinology & Metabolism. 2014 May 1;99(5):1807-15.

[105] Bellia A, Garcovich C, D'Adamo M, Lombardo M, Tesauro M, Donadel G, Gentileschi P, Lauro D, Federici M, Lauro R, Sbraccia P. Serum 25-hydroxyvitamin D levels are inversely associated with systemic inflammation in severe obese subjects. Internal and emergency medicine. 2013 Feb;8(1):33-40.

[106] Jorde R, Sneve M, Torjesen PA, Figenschau Y, Gøransson LG, Omdal R. No effect of supplementation with cholecalciferol on cytokines and markers of inflammation in overweight and obese subjects. Cytokine. 2010 May 1;50(2):175-80.

[107] Ward KA, Das G, Roberts SA, Berry JL, Adams JE, Rawer R, Mughal MZ. A randomized, controlled trial of vitamin D supplementation upon musculoskeletal health in postmenarchal females. The Journal of Clinical Endocrinology & Metabolism. 2010 Oct 1;95(10):4643-51.

[108] Holick MF. Vitamin D: photobiology, metabolism of action,

and clinical applications. Primer on the Metabolic Bone Diseases. 1999.

[109] Feldman D, Malloy PJ, Gross C. Vitamin D: biology, action, and clinical implications. InOsteoporosis 2001 Jan 1 (pp. 257-303). Academic Press.

[110] DeLuca HF. Overview of general physiologic features and functions of vitamin D. The American journal of clinical nutrition. 2004 Dec 1;80(6):1689S–96S.

[111] Bouillon R, Carmeliet G, Verlinden L, van Etten E, Verstuyf A, Luderer HF, Lieben L, Mathieu C, Demay M. Vitamin D and human health: lessons from vitamin D receptor null mice. Endocrine reviews. 2008 Oct 1;29(6):726-76.

[112] Mussolino ME, Gillum RF. Low bone mineral density and mortality in men and women: the Third National Health and Nutrition Examination Survey linked mortality file. Annals of epidemiology. 2008 Nov 1;18(11):847-50.

[113] Suzuki T, Yoshida H. Low bone mineral density at femoral neck is a predictor of increased mortality in elderly Japanese women. Osteoporosis international. 2010 Jan;21(1):71-9.

[114] Bischoff-Ferrari HA, Willett WC, Wong JB, Giovannucci E, Dietrich T, Dawson-Hughes B. Fracture prevention with vitamin D supplementation: a meta-analysis of randomized controlled trials. Jama. 2005 May 11;293(18):2257-64.

[115] Nieves J, Cosman F, Herbert J, Shen V, Lindsay R. High prevalence of vitamin D deficiency and reduced bone mass in multiple sclerosis. Neurology. 1994 Sep 1;44(9):1687-.

[116] Plotnikoff GA, Quigley JM. Prevalence of severe hypovitaminosis D in patients with persistent, nonspecific musculoskeletal pain. InMayo clinic proceedings 2003 Dec 1 (Vol. 78, No. 12, pp. 1463-1470). Elsevier.

[117] Bischoff-Ferrari HA, Giovannucci E, Willett WC, Dietrich T, Dawson-Hughes B. Estimation of optimal serum concentrations of 25-hydroxyvitamin D for multiple health outcomes. The American journal of clinical nutrition. 2006 Jun 1;84(1):18-28.

[118] Broe KE, Chen TC, Weinberg J, Bischoff-Ferrari HA, Holick MF, Kiel DP. A higher dose of vitamin D reduces the risk of falls in nursing home residents: a randomized, multiple-dose study. Journal of the American Geriatrics Society. 2007 Feb;55(2):234-9.

[119] Carthy EP, Yamashita W, Hsu A, Ooi BS. 1, 25-Dihydroxyvitamin D3 and rat vascular smooth muscle cell growth. Hypertension. 1989 Jun;13(6_pt_2):954-9.

[120] Michos ED, Melamed ML. Vitamin D and cardiovascular disease risk. Current Opinion in Clinical Nutrition & Metabolic Care. 2008 Jan 1;11(1):7-12.

[121] Kuneš J, Tremblay J, Bellavance F, Hamet P. Influence of environmental temperature on the blood pressure of hypertensive patients in Montreal. American journal of hypertension. 1991 May 1;4(5_Pt_1):422-6.

[122] Krause R, Bühring M, Hopfenmüller W, Holick MF, Sharma AM. Ultraviolet B and blood pressure. Lancet (British edition). 1998;352(9129):709-10.

[123] McAlpine D, Compston A. McAlpine's multiple sclerosis. Elsevier Health Sciences; 2005.

[124] Gale CR, Martyn CN. Migrant studies in multiple sclerosis. Progress in

neurobiology. 1995 Nov 1;47(4-5):425-48.

[125] Acheson ED, Bachrach CA, Wright FM. Some comments on the relationship of the distribution of multiple sclerosis to latitude, solar radiation, and other variables. Acta Psychiatrica Scandinavica. 1960 Nov;35(S147):132-47.

[126] Norman Jr JE, Kurtzke JF, Beebe GW. Epidemiology of multiple sclerosis in US veterans: 2. Latitude, climate and the risk of multiple sclerosis. Journal of chronic diseases. 1983 Jan 1;36(8):551-9.

[127] Goldberg P. Multiple sclerosis: vitamin D and calcium as environmental determinants of prevalence: (A viewpoint) part 2. biochemical and genetic factors. International Journal of Environmental Studies. 1974 Jan 1;6(2-3):121-9.

[128] Acheson ED, Bachrach CA, Wright FM. Some comments on the relationship of the distribution of multiple sclerosis to latitude, solar radiation, and other variables. Acta Psychiatrica Scandinavica. 1960 Nov;35(S147):132-47.

[129] Sutherland JM, Tyrer JH, Eadie MJ. The prevalence of multiple sclerosis in Australia. Brain. 1962 Mar 1;85(1):149-64.

[130] VanAmerongen BM, Dijkstra CD, Lips P, Polman CH. Multiple sclerosis and vitamin D: an update. European journal of clinical nutrition. 2004 Aug;58(8):1095-109.

[131] Pierrot-Deseilligny C, Souberbielle JC. Vitamin D and multiple sclerosis: an update. Multiple sclerosis and related disorders. 2017 May 1;14:35-45.

[132] Ascherio A, Munger KL, Simon KC. Vitamin D and multiple sclerosis. The Lancet Neurology. 2010 Jun 1;9(6):599-612.

[133] Garland CF, Garland FC. Do sunlight and vitamin D reduce the likelihood of colon cancer?. International journal of epidemiology. 1980 Sep 1;9(3):227-31.

[134] Garland FC, Garland CF, Gorham ED, Young JF. Geographic variation in breast cancer mortality in the United States: a hypothesis involving exposure to solar radiation. Preventive medicine. 1990 Nov 1;19(6):614-22.

[135] LEFKOWITZ ES, Garland CF. Sunlight, vitamin D, and ovarian cancer mortality rates in US women. International journal of epidemiology. 1994 Dec 1;23(6):1133-6.

[136] Young MR, Halpin J, Hussain R, Lozano Y, Djordjevic A, Devata S, Matthews JP, Wright MA. Inhibition of tumor production of granulocyte-macrophage colony-stimulating factor by 1 alpha, 25-dihydroxyvitamin D3 reduces tumor motility and metastasis. Invasion & metastasis. 1993 Jan 1;13(4):169-77.

[137] Evans SR, Shchepotin EI, Young HE, Rochon JA, Uskokovic MI, Shchepotin IB. 1, 25-dihydroxyvitamin D3 synthetic analogs inhibit spontaneous metastases in a 1, 2-dimethylhydrazine-induced colon carcinogenesis model. International journal of oncology. 2000 Jun 1;16(6):1249-303.

[138] FUJIOKA T, HASEGAWA M, ISHIKURA K, MATSUSHITA Y, SATO M, TANJI S. Inhibition of tumor growth and angiogenesis by vitamin D3 agents in murine renal cell carcinoma. The Journal of urology. 1998 Jul;160(1):247-51. Sundaram S, Sea A, Feldman S, Strawbridge R, Hoopes PJ, Demidenko E, Binderup L, Gewirtz DA. The combination of a potent vitamin D3 analog, EB 1089, with ionizing radiation

reduces tumor growth and induces apoptosis of MCF-7 breast tumor xenografts in nude mice. Clinical Cancer Research. 2003 Jun 1;9(6):2350-6.

[139] Holick MF. Vitamin D: its role in cancer prevention and treatment. Progress in biophysics and molecular biology. 2006 Sep 1;92(1):49-59.

[140] Feskanich D, Ma J, Fuchs CS, Kirkner GJ, Hankinson SE, Hollis BW, Giovannucci EL. Plasma vitamin D metabolites and risk of colorectal cancer in women. Cancer Epidemiology and Prevention Biomarkers. 2004 Sep 1;13(9):1502-8.

[141] John EM, Schwartz GG, Dreon DM, Koo J. Vitamin D and breast cancer risk: the NHANES I epidemiologic follow-up study, 1971-1975 to 1992. Cancer Epidemiology and Prevention Biomarkers. 1999 May 1;8(5):399-406.

[142] Wild S, Roglic G, Green A, Sicree R, King H. Global prevalence of diabetes: estimates for the year 2000 and projections for 2030. Diabetes care. 2004 May 1;27(5):1047-53.

[143] Martineau AR, Honecker FU, Wilkinson RJ, Griffiths CJ. Vitamin D in the treatment of pulmonary tuberculosis. The Journal of steroid biochemistry and molecular biology. 2007 Mar 1;103(3-5):793-8.

[144] Blondon M, Rodabough RJ, Budrys N, Johnson KC, Berger JS, Shikany JM, Raiesdana A, Heckbert SR, Manson JE, LaCroix AZ, Siscovick D. The Effect of Calcium plus vitamin D supplementation on the risk of venous thromboembolism in the Women's Health Initiative Randomized Controlled Trial. Thrombosis and haemostasis. 2015 May;113(5):999.

[145] Moscarelli L, Zanazzi M, Bertoni E, Caroti L, Rosso G, Farsetti S, Annunziata F, Paudice N, Salvadori M. Renin angiotensin system blockade and activated vitamin D as a means of preventing deep vein thrombosis in renal transplant recipients. Clinical nephrology. 2011 May 1;75(5):440-50.

[146] Lindqvist PG, Epstein E, Olsson H. Does an active sun exposure habit lower the risk of venous thrombotic events? AD-lightful hypothesis. Journal of Thrombosis and Haemostasis. 2009 Apr;7(4):605-10.

[147] Brot C, Vestergaard P, Kolthoff N, Gram J, Hermann AP, Sørensen OH. Vitamin D status and its adequacy in healthy Danish perimenopausal women: relationships to dietary intake, sun exposure and serum parathyroid hormone. British Journal of Nutrition. 2001 Aug;86(S1):S97-103.

[148] Bilezikian JP, Bikle D, Hewison M, Lazaretti-Castro M, Formenti AM, Gupta A, Madhavan MV, Nair N, Babalyan V, Hutchings N, Napoli N. Mechanisms in endocrinology: vitamin D and COVID-19. European journal of endocrinology. 2020 Nov 1;183(5):R133-47.

[149] Lau FH, Majumder R, Torabi R, Saeg F, Hoffman R, Cirillo JD, Greiffenstein P. Vitamin D insufficiency is prevalent in severe COVID-19. MedRxiv. 2020 Jan 1.

[150] Lanham-New SA, Webb AR, Cashman KD, Buttriss JL, Fallowfield JL, Masud T, Hewison M, Mathers JC, Kiely M, Welch AA, Ward KA. Vitamin D and SARS-CoV-2 virus/COVID-19 disease. BMJ Nutrition, Prevention & Health. 2020;3(1):106.

[151] Aslan MT, Aslan İÖ, Özdemir Ö. Letter to the Editor: Is Vitamin D One of the Key Elements in COVID-19 Days? J Nutr Health Aging. 2020;24(9):1038-1039. doi: 10.1007/s12603-020-1413-5. PMID: 33155635; PMCID: PMC7597430.

Section 3

Vitamin D and Dental Medicine

Chapter 7

Vitamin D and Dentistry

Elif Gül Aydın and Öner Özdemir

Abstract

Vitamin D deficiency is a pandemic issue due to decreased vitamin D intake from food and lessened sunlight exposure. Attention is drawn to vitamin D and its role learned in notable clinical disorders such as diabetes, cardiovascular disease and cancers including oral ones. Vitamin D is also very effective along with minerals in the protection of oral health. Vitamin D helps maintain the calcium-phosphate balance and contributes to the shaping of the bone. It is reported that with sufficient vitamin D level, the onset and progression of caries in the tooth structure can be stopped, the formation of caries can be reduced and enamel loss can be prevented. Vitamin D also affects the disease and health conditions of the periodontium. Anti-inflammatory and immuno-modulatory functions have a role in the pathogenesis of periodontal disorders. It can reduce bone resorption and suppress the inflammatory outcome related to periodontal diseases by increasing mineral density. Vitamin D has been linked with tooth decay, gingivitis, and tooth loss. Vitamin D, in particular, as a promising oral health-protective agent, is said to lessen the incidence of caries and periodontitis.

Keywords: Vitamin D, periodontitis, gingivitis, caries

1. Introduction

Vitamin D deficiency (**VDD**) owing to significant sunlight decrease in today's conditions and the use of sunscreens that increase in both summer and winter months is considered as a pandemic issue [1–3]. The amount of vitamin D (**vitD**) intake from food is very low. This amount cannot meet the daily vitD requirement for both adults and children [1].

Some of the oldest phytoplankton in the world (species that have existed for more than 750 years) have been reported to produce vitD when exposed to sun exposure. Among the species existing in the world, all species containing vertebrae need the sun for their vitD production [1]. The definition of rickets, which showed devastating bone deformities in children lack of sunlight, was made by Sniadecki in 1822. After approximately 100 years later, The US government had arranged an organization to explain and provide recommendations to parents about the favorable effects of sunlight exposure in order to prevent this disease. In those years, fortification of milk by adding vitD has been found to be quite effective in preventing rickets in the USA. However, they continued to supplement vitD into milk that expired due to the shortage in milk supply after the Second World War in Great Britain. The reason for this, they thought that the vitD added to the milk had extended the shelf life of the milk. Subsequently, vitD supplementation was banned in dairy products in Europe as a result of increasing hypercalcemia cases in infants [1].

IntechOpen

It is recognized that vitD levels in serum begin to decrease with age. The reason for this is explained as the decline in endogenous vitD synthesis and the surge in the time spent indoors due to the limitation of physical activity [2, 4].

2. Sources of vitamin D

The key source of vitD is the sunlight, and the level of 25-hydroxy vitD (25 (OH) D) in serum varies depending on the seasonal change of sunlight. Fatty fish like salmon, mackerel and herring, and fats from fish, containing cod liver oil, are among the rare foods that naturally comprise vitD. Milk, some juice products, some bread, yogurts and cheeses are supplied with vitD in the US. Furthermore, commercially available multivitamin preparations contain varying amounts of vitD and are offered for daily use to individuals [1, 2].

3. Synthesis of vitamin D

One of the fat-soluble secosteroids recognized as vitD is in control of the increased absorption of phosphate, magnesium and calcium in the gut. In humans, vitD3 (defined as cholecalciferol) and vitD2 (named as ergocalciferol) are identified as the most significant elements in this group. There are two varied ways of obtaining vitD: dietary and non-dietary substance by exposure to sunlight [1, 4].

Ultraviolet (**UV**)- B rays regulate vitD synthesis. Initially, pro- vitD 3 is formed by converting cholesterol to 7- dehydrocholesterol in the intestinal epithelium by oxidation. Then, it is transformed into pro- vitD 3 and transferred to the skin and pre- vitD 3 is produced by UV rays at wavelengths of 270 to 300 nm. The pre- vitD 3 isomerizes to vitD 3 and cholecalciferol in the heat-dependent reaction. Activation of vitD 3 occurs by two hydroxylations and 1α, 25-dihydroxy vitD 3 (calcitriol, the biologically active type of vitD) is formed [5].

4. The effects of VDD on musculoseletal system

Vitamins are organic compounds that play a role in basic metabolic reactions in our body. Serious problems can occur in the deficiencies of vitamins, since the mechanisms of basic metabolic events will be disrupted.

The serum level required for vitD (25 (OH) D) to be identified as deficient is 50 nmol/L or 20 ng/mL. Concentrations of 25 (OH) D between 51 and 74 nmol/L or 21–29 ng/mL are considered insufficient, while levels of 80 nmol/L or 30 ng/mL are thought to be sufficient [1, 6]. It is presumed that children require the same doses as adults. It is stated that vitD toxicity will not occur until 25 (OH) D levels reach up to 375 nmol/L or 150 ng/mL [1, 4].

The most lately reported recommendations for vitD consumption are 200 IU/day for children and adults up to the age of 50, 400 IU/day for 50–70 years, and 600 IU/day afterward. The increase in recommendations with age is a clear reflection of the fact that the efficiency of this synthesis decreases with age, although cutaneous synthesis appears to happen in most individuals [4].

Vitamin D has a vital biological role in the human body and helps continue normal growth and mineralization of bone and other calcified tissues, including teeth [2]. Vitamin D deficiency will result in growth delay and the characteristic signs and symptoms of rickets in children. In adults, VDD will accelerate and aggravate both osteopenia and osteoporosis and amplify the risk of fractures of bones. Muscle weakness has long been thought to be related with VDD. Vitamin D receptor (VDR) s are available in skeletal muscle, and VDD has been linked with proximal muscle weakness, enhanced body sway, and an augmented risk of falling. Vitamin D deficiency can also end up with skeletal mineralization disorder [1].

Vitamin D and VDR have increasing importance in recent years as they produce an important role in calcium and phosphorus metabolism as well as homeostasis. Furthermore, attention is drawn to vitD and VDR's role learnt in notable clinical disorders such as diabetes, cardiovascular disease and cancer [5, 7].

5. The effect of vitamin D and VDR in oral cancer

Oral cancer is defined as malignant neoplasia that occurs in the lips or oral cavity. Oral squamous cell carcinomas (OSCC) are important types consisting of more than 90% of all oral cancers [8]. In recent years, OSCC has generally been observed at increasing rates around the world. Widespread studies on the main risk factors for the development of oral cancers indicate that alcohol consumption and tobacco use increase the risk of oral cancer by 80%. Oral infection due to human papilloma virus (HPV) is defined as another important risk factor for oral infection, pharyngeal and oral cancers [9]. Eliminating significant risk factors, even after diagnosis of oral cancer, can improve prognosis and reduce the risk of recurrence [5].

OSCC growth is a multi-step progress that affects vital cellular pathways implicated in tumor development and growth. Various exogenous and endogenous incitements have been shown to lead to multifaceted molecular changes that contribute to cancer development. The anti-neoplastic activity of vitD (calcitriol) has been demonstrated in in vitro and in vivo studies in a wide variety of cancer-associated defects, containing head and neck cancer, and particularly in OSCC [10]. Also, it has the capacity to affect cytostatic chemotherapy and augment apoptosis induction in OSCC cells. Examination of the association between serum vitD level and VDR seems appropriate to guide supportive therapy for patients with pre-cancerous lesions and OSCC [5]. Although the anticancer influences of vitD have been demonstrated by various in vitro and in vivo studies, new data suggests that these influences are controlled by some other elements. Further studies are needed to assess the effects of the vitD system (both ligand and receptor) on the growth of oral cancer and the potential benefits of improving VDD on tumor growth and progression [5].

6. Vitamin D relation of oral and dental health

A balanced and good diet is necessary and essential for maintaining general body health as well as improving oral health [6]. While the importance of vitamins in general health has been highly researched and developed, their relationship with oral and dental health has not been fully elucidated. Vitamins act as a catalyzer for basic metabolic events in the body that are essential for growth, development, energy, and cell maintenance [11].

Minerals such as magnesium, calcium, and phosphorus, the basic structural components of the tooth, should be taken in sufficient levels with the diet. These minerals play a role by interacting with vitamins in strengthening the tooth structure. Especially vitD is related with calcium, magnesium, and zinc [6]. Several possible mechanisms have been suggested to clarify the role of vitD in decreasing the risk of caries.

One of these mechanisms is the regulation of serum calcium, phosphate and parathyroid hormone, which are necessary for the formation, calcification, mineralization and protection of teeth. Calcium and phosphate homeostasis is necessary for the formation, calcification, mineralization and maintenance of oral bone and teeth, as well as bone and hard tissue. Enamel and dentin defects- hypoplasia have been linked with hypocalcemia and hypophosphatemia [2, 7].

Dental caries and VDD affect children around the world. In children who had a VDD, changes in both enamel and dentin are observed. Therefore, vitD has a significant role in the formation of oral hard tissue, comprising tooth enamel and dentin, and affects primary teeth development [2].

Vitamin D has a significant role in odontogenesis [2, 12]. The mechanism by which vitD excites the mineralization of tooth enamel involves binding to VDR expressed in both tooth and bone cells. Vitamin D receptors direct the transcription of several target genes, most expressed by ameloblasts and odontoblasts [2, 7, 13]. VDR stimulates the formation of structural gene products in dentin, together with calcium-binding proteins and diverse extracellular matrix proteins. The gene encoding VDR is positioned on chromosome 12q13.11 and comprising several polymorphisms [14]. The VDR gene adjusts the biological role of major vitD metabolites, thus having a key role in the configuration of teeth, particularly in the mineralization of dentin and enamel. Consequently, enamel developmental deficiencies e.g., enamel hypoplasia, can take place in consequence of VDD. It was decided that vitD and VDR at the molecular level influence the tooth germ formation; supplies to the regulation of enamel and dentin structure and maturation; and organizes the phases of dental crown growth [2, 6].

Moreover, vitD adjusts and adapts both the innate and adaptive immune system. The immunological role of vitD is stimulation of the arrangement of some antimicrobial peptides, e.g. defensins and cathelicidin (LL-37), which defend against many pathogens, counting oral bacteria [2, 15]. Cathelicidin (LL-37 or hCAP-18) is controlled by vitD, which has both anti-endotoxin and antimicrobial properties [3].

In mineral deficiencies due to absorption disorders, increased tendency to bleeding, bone resorption, and early tooth loss occur [6]. The chewing process ensures that the person receives the highest possible amount of nutrients, and the number and distribution of teeth affect chewing efficiency. Since diet selection and nutritional status are affected in early tooth loss, deficiency occurs in the intake of vitamins, that is, the two situations create a synergistic effect on each other. During the development of the tooth, the hard tissues of the tooth are strongly affected by nutritional status and thus vitamin deficiency. It is stated that there is a positive correlation between malnutrition and enamel hypoplasia and caries in the primary dentition period in children [11]. In addition, deficiencies of these minerals cause delayed tooth eruption, bleeding gums, destruction patterns in alveolar bone, periodontal disease, enamel or dentin hypoplasia [6, 11].

Vitamin D is also very effective along with minerals in the protection of oral health. Vitamin D helps maintain the calcium-phosphate balance and contributes to the shaping of the bone. It also has important functions by showing anti-inflammatory effects. It is reported that with sufficient vitD level, the onset and progression of caries in the tooth structure can be stopped, the formation of caries can be reduced and enamel loss can be prevented [2, 6, 16].

In the formation of tooth decay, the acid that is produced by bacterial fermentation of the residues on the tooth surface that are not brushed after eating sugary foods lowers the pH below 7 and plays a role in the destruction of the tooth hard tissues. However, it has been recently revealed that dental caries can be reduced with UV- B rays and vitD supplements. Considering the helpful effects of vitD on dental caries, it is thought to be effective in reducing the overall prevalence, especially in children at risk of early caries [2, 6]. Early childhood caries (**ECC**) were described as the presence of one or more caries, missing (due to caries) or filled (DMFT: decay, missing, filled) tooth surface in any primary teeth in young children under six years old, is one of the most common chronic diseases and can have adverse effect on individual's overall health [2, 17].

Early childhood caries affect the nutritional status and general health of the child. It is stated that children with ECC may have malnutrition, iron deficiency anemia and VDD [2, 16]. When the relationship between vitD intake and caries is evaluated, it is determined that the incidence of tooth decay is higher in children with low vitD or children of mothers with low vitD during pregnancy. There is an association between vitD levels in early childhood (up to 8 years old) and DMFT scores. When serum vitD concentrations are more than 50 nmol in early adolescents (10–11 years) considerably less caries is detected in permanent first molars has been found. Similarly, in children aged 6 to 17 years, they found a 0.66 decrease in DMFT for every 10 ng/ml of serum vitD level increase. In general, malnutrition and shortage in vitamin intake due to malnutrition augments the incidence of enamel hypoplasia in children [2, 11, 18].

Vitamin D use may have a role in the protection of caries early in life. It is thought to be a promising caries prevention agent, given that vitD supplementation is connected with a 47% reduction in caries in children according to meta-analysis studies [16]. Vitamin D deficiency during pregnancy (a vital period for tooth growth) is related with developmental defects; especially enamel hypoplasia and caries susceptibility. Also, vitD intake during pregnancy diminishes the risk of enamel defects and hypoplasia in babies and is associated with better eruption of deciduous teeth [2, 11].

Improving vitD levels in children from an early stage of life appears to be an important task. This requires awareness from pregnancy. Pregnant women should have their vitD levels tested routinely during the first trimester of pregnancy and the risk of VDD, VDD and vitD ingestion should be evaluated. Prenatal vitD levels appear to influence the development of primary dentition and ECC [2, 11, 18].

Vitamin D is an essential hormone for the absorption of calcium, magnesium and phosphorus from the intestine, which is necessary for the appropriate mineralization of bones and teeth. In addition, covering the surfaces of the implants with vitD during implant application, which is one of the dental procedures, increases osteointegration. Moreover, applying vitD3 intraperitoneally speeds up orthodontic tooth movement, and even patients receiving vitD and bisphosphonate therapy can obtain orthodontic treatment [6].

7. Vitamin D and periodontal health

Vitamin D also affects the disease and health conditions of the periodontium. Anti-inflammatory and immunomodulatory functions have a role in the pathogenesis of periodontal disorders [3]. It can reduce bone resorption and suppress the inflammatory outcome related to periodontal diseases by increasing mineral density [6, 11].

There is a positive correlation between increased mineral density and decreased bone resorption in the mandibular bone and taking vitD and calcium and magnesium supplements. It is also reported that loss of attachment level is associated with decreased serum vitD levels. It is stated that in individuals with sufficient vitD, periodontal tissues are healthier, and accordingly, gingivitis formation, bleeding during probing, attachment, bone and tooth loss are reduced [11].

In studies conducted on women's level of vitD in their saliva and serum, a statistically significant relationship was found between gingivitis and periodontitis during their life, pregnancy, menopause and postmenopausal periods [19, 20]. The prevalence of periodontal disease was higher in individuals with low vitD levels [11].

Besides these beneficial effects on bone metabolism, it has been found that periodontitis accelerates the healing with its direct antibiotic effect on periodontal pathogens. Vitamin D reduces inflammatory mediators causing periodontal destruction. Having a diet rich in vitD after periodontal surgical procedures contributes to the faster and easier recovery of periodontal tissues. The quality of the host immune response is highly correlated with healthy and proper nutrition. It plays an important role not only in the prevention of periodontal diseases, but also in facilitating the recovery of tissues in the existing periodontal disease conditions. One of the most important functions of vitD in the immune system is that it has a stimulating effect on human cathelicidin (LL-37). LL-37 has both antimicrobial and anti-endotoxin functions. Vitamin D excites cathelicidin in oral epithelial cells and children with high dental caries activity had low LL-37 levels. Many epithelial antimicrobial peptides, including LL-37, have been termed the guardian of the oral cavity and detected to play important roles in oral health. LL-37 also has significant benefits in decreasing the risk of gingivitis. Maternal VDD also increases the DMFT score in children of 12–35 months old. As a result, vitD may be useful in the treatment of periodontitis due to its direct effects on bone metabolism and potential anti-inflammatory effects on periodonto-pathogens [6, 15].

As diet plays a dominant modifier in the development of periodontal disorders, dentists should inform patients on how good diet influences the supporting the formation of teeth, e.g. the significance of ingesting healthy foods rich in magnesium and vitD in thwarting dental caries [6].

There is common agreement on the effects of vitamin deficiencies or supplementation on oral health, but scientific data is still at a level that needs to be investigated. In particular, multivitamin supplements or the mixture of two or more vitamins lead to more bias as it is not likely to determine the single help of each vitamin.

8. Conclusion

Vitamin D has been linked with tooth decay, gingivitis, and tooth loss. Vitamin D, in particular, as a promising oral health-protective agent, is said to lessen the incidence of caries and periodontitis, leading to a low-precision result. In order to prevent tooth decay, which is a serious public health problem, existing structural defects in teeth (enamel and dentin hypoplasias) and to maintain oral health, the awareness of health care providers should be increased. It seems to be an issue that should not be overlooked, especially from the early stages of life, to control vitD levels for oral health.

Author details

Elif Gül Aydın[1]* and Öner Özdemir[2]

1 Department of Pediatric Dentistry, Faculty of Dentistry, Sakarya University, Adapazari/Sakarya, Turkey

2 Department of Pediatrics, Division of Allergy and Immunology, Sakarya University, Faculty of Medicine, Training and Research Hospital, Adapazari/Sakarya, Turkey

*Address all correspondence to: elifgul36@hotmail.com

References

[1] HOLICK, Michael F.; CHEN, Tai C. Vitamin D deficiency: a worldwide problem with health consequences. The American journal of clinical nutrition, 2008, 87 (4):1080-1086

[2] ALMOUDI, Manal Mohamed, et al. Dental caries and vitamin D status in children in Asia. Pediatrics International, 2019, 61 (4): 327-338.

[3] MOLLOY, E. J.; MURPHY, N. Vitamin D, Covid-19 and children. Ir Med J, 2020, 113 (4): 64

[4] HEANEY, Robert P. Vitamin D in health and disease. Clinical Journal of the American Society of Nephrology, 2008, 3 (5): 1535-1541

[5] FATHI, Nazanin, et al. Role of vitamin D and vitamin D receptor (VDR) in oral cancer. Biomedicine & Pharmacotherapy, 2019, 109: 391-401

[6] UWITONZE, Anne Marie, et al. Oral manifestations of magnesium and vitamin D inadequacy. The Journal of steroid biochemistry and molecular biology, 2020, 200: 105636.

[7] FATTURI, Aluhê Lopes, et al. The relationship between molar incisor hypomineralization, dental caries, socioeconomic factors, and polymorphisms in the vitamin D receptor gene: a population-based study. Clinical oral investigations, 2020, 24 (11): 3971-3980

[8] Gandini S, Gnagnarella P, Serrano D, Pasquali E, Raimondi S. Vitamin D receptor polymorphisms and cancer. Adv Exp Med Biol. 2014;810:69-105

[9] CHATURVEDI, Anil K. Epidemiology and clinical aspects of HPV in head and neck cancers. Head and neck pathology, 2012, 6 (1): 16-24.

[10] GRIMM, Martin, et al. Serum vitamin D levels of patients with oral squamous cell carcinoma (OSCC) and expression of vitamin D receptor in oral precancerous lesions and OSCC. *Medicina oral, patologia oral y cirugia bucal*, 2015, 20 (2): 188-195.

[11] CAGETTI, Maria Grazia, et al. The role of vitamins in oral health. A systematic review and meta-analysis. International journal of environmental research and public health, 2020, 17 (3): 938.

[12] ZHANG, Xueming, et al. Regulation of enamel and dentin mineralization by vitamin D receptor. In: *Comparative Dental Morphology*. Karger Publishers, 2009. p. 102-109.

[13] BERDAL, A., et al. Ameloblasts and odontoblasts, target-cells for 1, 25-dihydroxyvitamin D3: a review. International Journal of Developmental Biology, 2003, 39 (1): 257-262.

[14] HOLLA, Lydie Izakovicova, et al. Vitamin D receptor TaqI gene polymorphism and dental caries in Czech children. Caries research, 2017, 51 (1): 7-11.

[15] GYLL, Johanna, et al. Vitamin D status and dental caries in healthy Swedish children. Nutrition journal, 2018, 17 (1): 1-10.

[16] HUJOEL, Philippe P. Vitamin D and dental caries in controlled clinical trials: systematic review and meta-analysis. Nutrition reviews, 2013, 71 (2): 88-97.

[17] Pitts NB, Baez RJ, Diaz-Guillory C, Donly KJ, Alberto Feldens C, McGrath C, Phantumvanit P, Seow WK, Sharkov N, Songpaisan Y, Tinanoff N, Twetman S. Early Childhood Caries: IAPD Bangkok Declaration. J Dent Child (Chic). 2019;86(2):72.

[18] SINGLETON, R., et al. Association of maternal vitamin D deficiency with

early childhood caries. Journal of dental research, 2019, 98 (5): 549-555.

[19] WOELBER, Johan Peter, et al. An oral health optimized diet can reduce gingival and periodontal inflammation in humans-a randomized controlled pilot study. BMC oral health, 2017, 17 (1): 1-8.

[20] MILLEN, Amy E., et al. Vitamin D status and 5-year changes in periodontal disease measures among postmenopausal women: the Buffalo OsteoPerio Study. Journal of periodontology, 2014, 85 (10): 1321-1332.

Chapter 8

The Importance of Vitamin D for Periodontal Tissues

Egle Jagelaviciene

Abstract

There are many causes of vitamin D deficiency, which determines pathogenesis of many diseases, including periodontal ones. Constant low uptake or deficiency of vitamin D results in progression of periodontal diseases and jaw bone metabolism - leads to change of bone mineral density, causes resorption in alveolar bone, tooth loss, changes of masticatory function and osteoporosis. The clinical studies strive to link vitamin D with gingivitis and periodontitis and prove its therapeutic and preventive role, because of vitamin D immunomodulatory, anti-inflammatory and antiproliferative effects for periodontal tissues and best treatment outcome. The purpose of this chapter is to analyze the importance of vitamin D on the pathogenesis of periodontal diseases, its role on regulation of the immune system and defense mechanism, influence on jawbone quality and on the correlation between vitamin D concentration in plasma and periodontal diseases.

Keywords: vitamin D, vitamin D deficiency, periodontal disease, jawbone, bone mineral density

1. Introduction

One billion people on the planet were diagnosed with vitamin D deficiency during the last decade [1]. Opinion, advocating important role of vitamin D and its deficiency in significant number of individuals, prevails within the society, a lot of information is available regarding its use, doses, sources, etc. However, each individual may have different vitamin D needs and the consumption of it should be monitored by testing individual serum levels of D_2 (of alimentary origin) and D_3 (synthesized in the skin), thus evaluating total level of vitamin D [2]. There are many causes of vitamin D deficiency, which is finally diagnosed if serum level of $25OHD_3$ is less than 20 ng/mL [3, 4]. This determines pathogenesis of many diseases, including periodontal ones, resulting in loss of masticatory function.

Periodontium (PT) consists of gingiva, periodontal ligament, cementum and alveolar bone. This is functional unit, maintaining homeostasis – the connection between tooth and gingiva makes up a unified whole, preventing penetration of microorganisms, chemical substances, capable to induce inflammation of periodontal tissues (PTs). The periodontal ligament and bone keep tooth inside the alveolar socket, distribute mechanical load of mastication. PT has its own blood supply, neural regulation and defensive mechanisms. Soft and mineralized dental plaque is initiative risk factor of periodontal diseases (PD) – bacterial biofilm and its adhesion to tooth surface induces response of PTs, but in general, diseases are caused by many predisposing factors. PD initially manifest as gingivitis, which, if untreated, spreads deeper within PT: causing attachment loss, periodontal pocket formation, alveolar bone resorption and tooth loss over time [5, 6]. Increasing number of studies proves importance of vitamin D in prevention and management of oral diseases [7]. Clinical studies strive to link vitamin D with PD and prove its therapeutic and preventive role. Vitamin D is secosteroidal hormone, playing important role in the treatment of gingivitis and periodontitis because of its anti-inflammatory and antibacterial effect on PTs as well as its immunomodulatory, differentiating, anti-proliferative and regulative effect on autoimmune processes, cellular apoptosis and participation in bone metabolism [3, 7–10]. Disintegration and renewal processes of bone depend on metabolism, as constant interchange of mineral substances between bone and blood plasma, where an active form of vitamin D is circulating, takes place [11]. One of the main functions of vitamin D is maintaining of blood levels of calcium and phosphorus by regulating absorption of these substances inside the bowels and reabsorption in kidneys and by enhancing remodeling processes [12, 13]. Bone is like a living and continuously changing organ where resorption and regeneration, i.e. remodelation, take place [14]. For this reason, the old bone is not accumulating and adaptation to changing mechanical forces develops. Jawbone support the teeth in alveolar sockets, skeletal bones protect internal organs and acts as depot of mineral substances especially calcium (also is necessary for normal muscle function) [15]. Osteoporotic (OP) changes of skeletal bones occur because of impaired mineralization due to long term decreased uptake of vitamin D and calcium, increasing risk of fractures, accelerated jawbone resorption causes adentia [16, 17].

2. Vitamin D metabolism

There are 4 forms of vitamin D (calciferol) – lamisterol (vit. D_1), ergocalciferol (vit. D_2), cholecalciferol (vit. D_3) and dihydrotachysterol (vit. D_4), 2 of which being the most important – D_2 and D_3. Under the influence of UV radiation, ergosterol (plant based) and cholesterol (synthetized from 7-dehydrocholesterol of animal origin) are transformed into vitamin D_2 and D_3 respectively [1, 18]. Major part of vitamin D, around 90%, is synthesized in epidermis under the effect of the sun, while the rest is absorbed in small intestine together with food, nowadays being enriched with vitamin D with increasing frequency [19, 20]. Hydroxylation of vitamin D is a two-stage process, taking place in liver and kidneys. Thus renal and liver diseases impair metabolism of vitamin D. Enzyme 25-hydroxylase transforms vitamin D_3 into 25-hydroxyvitamin D_3 25(OH)D_3 in liver, which is the main metabolite of vitamin D_3, circulating in blood [21]. Recently it was proved that when inflammation occurs gingival fibroblasts and periodontal cells are capable of producing 25-hydroxylase and it appears to be a new extrahepatic site of 25(OH)D_3 synthesis [21]. Further, 25-hydroxyvitamin D_3 is hydroxylated in kidneys by means of 1 α-hydroxylase into 1,25-dihydroxyvitamin D (1,25$(OH)_2D_3$), calcitriol, active form of vitamin D, which is active hormone, participating in calcium absorption in intestines, important for both specific and nonspecific immune response against bacterial infections of oral cavity and other organs [2, 7, 21, 22]. Calcitriol binds to vitamin D-binding protein (DBP) and is transported to the cells of target tissues [23]. Synthesis of 1α-hydroxylase starts after receptors of cellular membranes have been influenced by microorganisms. Calcitriol is activated after binding to vitamin D receptors (VDR) of nuclei of immune and epithelial cells [7, 23–25]. VDR can be found in many human tissues, regulating activity of more than 200 genes in direct or indirect way [26, 27]. Numerous distribution of VDR in tissues determines complex effect of vitamin D, whereas deficiency determines disorders [26–28]. Polymorphism of VDR gene is related to many infectious diseases, including PD

[28–30]. Polymorphism of VDR gene and exact mechanism of periodontitis remain unclear so far. There is no link established between polymorphism of VDR genes and aggressive form of periodontitis [31, 32].

3. The role of vitamin D in immune response of periodontal tissues

Marginal gingival epithelium (GE) descends from free inner margin towards root apex and transits to sulcular epithelium – semi permeable membrane. Sulcular epithelium attaches to tooth by means of loose connections, creating favorable conditions for bacterial invasion from dental plaque [33]. Thin and non-keratinized epithelium forms a junctional epithelium (JE), laying at the bottom of gingival sulcus. JE is a narrow structure of 1–2 mm with good regenerative properties, connected to tooth by layer of organic substance. Its cubic and flat cells have gaps and attach to tooth and with each other by means of hemidesmosoms and have 2 basal membranes: internal, near the tooth, and the outer one on the other side, contacting with subepithelial tissue. Disruption of the bonds between enamel cuticle and JE leads to inflammatory processes. This anatomical unit plays a barrier function, which is supported by gingival fluid, flushing gingival sulcus – blood filtrate, containing lots of various protective cells (neutrophilic leucocytes, lymphocytes, monocytes, and macrophages), specific antibodies, immunoglobulins, cytokines, proteins, enzymes, epithelial cells and bacteria. The amount of gingival fluid can change due to circadian rhythms and depends on the health of PTs, oral hygiene, mechanic impact while mastication, medications used, etc. [34, 35]. Plasma proteins strengthen junctional epithelium-enamel bonds and namely calcitriol, affecting nonspecific immunity, activates synthesis of proteins, necessary for small adherens, gap and desmosome epithelium intercellular junctions, activates hydrogen peroxide secretion in monocytes, stimulates the synthesis of antimicrobial peptides, chemotaxis, production of cytokines and chemokines, cellular reproduction, vascular permeability, wound healing, and neutralization of bacterial endotoxins [7, 25, 36]. Hence 1,25(OH)2D_3 enhances antibacterial defense of GE [25, 36, 37].

Immune response can be nonspecific and specific. After bacteria have entered the periodontal tissues, defensive mechanism starts – immune response, during which the foreign substance is neutralized and eliminated or memorized. Neutrophilic leucocytes play important role in nonspecific immune response. It is interesting, that these cells are always found in gingival sulcus and this is the only site in organism, where neutrophilic leucocytes can freely migrate from organism outwards. During the bacterial invasion into PTs, chemotactic mechanisms are activated and neutrophilic leucocytes start migrating from blood vessels into inflamed tissues. Right here, together with macrophages, they take part in phagocytosis, thus fighting with different antigens. Neutrophilic leucocytes, monocytes and activated macrophages produce immune mediators (IL-1β, IL-1ra, IL-6, IL-10, IL-12, TNF-α, PGE2, MMP, Interferon γ (IFNγ)) and chemokines [37]. Vitamin D protects the organism from excessive immune response by decreasing the secretion of IL-1, IL-6, IL-8, IL-12, TNF-α cytokines, decreases production of matrix metalloproteinase (MMP) in leucocytes [33, 38]. MMP – enzymes, participating in alterations of intercellular tissues. Blood plasma levels of MMP-3, MMP-8 and MMP-9 increase with PD [39]. Very high level of MMP-9 is detected in cases of rapidly progressing periodontitis, but it can decrease up to 69% taking even little doses of vitamin D for extended period of time [40, 41].

Blood monocytes, after migration into connective tissues, transform into macrophages, which are very important for both, cellular and humoral immunity, as they have surface receptors, reacting with any foreign substance [42]. In the process of phagocytosis, immunoglobulins and serum complement envelope foreign substance. Such formation enters phagocytic vacuoles and is destroyed by lysosome enzymes. Afterwards these substances are transferred to lymphocytes, determining further immune response [42]. Products of tissue breakdown, histamine and complement system enhances phagocytosis. Specific immune response manifests later. Antibodies circulate in blood, T and B lymphocytes react only to specific antigen. Lymphocytes are often related to Langerhans cells of oral epithelium, producing cytokines, e.g., IL-1, activating T lymphocytes, enhancing proliferation and production of antibodies. Active T lymphocytes have cytotoxic effect. Keratinocytes of oral epithelium produce IL-1 and IL-8, regulating the amount of lymphocytes and polymorphonuclear leucocytes [42]. Impaired specific immunity is responsible for resorption, osteoclast genesis and inflammatory processes of bone, thus causing autoimmune diseases. Calcitriol suppresses progression of OP and PD with signs of autoimmune diseases.

Active hormonal form of vitamin D, $1,25(OH)_2D_3$, directly regulates antimicrobial immune response, modulates cytokine production and stimulates secretion of antimicrobial peptides by monocytes-macrophages and activates release of hydrogen peroxide in monocytes, thus exhibiting anti-inflammatory and antimicrobial properties [7, 43, 44]. Monocytes not only produce cytokines, but TNF-α as well, they release substances, activating lymphocytes and interacting with them as antigen-presenting cell (APC), destroy PTs, accelerate proliferation, differentiation and activation of osteoclasts, move in tissues in chemotactic way and participate in phagocytosis. Antimicrobial peptides play important role in nonspecific immunity against periodontitis causing agents. Antimicrobial peptides, β-defensines and especially cathelicidine LL-37 take part in neutralization of bacterial endotoxins, healing of wounds, regulate cell multiplication, blood vessel permeability, cytokine and chemokine production and chemotaxis, have prolonged antimicrobial activity and neutralize lipopolysaccharides as well [3, 7, 23, 25, 45, 46]. Activity of defensines depends on vitamin D levels [45, 46]. β-defensines show antimicrobial activity on PD bacteria– *Actinobacilus actinomycetemcomitans, Porphyromonas gingivalis, Fusobacterium nucleatum, Candida* and papilloma viruses [47]. APCs, including macrophages and dendritic cells, transform the main $25(OH)D_3$ form circulating in blood into active $1,25(OH)_2D_3$, and, via VDR, induce cellular response and regulate transcription. Antimicrobial activity via VDR is associated with cathelicidine hCAP-18 gene [48]. Cathelicidine has wide antimicrobial activity against gram-positive and gram-negative bacteria, some fungi and viruses [3]. Treatment with vitamin D increases cathelicidine mRNA level in keratinocytes, neutrophils and macrophages [3, 44]. Irritation of macrophage receptors with pathogens increases synthesis of $1,25(OH)_2D_3$, activity in macrophages and production of antibacterial proteins, cathelicidine and β-defensines, increases [43]. Therefore, it is supposed that vitamin D deficiency determines weak antibacterial response and tendency to infections [49].

During specific immune response, $1,25(OH)_2D_3$ affects B and T lymphocytes [7]. The latter release cytokines (interleukine-1, TNF-α, macrophage activating factor, macrophage migration inhibitory factor), stimulating resorption of dental supportive tissues (due to increased number of osteoclasts) and decay of extracellular matrix; release immunoglobulins; destroy pathogens, transferred by macrophages and dendritic cells and participate in production of antibodies. Such immune response mechanism enhances pathogenesis of PTs and aggravates the course of disease [16, 21, 33]. $1,25(OH)_2D_3$ suppresses proliferation, maturation and differentiation of dendritic cells [50]. T lymphocytes are one of the dominating cells in the beginning of PTs pathologic process and its regulator; immature dendritic cells stimulate their tolerance, whereas mature dendritic cells activate them [51]. $1,25(OH)_2D_3$ decreases the number of APCs and ability of T lymphocyte to stimulate monocytes-macrophages [52]. The main target is T helpers. Vitamin D can contribute to formation of acquired immune response by selective stimulation of the specific T helpers [53]. B lymphocytes interact with macrophages and become plasmocytes, releasing Ig, which adhere to antigens. Such antigen–antibody complex activates complement system, initiating production of cytotoxic molecules, increasing blood vessel permeability, acting as chemotactic agents for polymorphonuclear leucocytes and macrophages. Vitamin D inhibits T lymphocyte proliferation, release of immunoglobulins and transformation of B lymphocytes into plasmocytes, hereby suppressing specific immune response, release of IL-1, IL-6, IL-8, IL-12 cytokines and alpha TNF-α [16, 21, 52]. IL-1, IL-6 and TNF-α are potential activators of osteoclasts and supporters of inflammation. IL-1 is released not only by afore mentioned monocyte-macrophages, but by endothelial and epithelial cells, fibroblasts and lymphocytes as well. This substance supports inflamation, stimulates production, differentiation and activation of osteoclasts, leading to resorption of alveolar bone, release of enzymes splitting extracellular matrix and release of E2 prostaglandin, enhancing relaxation of blood vessels and edema in PTs [13]. IL-6 activates synthesis of C reactive protein and glucose metabolism [54]. It is proven, that increase of vitamin D serum levels leads to decrease of IL-6 and leptin (factor indicating inflammation) levels, increase of adiponectin (cytokine inhibitor) and IL-8 levels [54, 55]. IL-8 activates neutrophil chemotaxis and is found in normal PTs. Its levels increase with the progression of inflammatory processes, therefore polymorphonuclear neutrophils are the first to react to inflammation. Its deficiency is related to severe forms of periodontitis. As the amount of pathogens increases, IL-8 levels and number of neutrophils increase as well, causing destruction of PTs [6]. Vitamin D acts on periopathogens, inhibits inflammation of PT and decreases IL-8 expression in periodontal ligament [55]. It can be concluded, that vitamin D plays important role in defensive mechanisms of PT and vital for the health of both soft and hard PTs.

4. Change in the concentration of 25-hydroxyvitamin D in plasma by periodontal diseases

There is no unanimous attitude towards the relation between these two factors as there exist differences between populations, test methodology and occurring limitations of the tests. When analyzing the relation between vitamin D, as protective factor, and PD, different criteria of vitamin D and examination of PTs are applied: average plasma level of vitamin D, dosage applied or any other certain diagnostic criteria. Status of PTs is evaluated according to the periodontal pocket depth, clinical attachment level, clinical attachment loss, attachment gain, alveolar bone loss, bone defects in oral cavity or any other selected criteria, such as short/long term results of periodontal surgery [56]. If only one side of oral cavity is examined, data cannot be accurate and the amount of information is lost. Studies can cover general population or part of it, e.g., smoking individuals, individuals of different age, with different PD, etc. Scientific base of linking these two factors and widening of the knowledge is possible due to widely chosen evaluative protocols and indicators. For example, smoking is risk factor for PD, but with the additional deficiency of vitamin D, destruction of PTs is more severe and more cases are identified [57]. Individuals over 50 year with low vitamin D levels have greater periodontal attachment loss than ones with high levels [58]. PTs in most cases are healthier and risk is lower in individuals with sufficient levels of vitamin D, but it is not successfully proved in all the cases, leading to the controversial interpretation of the results obtained [56, 58–61]. It is becoming clear, that performing blood tests and monitoring vitamin D levels it is possible to suspect that individual is suffering from chronic periodontitis and condition of PTs is poor, especially in older population [56, 62, 63]. It can be one of additional diagnostic possibilities.

In case of acute inflammation, serum levels of 25-hydroxyvitamin D are increasing, as periodontal cells are producing it in the site of inflammation as anti-inflammatory agent. Serum levels of 25-hydroxyvitamin D usually are lower in cases of chronic inflammation. Such correlation might be explained that because of low serum levels of vitamin D, ability of epithelium to fight against pathogens is impaired and inflammation develops. Optimal serum level of 25-hydroxyvitamin D for prophylactic and therapeutic purposes should be 90-100 nmol/l, but it is not definitely clear what should be the daily dose of vitamin D in order to achieve these levels [13]. Gingival bleeding are the sign of both, acute and chronic PD. Decreased level of 25-hydroxyvitamin D correlates with worsened health status of PTs; course of chronic gingivitis (with insufficient serum levels) and intensified gingival bleeding [36, 58]. Gingival bleeding during the probing is observed by 20% less in patients with high serum levels of 25(OH)D, those with sufficient ($\geq$ 50 nmol/L) levels of vitamin are less likely to develop PD by 33% and by 42% are less likely to have more than 50% of gingival bleeding [60, 64]. Prolonged combined supplementation of vitamin D and calcium decreases bleeding on probing, changes the clinical attachment level and pockets depth [65]. The tendency to severe periodontitis may decrease up to 33% with daily dose of 800 IU of vitamin D [62]. Exacerbation of gingival bleeding is observed during pregnancy, thus there are data, concerning the influence of vitamin D during this period (if 25(OH) D level < 75 nmol/L) [36]. Without timely evaluation of all these data, periodontitis of more severe form develops, as correlation between increased serum levels of vitamin D_3 and severity of PD exists, though it is not always confirmed [36, 66, 67]. There are cases described when serum level of 1,25(OH)D increases significantly following the periodontal treatment [68]. Besides, increased serum level of 25(OH)D is common in patients with aggressive periodontitis (AP)- disease of PTs, affecting young individuals, characterized by rapid destruction of PT and tooth loss. Significantly higher vitamin D binding protein (DBP), IL-6, procalctonine and 25(OH)D_3 plasma levels and higher counts of leucocytes and neutrophils are found in patients with this PD [69]. Level of 25(OH)D_3 increases due to activation of 25-hydroxylase in periodontal cells in acute inflammation of PTs, and decrease in chronic one [67]. Due to production of this enzyme in cases of AP, levels of 25(OH)D_3 in gingival sulcus is up to 300 times higher than in blood plasma [21]. DBP is plasma protein and is synthesized by hepatocytes [70]. It is the main carrier of 25(OH)D_3 in the plasma, directly affecting cellular functions, including activity of macrophages [71, 72]. DBP bound to the cell surface, B-lymphocytes, T-lymphocytes, monocytes, neutrophils [70]. The amount of this protein is related to the severity degree of illness with direct relation to neutrophil – increased number of neutrophils and IL-6 can contribute to increased plasma levels of DBP by active periodontitis. DBP is the most important "during inflammation since it induces selective recruitment of neutrophils" [70]. Activated neutrophils can excrete DBP, which expression is regulated by IL-6, participating in immune response [69]. Thus detection of plasma levels of DBP could confirm correlation between it and periodontal inflammation. Anti-inflammatory effect depends on the dose of vitamin supplement. Safe and effective anti-inflammatory dose of 500–2000 IU of vitamin D is recommended. Results are noted earlier when higher dose of 2000 IU is used [73].

5. Conclusion

In conclusion, vitamin D is very unique substance due to its abilities, functions and participation in various processes. Its optimal serum levels could prevent occurrence of numerous diseases, including such common diseases throughout the world as chronic periodontal diseases, which are social problems, compromising individual's quality of life.

Conflict of interest

The author declares no conflict of interest.

Author details

Egle Jagelaviciene
Department of Dental and Oral Pathology, Lithuanian University of Health Sciences (LUHS), Kaunas, Lithuania

*Address all correspondence to: egle.jagelaviciene@lsmuni.lt

References

[1] Gailytė I. Jaunų sveikų vyrų vitamino D koncentracijos, kūno sandaros, endokrininės ir psichologinės būklės bei gyvenimo kokybės sąsajos (Associations Between Vitamin D Concentracion, Body Composition, Endocrine and Psychological State and Life Quality in Young Healthy Men. [thesis]. Kaunas, Lietuvos Sveikatos Mokslų Universitetas; 2013.

[2] Holman P. Vitamin D Day November 2nd – Help Stop Vitamin D Deficiency. Woodstock. 2013.10.31

[3] Holick MF, Binkley NC, Bischoff-Ferrari HA, Gordon CM, Hanley DA, Heaney RP, et al. Evaluation, treatment, and prevention of vitamin D deficiency: an Endocrine Society clinical practice guideline. Journal of Clinical Endocrinology & Metabolism. 2011;96(7):1911-30. DOI: 10.1210/jc.2011-0385

[4] Glade MJ. Vitamin D: Health panacea or false prophet? Nutrition 2013;29:37-41. DOI: 10.1016/j.nut.2012.05.010

[5] Amin E. Hatem. Epidemiology and Risk Factors of Periodontal Disease. In Intechopen.com/books, editor. 2011;03:213-222. DOI:10.5772/29272

[6] Bikle DD. Vitamin D and the immune system: Role in protection against bacterial infection. Current Opinion in Nephrology and Hypertension. 2008;17: 348-352. DOI: 10.1097/MNH.0b013e3282ff64a3

[7] Schwalfenberg GK. A review of the critical role of vitamin D in the functioning of the immune system and the clinical implications of vitamin D deficiency. Molecular Nutrition & Food Research. 2011 Jan;55(1):96-108. DOI: 10.1002/mnfr.201000174

[8] Muszkat P, Camargo MB, Griz LH, Lazaretti-Castro M. Evidence-based non-skeletal actions of vitamin D. Arquivos Brasileiros de Endocrinologia & Metabologia. 2010;54(2):110-7. DOI: 10.1590/s0004-27302010000200005.

[9] Krishnan AV, Feldman D. Mechanisms of the anti-cancer and antiinflammatory actions of vitamin D. *Annual Review of Pharmacology and Toxicology*. 2011;51:311-36. DOI: 10.1146/annurev-pharmtox-010510-100611.

[10] Gropper SS, Smith JL, Groff JL, editors. Advanced Nutrition and Human Metabolism. 5. Belmont, CA: Wadsworth, Cengage Learning; 2009. Calcium; p. 431-443.

[11] Praškevičius A, Burneckienė J. Kaulų, dantų, seilių biochemija (Biochemistry of bones, teeth and saliva). Kaunas: KMU Press; 2000. p.44.

[12] Amano Y, Komiyama K, Makishima M. Vitamin D and periodontal disease. Journal of Oral Science. 2009 Mar;51(1):11-20. DOI: 10.2334/josnusd.51.11

[13] Hildebolt CF. Effect of vitamin D and calcium on periodontitis. Journal of Periodontology. 2005 Sep;76(9):1576-87. DOI: 10.1902/jop.2005.76.9.1576.

[14] Lopata G. Dabartinis požiūris į kaulinio audinio remodeliaciją (Current approaches to bone remodeling). Lietuvos endokrinologija. 2003;11(1,2,3):82-8.

[15] Berchtold MW, Brinkmeier H, Muntener M. Calcium ion in skeletal muscle: its crucial role for muscle function, plasticity, and disease. Physiological Reviews. 2000;80(3):1215-65. DOI: 10.1152/physrev.2000.80.3.1215

[16] Stein SH, Tipton DA. Vitamin D and its impact on oral health-an update. The Journal of *the Tennessee Dental Association*. 2011 Spring;91(2):30-3; quiz 34-5.

[17] Palacios C, Joshipura K, Willett W. Nutrition and health: guidelines for dental practitioners. Oral Dis. 2009 Sep;15(6):369-81.DOI:10.111 1/j.1601-0825.2009.01571.

[18] Available from: https://lt.wikipedia.org/wiki/Vitamin_D[internet]. [Accessed: 2020.12.20]

[19] Zittermann A, Gummert J F. Nonclassical Vitamin D Action. Nutrients 2010, 2(4), 408-425. DOI:10.3390/nu2040408

[20] DeLuca HF. Overview of general physiologic features and functions of vitamin D. American Journal of Clinical Nutrition. 2004;80 (6 Suppl):1689S–96S. DOI: 10.1093/ajcn/80.6.1689S

[21] Liu K, Meng H, Hou J. Activity of 25-hydroxylase in human gingival fibroblasts and periodontal ligament cells. PLoS One. 2012;7(12):e52053. DOI: 10.1371/journal.pone.0052053

[22] Bikle DD. Vitamin D Metabolism and Function in the Skin. Molecular and Cellular Endocrinology.2011 Dec 5; 347(1-2): 80-89. DOI: 10.1016/j.mce.2011.05.017

[23] Chun RF, Adams JS, Hewison M. Back to the future: a new look at 'old' vitamin D. Journal of Endocrinology. 2008;198(2):261-9. DOI: 10.1677/JOE-08-0170

[24] Van der Velden U, Kuzmanova D, Chapple I.L. Micronutritional approaches to periodontal therapy. J. Clin.Periodontol. 2011; 38 (Suppl. 11), 142-158. DOI: 10.1111/j.1600-051X.2010.01663.x

[25] McMahon L, Schwartz K, Yilmaz O, Brown E, Ryan LK, et al. Vitamin D-mediated induction of innate immunity in gingival epithelial cells. *Infection and Immunity*. 2011;79:2250-2256. DOI: 10.1128/IAI.00099-11

[26] Nagpal S, Na S, Rathnachalam R. Noncalcemic actions of vitamin D receptor ligands. Endocrine Reviews. 2005;26(5):662-87. DOI: 10.1210/er.2004-0002

[27] Holick MF. Vitamin D deficiency. New England Journal of Medicine. 2007;357:266-281.

[28] Bellamy, R, Ruwende, C, Corrah T, McAdam K P, Thursz M, Whittle H C, Hill A V. Tuberculosis and chronic hepatitis B virus infection in Africans and variation in the vitamin D receptor gene. Journal of Infectious Diseases. 1999; 179, 721-724. DOI: 10.1086/314614

[29] Park K S, Nam J H, Choi J. The short vitamin D receptor is associated with increased risk for generalized aggressive periodontitis. Journal of Clinical Periodontology. 2006; 33, 524-528. DOI. org/10.1111/j.1600-051X.2006.00944.x

[30] de Brito Junior R B, Scarel-Caminaga R M, Trevilatto P C, de Souza A P, Barros S P. Polymorphisms in the vitamin D receptor gene are associated with periodontal disease. Journal of Periodontology. 2004; 75, 1090-1095. DOI: 10.1902/jop.2004.75.8.1090

[31] Deng H1, Liu F, Pan Y, Jin X, Wang H, Cao J.BsmI, TaqI, ApaI, and FokI polymorphisms in the vitamin D receptor gene and periodontitis: a meta-analysis of 15 studies including 1338 cases and 1302 controls. Clinical Periodontology. 2011;38(3):199-207. DOI: 10.1111/j.1600-051X.2010.01685.x

[32] Li-li Chen,* Hao Li,† Peng-peng Zhang,* and Shu-mei Wang* Association Between Vitamin D Receptor Polymorphisms and Periodontitis: A Meta-Analysis. Journal of Periodontology 2012;83:1095-1103. DOI: 10.1902/jop.2011.110518

[33] Jagelaviciene E, Vaitkeviciene I, Silingaite D, Sinkunaite E, Daugelaite G. The Relation between Vitamin D and

Periodontal Pathology. Medicina 2018; 55(2). DOI: 10.3390/medicina54030045

[34] Newman MG, Takei HH, Carranza FA. Carranza's Clinical Periodontology. 9th ed. W.B. Saunders company, USA; 2002.

[35] Vaitkeviciene I, Jagelaviciene E, Vaitkevicius R. Įvadas į periodontologijos kursą (Introduction to the course of periodontology). LSMU, Leidybos namai, Kaunas, 2019.

[36] Boggess KA, Espinola JA, Moss K, Beck J, Offenbacher S, Camargo CA Jr Vitamin D status and periodontal disease among pregnant women. Journal of Periodontology. 2011 Feb;82(2):195-200. DOI: 10.1902/jop.2010.100384

[37] Kornman K S, Page R C, Tonetti M S. The host response to the microbial challenge in periodontitis: assembling the players. Periodontology 2000. 1997 Jun;14:33-53. DOI: 10.1111/j.1600-0757.1997.tb00191.x

[38] Coussens A, Timms PM, Boucher BJ, Venton TR, Ashcroft AT, Skolimowska KH, et al. 1alpha,25-dihydroxyvitamin D3 inhibits matrix metalloproteinases induced by *Mycobacterium tuberculosis* infection. Immunology 2009; 127:539-48. DOI: 10.1111/j.1365-2567.2008.03024.x

[39] Marcaccini AM, Novaes AB Jr, Meschiari CA, Souza SL, Palioto DB, Sorgi CA, et al. Circulating matrix metalloproteinase-8 (MMP-8) and MMP-9 are increased in chronic periodontal disease and decrease after non-surgical periodontal therapy. Clinica Chimica Acta 2009; 409:117-22. DOI: 10.1016/j.cca.2009.09.012

[40] Lorencini M, Silva JA, de la Hoz CL, Carvalho HF, Stach-Machado DR. Changes in MMPs and inflammatory cells in experimental gingivitis. Histology and *Histopathology.* 2009; 24:157-66. DOI: 10.14670/HH-24.157

[41] Timms PM, Mannan N, Hitman GA, Noonan K, Mills PG, Syndercombe-Court D, et al. Circulating MMP9, vitamin D and variation in the TIMP-1 response with VDR genotype: mechanisms for inflammatory damage in chronic disorders? QJM: An International Journal of Medicine. 2002;95:787-96. DOI.org/10.1093/qjmed/95.12.787

[42] Vaitkeviciene I, Jagelaviciene E, Vaitkevicius R. Burnos gleivinė: sandara, funkcijos ir tyrimas (Oral mucosa: structure, functions and examination). LSMU, Leidybos namai, Kaunas, 2015.

[43] Liu PT, Stenger S, Li H et al. Toll-like receptor triggering of a vitamin D-mediated human anti-microbial response. Science 2006;311:1770-1773. DOI: 10.1126/science.1123933

[44] Wang TT, Nestel FP, Bourdeau V et al. Cutting edge: 1, 25-dihydroxyvitamin D3 is a direct inducer of antimicrobial peptide gene expression. Journal of Immunology. 2004;173:2909-2912. DOI: 10.4049/jimmunol.173.5.2909

[45] Weber G, Heilborn JD, Chamorro Jimenez CI. et al. Vitamin D induces the antimicrobial protein hCAP18 in human skin. Journal of Investigative Dermatology. 2005;124:1080-1082. DOI: 10.1111/j.0022-202X.2005.23687.x

[46] Yim S, Dhawan P, Ragunath C, Christakos S, Diamond G. Induction of cathelicidin in normal and CF bronchial epithelial cells by 1,25-dihydroxyvitamin). Journal of Cystic Fibrosis. 2007;6:403-410. DOI: 10.1016/j.jcf.2007.03.003

[47] Zhou C, Assem M, Tay JC, Watkins PB, Blumberg B, Schuetz EG, Thummel KE 2006 Steroid and xenobiotic receptor and vitamin D receptor crosstalk mediates CYP24 expression and drug-induced

osteomalacia. Journal of Clinical Investigation 116:1703-1712. DOI: 10.1172/JCI27793

[48] Martineau AR, Wilkinson KA, Newton SM et al. IFN gamma and TNF-independent vitamin D-inducible human suppression of mycobacteria: the role of cathelicidin LL-37. Journal of Immunology. 2007;178:7190-7198. DOI: https://doi.org/10.4049/jimmunol.178.11.7190

[49] Hewison M. Antibacterial effects of vitamin D. Nature Reviews Endocrinology. 2011;7:337-345. DOI: 10.1038/nrendo.2010.226

[50] Gauzzi MC, Purifacto C, Donato K et al. Suppressive effect of 1 alpha,25-hydroxyvitamin D3 on type I IFN-mediated monocyte differentiation into dendritic cells: impairment of functional activities and chemotaxis. Journal of Immunology. 2005;174:270-276. DOI: 10.4049/jimmunol.174.1.270

[51] Abiko Y, Saitoh M, Nishimura M, Yamazaki M, Sawamura D, Kaku T (2007) Role of β-defensins in oral epithelial health and disease. Medical Molecular Morphology. 40, 179-184.

[52] Almerighi C, Sinistro A, Cavazza A et al. 1a,25-hydroxyvitamin D3 inhibits CD-40L-induced pro-inflammatory and immunomodulatory activity. Cytokine. 2009;45:190-197. DOI: 10.1016/j.cyto.2008.12.009

[53] Nithya Anand, S. C. Chandrasekaran, and Narpat Singh Rajput. Vitamin D and periodontal health: Current concepts. *Journal* of *Indian Society of* Periodontology. 2013 May-Jun; 17(3): 302-308. DOI: 10.4103/0972-124X.115645

[54] Teles FR, Teles RP, Martin L, Socransky SS, Haffajee AD. Relationships among interleukin-6, tumor necrosis factor-α, adipokines, vitamin D, and chronic periodontitis. Journal of Periodontology. 2012 Sep;83(9):1183-91. DOI: 10.1902/jop.2011.110346

[55] Tang X, Pan Y, Zhao Y. Vitamin D inhibits the expression of interleukin-8 in human periodontal ligament cells stimulated with Porphyromonas gingivalis. Archives of Oral Biology. 2013 Apr;58(4):397-407. DOI: 10.1016/j.archoralbio.2012.09.010

[56] Pinto JPNS, Goergen J, Muniz FWMG, Haas AN. Vitamin D levels and risk for periodontal disease: A systematic review. Journal of Periodontal Research. 2018;1-8. DOI: 10.1111/jre.12531

[57] Lee HJ, Je DI, Won SJ, Paik DI, Bae KH. Association between vitamin D deficiency and periodontal status in current smokers. Community Dentistry and Oral Epidemiology. 2015;43:471-478. DOI: 10.1111/cdoe.12173

[58] Dietrich T, Joshipura KJ, Dawson-Hughes B, Bischoff-Ferrari HA. Association between serum concentrations of 25-hydroxyvitamin D3 and periodontal disease in the US population. American Journal of Clinical Nutrition. 2004;80:108-113. DOI: 10.1093/ajcn/80.1.108

[59] Millen AE, Andrews CA, LaMonte MJ, et al. Vitamin D status and 5-year changes in periodontal disease measures among postmenopausal women: the Buffalo OsteoPerio Study. Journal of Periodontology. 2014;85:1321-1332. DOI: 10.1902/jop.2014.130686

[60] Millen AE, Hovey KM, LaMonte MJ, et al. Plasma 25-hydroxyvitamin D concentrations and periodontal disease in postmenopausal women. Journal of Periodontology 2013;84:1243-1256. DOI: 10.1902/jop.2012.120445

[61] Zhan Y, Samietz S, Holtfreter B, Hannemann A, Meisel P, Nauck M, Völzke H, Wallaschofski H, Dietrich T,

Kocher T. Prospective Study of Serum 25-hydroxy Vitamin D and Tooth Loss. J Dent Res. 2014 Jul; 93(7): 639-644. DOI: 10.1177/0022034514534985

[62] Alshouibi EN, Kaye EK, Cabral HJ, Leone CW, Garcia RI. VitaminD and periodontal health in older men. Journal of Dental Research. 2013;92:689-693. DOI: 10.1177/0022034513495239

[63] Wang Y, Sugita N, Yoshihara A, et al. Peroxisome proliferator-activated receptor (PPAR) γ polymorphism, vitamin d, bone mineral density and periodontitis in postmenopausal women. Oral Dis. 2013;19:501-506.DOI: 10.1111/odi.12032

[64] Dietrich T, Nunn M, Dawson-Hughes B, Heike A, Bischoff-Ferrari H. Association between serum concentrations of 25-hydroxyvitamin D and gingival inflammation. American Journal of Clinical Nutrition. 2005;82:575-80. DOI: 10.1093/ajcn.82.3.575

[65] Garcia MN, Hildebolt CF, Miley DD, Dixon DA, Couture RA, et al. One-year effects of vitamin D and calcium supplementation on chronic periodontitis. Journal of Periodontology.2011; 82: 25-32. DOI: 10.1902/jop.2010.100207

[66] Liu K, Meng H, Lu R, Xu L, Zhang L, Chen Z, Shi D, Feng X, Tang X. Initial periodontal therapy reduced systemic and local 25-hydroxyvitamin D(3) and interleukin-1beta in patients with aggressive periodontitis. Journal of Periodontology. 2010 Feb;81(2):260-6. DOI: 10.1902/jop.2009.090355

[67] Liu K, Meng H, Tang X, Xu L, Zhang L, et al. Elevated plasma calcifediol is associated with aggressive periodontitis. Journal of Periodontoogy.l 2009;80: 1114-1120. DOI: 10.1902/jop.2009.080675

[68] Antonoglou G, Knuuttila M, Niemelä O, Hiltunen L, Raunio T, Karttunen R, Vainio O, Ylöstalo P, Tervonen T. Serum 1,25(OH)D Level Increases After Elimination of Periodontal Inflammation in T1DM Subjects. Journal of Clinical Endocrinology and Metabolism. 2013; 98: 3999-4005. DOI: 10.1210/jc.2013-1906

[69] Zhang X, Meng H, Sun X, Xu L, Zhang L, Shi D, et al. Elevation of vitamin D-binding protein levels in the plasma of patients with generalized aggressive periodontitis. Journal of Periodontal Research. 2013 Feb;48(1):74-9. DOI: 10.1111/j.1600-0765.2012.01505.

[70] Richard R. Kew. The Vitamin D Binding Protein and Inflammatory Injury: A Mediator or Sentinel of Tissue Damage? Frontiers in Endocrinology (Lausanne). 2019 Jul 10;10:470. DOI: 10.3389/fendo.2019.00470

[71] Speeckaert M, Huang G, Delanghe JR,Taes YE. Biological and clinical aspects of the vitamin D binding protein (Gc-globulin) and its polymorphism. Clinica Chimica Acta 2006;372:33-42. DOI: 10.1016/j.cca.2006.03.011

[72] White P, Cooke N. The multifunctional properties and characteristics of vitamin D-binding protein. Trends Endocrinol Metab 2000;11:320-327. DOI: 10.1016/s1043-2760(00)00317-9

[73] Hiremath VP, Rao CB, Naiak V, Prasad KV. Anti-inflammatory effect of vitamin D on gingivitis: a dose response randomised controlled trial. Indian J Public Health. 2013 Jan-Mar;57(1):29-32. DOI: 10.4103/0019-557X.111365

Section 4

Vitamin D and Other Diseases

Chapter 9

Vitamin D and Diabetic Foot

Antony Macido

Abstract

Approximately 15% of patients with diabetes mellitus (DM) are prone to developing diabetic foot ulcers (DFU) in their lifetime. The term vitamin D status or 25-hydroxyvitamin D [25(OH)D] levels are used interchangeably to represent the status of vitamin D in individuals throughout this paper. Evidence suggests a relationship between 25(OH)D levels and DFU. However, very minimal data is available on the association between DFU and vitamin D deficiency. After a careful review of the literature, it was inferred that vitamin D could be associated with DFU and diabetic foot infections. Available evidence on vitamin D and DFU suggests a negative correlation between 25(OH)D levels and the presence of DFU. Evidence also supports a negative relationship between 25(OH)D levels and diabetic foot infections. Further large-scale randomized controlled studies need to be done to confirm the relationship between 25(OH)D levels and DFU including the use of vitamin D in the management of DFU and diabetic foot infections.

Keywords: Vitamin D, 1,25-dihydroxyvitamin D, diabetic foot ulcers, diabetic foot infections

1. Introduction

The role of serum vitamin D in diabetes mellitus (DM) and in the complications related to DM is an area of interest among researchers in the recent past [1, 2]. Diabetic foot complications including diabetic foot ulcers (DFU) and diabetic foot infections are often common with vitamin D deficiency [3]. The global prevalence of diabetic foot complication is 6.3% [4]. Almost 15% of patients with DM can develop DFU in their lives [1]. Infection of DFU is one of the common causes of hospitalization related to DM and accounts for 20% of admissions to hospitals [5]. Recurrence rates are very high with DFU although the recurrence rates have decreased recently [6].

DFU accounts for growing economic burden, while increasing the morbidity and mortality globally. It is estimated that the global economic burden of caring for DFU is more than $1.5 billion per year [7]. Every 30 seconds someone loses a lower extremity from DM in the world [8]. The five-year mortality in patients with DFU is 2.5 times higher than patients with DM but has no DFU [9].

There is growing evidence on the relationship between DFU and vitamin D levels. Nevertheless, data is scarce on the association between vitamin D deficiency and DFU [2]. Evidence suggests a negative correlation between DFU and vitamin D levels. There is growing evidence on a negative relationship between diabetic foot infections and vitamin D levels. Further large-scale randomized controlled studies are needed to solidify the evidence of the correlation between DFU and vitamin D levels. Before evaluating the significance of vitamin D in diabetic foot complications it is essential to review the effects of vitamin D in diabetic foot complications including the non-skeletal effects of vitamin D.

2. Non-skeletal effects of vitamin D

Vitamin D is a fat-soluble vitamin that has effects that are not confined to the skeleton. Vitamin D aids in glucose metabolism, angiogenesis, and migration of inflammatory cells [10]. 1,25-$(OH)_2D$ is the active form of vitamin D and it acts as a ligand for an intracellular receptor and transcription factor VDR [11, 12]. Vitamin D in the form of 1,25-$(OH)_2D$ exerts prodifferentiative and antiproliferative effects on the cutaneous keratinocytes [13], which in turn helps in defense against toxins and pathogens while helping to prevent water loss from the skin [11]. Vitamin D receptor is essential for differentiation, migration, and self-renewal of epidermal stem cells in wound healing [14].

3. Diabetic foot ulcers

International Working Group on the Diabetic Foot (IWGDF) defines DFU as a foot ulcer in persons with previously diagnosed or currently diagnosed DM and is usually accompanied by peripheral artery disease (PAD) and/or neuropathy in the lower extremity. Diabetic foot is defined as an ulceration, infection, or destruction of tissues of the foot of an individual with previously or currently diagnosed DM, usually accompanied by PAD and/or neuropathy in the lower extremity. A foot ulcer involves a break of the skin of the foot involving the entire epidermis and the dermis in part [15]. Diabetic foot ulcers can be located in different areas of the foot. Almost 25% of DFU are plantar ulcers that are localized to the forefoot [16].

4. Risk factors for developing DFU

Peripheral vascular disease and diabetic neuropathy are the important risk factors associated with the development of DFU [17]. Foot deformities and prior history of DFU are also risk factors associated with the development of DFU [18]. Inflammation along with oxidative stress have been postulated in the development of DFU [19]. Vitamin D deficiency is labeled as an independent risk factor in the development of diabetic neuropathy [20].

5. Vitamin D deficiency as a risk factor for diabetic foot ulcers/infections

Significantly low levels of vitamin D can be seen with diabetic foot complications [3]. Although vitamin D deficiency is common in DM, the magnitude of hypovitaminosis D is noticed to be more significant with infected DFU [21–23]. Vitamin D deficiency can in turn increase inflammatory cytokines and delay wound healing in patients with DFU [23]. An antimicrobial peptide called cathelicidin has an important role in wound healing process [24, 25]. In fact, 1,25-$(OH)_2D$ can increase the genes capable of inducing cathelicidin production [26]. The literature on vitamin D deficiency and diabetic foot can be synthesized as follows.

6. Literature review

Although there is literature available on the association between vitamin D and diabetic foot, only a few randomized controlled studies and metanalyses are available. A metanalysis by Iannuzzo et al. [27] reported that vitamin D deficiency was associated with PAD and may be an independent risk factor for developing PAD. Adults with diabetes and severe vitamin D deficiency are three times more likely to develop a diabetic foot ulcer than similar patients with sufficient vitamin D levels [28]. The Dai et al. [28] study is the first meta-analysis demonstrating the association between serum vitamin D levels and DFU.

A double-blind, randomized controlled clinical trial by Razzaghi et al. [29] showed that vitamin D supplementation can aid in the healing of DFU possibly from its effect of improved glycemic control. The study revealed reasonable decrease in ulcer depth, width, and length in the experiment group with vitamin D therapy [29]. The Tiwari et al. [22] study identified a cutoff value for vitamin D levels (25(OH)D < 25 nmol/l) in diabetic patients that put them at risk to develop diabetic foot infections. The study was a prospective cohort research but not randomized. Another non-randomized prospective cohort hospital-based study by Zubair et al. [2] revealed that patients with DFU had a median lower plasma level of 25(OH)D than the control group.

There is more than a dozen of other non-randomized studies that evaluated the prevalence of vitamin D deficiency and the potential use of vitamin D in diabetic foot complications. Majority of these studies reported low vitamin D levels in patients with DFU when compared to their counterparts with no DFU [3]. This strong association between vitamin D deficiency and DFU may not imply causation or correlation. However, this relationship of vitamin D deficiency and the presence of DFU may have implications in the clinical management of DFU [3]. Surprisingly, a study by Afarideh et al. [30] revealed increased levels of circulating 25 (OH)D with active chronic DFU. The authors claim that this is the only study that showed the conflicting finding of increased vitamin D levels in patients with DFU [30].

7. Vitamin D deficiency and supplementation

According to The Endocrine Society, vitamin D deficiency implies a serum 25(OH)D of less than 20 nanograms per milliliter (ng/ml). The recommended assay for diagnosing vitamin D deficiency is the measurement of serum 25(OH)D. Vitamin D deficiency can be treated with either vitamin D3 or vitamin D2 [31]. Vitamin D supplementation needs to be tailored according to the age, sex, presence of comorbidities, etc. Vitamin D deficiency in adults need to be treated with 50,000 IU of vitamin D2 or D3 once a week for a duration of eight weeks or its equivalent vitamin D2 or vitamin D3 as daily doses to achieve a serum 25 (OH) D level of more than 30 ng/ml, followed by 1500–2000 IU daily for maintenance therapy [31]. There are no current recommendations on vitamin D dosage for individuals with DM or individuals with DFU who also have vitamin D deficiency.

8. Conclusion

There is insufficient data on the significance of vitamin D in DFU. There are no guidelines or standardized measures available on routine evaluation of vitamin D levels and vitamin D supplementation in DFU or infected DFU. Data available on

DM and DFU do not comment on the recommendations on vitamin D use in the prevention and treatment of DFU. Literature does not support the routine use of vitamin D in the treatment and prevention of diabetic foot infections. The literature available on the different types of DM and the role of vitamin D in the development of DFU is scarce. Further research is needed to confirm the relationship between DFU and vitamin D including the use of vitamin D in the management of DFU and diabetic foot infections. Provided the beneficial effects on wound healing, identification and treatment of vitamin D deficiency could improve or prevent diabetic foot complication outcomes [3]. Despite the lack of strong evidence to recommending vitamin D in DM and DFU, routine vitamin D supplements in patients with DM and DFU should be considered for its other benefits.

Author details

Antony Macido
Keck Medical Center of USC, University of Southern California,
Los Angeles, California, USA

*Address all correspondence to: amacido@gmail.com

References

[1] Leone, S., Pascale, R., & Esposito, S. (2012). Epidemiology of diabetic foot. Infezioni in Medicina, *20*(Suppl. 1), 8-13.

[2] Zubair, M., Malik, A., Meerza, D., & Ahmad, J. (2013). 25-Hydroxyvitamin D [25(OH)D] levels and diabetic foot ulcer: Is there any relationship? Diabetes & Metabolic Syndrome, *7*(3), 148-153. doi:10.1016/j.dsx.2013.06.008

[3] Yammine, K., Hayek, F., & Assi, C. (2020). Is there an association between vitamin D and diabetic foot disease? A meta-analysis. The International Journal of Tissue Repair and Regeneration, *28*(1), 90-96. 10.1111/wrr.12762

[4] Zhang, P., Lu, J., Jing, Y., Tang, S., Zhu, D., & Bi, Y. (2017). Global epidemiology of diabetic foot ulceration: A systematic review and meta-analysis. Annals of Medicine, *49*(2), 106-116. doi:10.1080/07853890.2016.1231932

[5] Frykberg, R. G., Wittmayer, B., & Zgonis, T. (2007). Surgical management of diabetic foot infections and osteomyelitis. Clinics in Podiatric Medicine and Surgery, *24*(3), 469-482. doi:10.1016/j.cpm.2007.04.001

[6] Fu, X. L., Ding, H., Miao, W. W., Mao, C. X., Zhan, M. Q., & Chen, H. L. (2019). Global recurrence rates in diabetic foot ulcers: A systematic review and meta-analysis. Diabetes/Metabolism Research and Reviews, *35*(6), e3160. doi: 10.1002/dmrr.3160

[7] Hicks, C. W., Selvarajah, S., Mathioudakis, N., Perler, B. A., Freischlag, J. A., Black 3rd, J. H., & Abularrage, C. J. (2014). Trends and determinants of costs associated with the inpatient care of diabetic foot ulcers. Journal of Vascular Surgery, *60*(5), 1247-1254. 10.1016/j.jvs.2014.05.009

[8] Khatib, O., & Tabatabaei-Malazy, O. (2007). Prevention and public approach to diabetic foot. Iranian Journal of Diabetes and Metabolism, *7*(2), 123-133. Retrieved from http://ijdld.tums.ac.ir/browse.php?a_id=276&sid=1&slc_lang=en

[9] Armstrong, D. G., Boulton, A. M., & Bus, S. A. (2017). Diabetic foot ulcers and their recurrence. New England Journal of Medicine, *376*(24), 2367-2375. doi:10.1056/NEJMra1615439

[10] McGuire, J., & Sheltzer, A. (2019). A Clinical Approach to Nutrition and Wound Healing: A patient's diet matters. Podiatry Management, *38*(9), 87-94.

[11] Rosen, C. J., Adams, J. S., Bikle, D. D., Black, D. M., Demay, M. B., Manson, J. E., Kovacs, C. S. (2012) The nonskeletal effects of vitamin D: An Endocrine Society scientific statement. Endocrine Reviews, 33(3): 456-492. doi:10.1210/er.2012-1000

[12] Vanchinathan, V. & Lim, H. W. (2012). A dermatologist's perspective on vitamin D. Mayo Clinic Proceedings, *87*(4), 372-380. doi:10.1016/j.mayocp.2011.12.010

[13] Bikle, D., Chang, S., Crumrine, D., Elalieh, H., Man, M., Choi, E., Elias, P. (2004) 25 Hydroxyvitamin D 1 α-hydroxylase is required for optimal epidermal differentiation and permeability barrier homeostasis. Journal of Investigative Dermatology, 122(4): 984-992. doi:10.1111/j.0022-202X.2004.22424.x

[14] Oda, Y., Hu, L., Nguyen, T., Fong, C., Zhang' J., Guo, P., & Bikle, D. D. (2018). Vitamin D receptor is required for proliferation, migration, and differentiation of epidermal stem cells and progeny during cutaneous wound repair. Journal of Investigative Dermatology, *138*(11), 2423-2431. doi: 10.1016/j.jid.2018.04.033

[15] van Netten, J. J., Bus, S. A., Apelqvist, J., Lipsky, B. A., Hinchliffe, R. J., Game, F., Rayman, G., Lazzarini, P. A., Forsythe, R. A., Peters, E. J. G., Senneville, E., Vas, P., Monteiro-Soares, M., & Schaper, N. C. (2020). Definitions and criteria for diabetic foot disease. Diabetes/Metabolism Research and Reviews, *36*(S1), 1-6. doi: 10.1002/dmrr.3268

[16] Örneholm, H., Apelqvist, J., Larsson, J., & Eneroth, M. (2017). Recurrent and other new foot ulcers after healed plantar forefoot diabetic ulcer. Wound Repair & Regeneration, *25*(2), 309-315. doi:10.1111/wrr.12522

[17] Sinwar, P. D. (2015) The diabetic foot management: Recent advance. International Journal of Surgery, 15: 27-30. doi:10.1016/j.ijsu.2015.01.023

[18] Monteiro-Soares, M., Boyko, E., Ribeiro, J., Ribeiro, I., Dinis-Ribeiro, M. (2012) Predictive factors for diabetic foot ulceration: A systematic review. Diabetes/Metabolism Research & Reviews, 28(7): 574-600. doi:10.1002/dmrr.2319

[19] Sytze Van Dam, P., Cotter, M. A., Bravenboer, B., Cameron, N. E. (2013). Pathogenesis of diabetic neuropathy: Focus on neurovascular mechanisms. European Journal of Pharmacology, 5: 180-186. doi: 10.1016/j.ejphar.2013.07.017

[20] He, R., Hu, Y., Zeng, H., Zhao, J., Zhao, J., Chai, Y., Lu, F., Liu, F., & Jia, W. (2017). Vitamin D deficiency increases the risk of peripheral neuropathy in Chinese patients with type 2 diabetes. *Diabetes/Metabolism Research & Reviews*, *33*(2), n/a. doi:10.1002/dmrr.2820

[21] Kota, S. K., Meher, L. K., Jammula, S., & Modi, K. D. (2013). Inflammatory markers in diabetic foot and impact of vitamin D deficiency. Endocrine Abstracts, *31*, 198. doi:10.1530/endoabs.31.P198

[22] Tiwari, S., Pratyush, D. D., Gupta, B., Dwivedi, A., Chaudhary, S., Rayicherla, R. K., & ... Singh, S. K. (2013). Prevalence and severity of vitamin D deficiency in patients with diabetic foot infection. British Journal of Nutrition, *109*(1), 99-102. doi:10.1017/S0007114512000578

[23] Tiwari, S., Pratyush, D. D., Gupta, S. K., & Singh, S. K. (2014). Vitamin D deficiency is associated with inflammatory cytokine concentrations in patients with diabetic foot infection. The British Journal of Nutrition, *112*(12), 1938-1943. doi:10.1017/S0007114514003018

[24] Gonzalez-Curiel, I., Trujillo, V., Montoya-Rosales, A., Rincon, K., Rivas-Calderon, B., deHaro-Acosta, J., &... Rivas-Santiago, B. (2014). 1,25-dihydroxyvitamin D3 induces LL-37 and HBD-2 production in keratinocytes from diabetic foot ulcers promoting wound healing: An in vitro model. Plos One, *9*(10), e111355. doi:10.1371/journal.pone.0111355

[25] Zhang, Y., Wu, S., & Sun, J. (2013). Vitamin D, vitamin D receptor, and tissue barriers. *Tissue Barriers*, *1*(1), e 23118. doi:10.4161/tisb.23118

[26] Schauber, J., Dorschner, R. A., Coda, A. B., Büchau, A. S., Liu, P. T., Kiken, D., & ... Gallo, R. L. (2007). Injury enhances TLR2 function and antimicrobial peptide expression through a vitamin D-dependent mechanism. The Journal of Clinical Investigation, *117*(3), 803-811. doi:10.1172/JCI30142

[27] Iannuzzo, G., Forte, F., Lupoli, R., & Di Minno, M. (2018). Association of vitamin D deficiency with peripheral arterial disease: A meta-analysis of literature studies. The Journal of

Clinical Endocrinology & Metabolism, *103*(6), 2107-2115. doi:10.1210/jc.2018-00136

[28] Dai, J., Jiang, C., Che, H., & Chai, Y. (2019). Vitamin D and diabetic foot ulcer: A systematic review and meta-analysis. Nutrition and Diabetes, *9*(1), 8. doi:10.1038/s41387-019-0078-9

[29] Razzaghi, R., Pourbagheri, H., Momen-Heravi, M., Bahmani, F., Shadi, J., Soleimani, Z., & Asemi, Z. (2017). The effects of vitamin D supplementation on wound healing and metabolic status in patients with diabetic foot ulcer: A randomized, double-blind, placebo-controlled trial. Journal of Diabetes and its Complications, *31*(4), 766-772. doi:10.1016/j.jdiacomp.2016.06.017

[30] Afarideh, M., Ghanbari, P., Noshad, S., Ghajar, A., Nakhjavani, M., & Esteghamati, A. (2016). Raised serum 25-hydroxyvitamin D levels in patients with active diabetic foot ulcers. The British Journal of Nutrition, *115*(11), 1938-1946. doi:10.1017/S0007114516001094

[31] Holick, M. F., Binkley, N. C., Bischoff-Ferrari, H. A., Gordon, C. M., Hanley, D. A., Heaney, R. P., & ... Weaver, C. M. (2011). Evaluation, treatment, and prevention of vitamin D deficiency: An Endocrine Society clinical practice guideline. The Journal of Clinical Endocrinology and Metabolism, *96*(7), 1911-1930. doi:10.1210/jc.2011-0385

Chapter 10

The Role of Vitamin D in Neurodegeneration and Other Pathological Processes of the Central Nervous System

Carl Nikolaus Homann

Abstract

The nervous system is the most complex organ in the human body, and it is the most essential. However nerve cells are particularly precious as, only like muscle cells, once formed, they do not replicate. This means that neural injuries cannot easily be replaced or repaired. Vitamin D seems to play a pivotal role in protecting these vulnerable and most important structures, but exactly how and to what extend is still subject to debate. Systematically reviewing the vast body of research on the influence of Vitamin D in various neuropathological processes, we found that Vitamin D particularly plays a mitigating role in the development of chronic neurodegeneration and the measured response to acutely acquired traumatic and non-traumatic nerve cells incidents. Adequate serum levels of Vitamin D before the initiation of these processes is increasingly viewed as being neuroprotective. However, comprehensive data on using it as a treatment during the ongoing process or after the injury to neurons is completed are much more ambiguous. A recommendation for testing and supplementation of insufficiencies seems to be well-founded.

Keywords: Vitamin D, nervous system, neurodegeneration, nerve cell damage, traumatic brain injury, acquired brain injury, metabolic encephalopathy, toxic encephalopathy, meningitis, stroke, autoimmune processes, neurooncoloy, Parkinson's disease, Alzheimer's disease

1. Introduction

The nervous system is the most complex organ in the human body. The brain, as the nervous system's command center, is fundamental to the human experience as it produces our every thought, action, memory, and feeling. In short, it is our apparatus to take in and react to phenomena of the inner and outside world. For this task, the brain has a highly interconnected network of approximately one hundred billion neurons at its disposal.

These cells, however, are particularly vulnerable. Compared to other cells, neurons have markedly higher energy demands. Also, as they neither have a backup energy source nor adequate energy stores, they depend on a continuous supply of glucose and oxygen by the blood. Any misalignment between demand and supply potentially contributes to permanent damage or cell death. Damage to brain cells can occur through events even before birth, as in congenital disorders caused by genetic abnormalities or perinatal exposure to noxious conditions. Causative conditions after birth can be divided into acquired, traumatic or non-traumatic, and neurodegenerative. Traumatic injuries commonly arise from exposure to external mechanical forces, as in traffic accidents, falls, and assaults [1]. Non-traumatic injuries derive from either an internal or external source and can be classified according to etiology into neurovascular, neoplastic, metabolic, neurotoxic, infectious, or autoimmune inflammatory (**Figure 1**). Only a few epidemiological studies provide proportional figures regarding traumatic and non-traumatic brain injuries. In one population-based survey on annual incidences of acquired brain injuries in Massachusetts [2], the outpatient diagnosis was most frequently related to traumatic causes (97%). Of the 3% of non-traumatic etiologies 39% were infections, in 25% metabolic or toxic conditions, 22% neoplastic, and 14% vascular brain diseases. The most severe cases were admitted to ICU, for which the authors calculated a ratio of 19% traumatic and 81% non-traumatic causes. The latter were predominantly of vascular origin (63%), followed by toxic-metabolic (30%) and infectious conditions (7%).

Whereas traumatic assaults primarily cause tearing and breaking of cells and structural tissue injuries, non-traumatic incidents tend to affect the metabolic functioning on a subcellular basis that either acutely or chronically lead to malfunction and cell destruction.

Neurons are also especially precious as, only like muscle cells, once formed, they do not replicate. This means that abnormalities in the development or injuries later in life cannot easily be replaced or repaired. Vitamin D (VD) appears to play a critical role in safeguarding these delicate and vital structures. VD deficiency affects a broad range of adult brain disorders with various etiologies and causative pathomechanisms, according to emerging evidence [3, 4], but it is also essential for neuronal growth and pruning in neonates and children [5].

This review examines, for each of the primary injury categories (**Figure 1**), the evidence for VD's role in the resilience to neuronal damage. It mainly focuses on

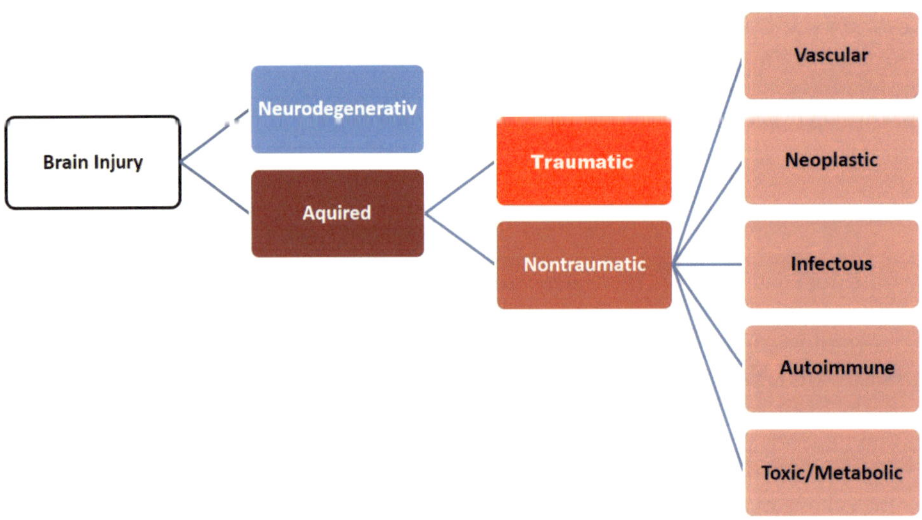

Figure 1.
Classification of brain injuries in adult life.

the importance of maintaining adequate VD blood levels before the initiation of these processes, the use of VD as treatment during the ongoing process, and as a remedy after the injury to neurons has been completed. For conciseness, it explicitly concentrates on adult diseases and excludes congenital disorders.

2. Role of Vitamin D in specific neurolopathological processes

2.1 Vitamin D and traumatic neuronal injury

Traumatic brain injury (TBI) may have a wide range of mental and physical consequences. Depending on the gravity, type, and location of impact, symptoms can vary in severity and duration from mild intermittent attention deficits to coma, from discrete transient headaches to permanent and complete incapacity or death.

Traumatic brain injury (TBI) occurs at an incidence rate of 235–556/10 million [6, 7]. Thus, it is one of the most common neurological diseases, and it is also one of the leading causes of morbidity and death among civilians and military personnel worldwide [1]. The mortality rate in severe TBI cases can be as high as 40%. Survivors, on the other hand, have a disability rate of 55–77% [1, 8, 9], resulting in a decrease in quality of life and high socioeconomic costs [10].

TBI is generally divided into two stages: primary and secondary injury. These two stages overlap to some extent [11]. Primary brain injury occurs at the moment of the initial trauma when mechanical forces cause acute and permanent damage to the brain parenchyma. The subsequent secondary brain injury usually starts quickly but may progress slowly over months or years [11]. It is, to a large extend, caused by microparticles released from damaged tissues that trigger hemostatic, ischemic, and inflammatory processes. This eventually leads to lasting secondary biochemical and cellular alterations. Depolarization, excitotoxicity, disruption of calcium homeostasis, free-radical generation, blood–brain barrier disruption, ischemic injury, edema formation, and intracranial hypertension are some of the most frequently cited mechanisms at play [12]. It is widely believed that treatments that can mitigate this cascade of events can considerably improve TBI outcomes [11, 12].

VD is thought to have a positive effect on this mechanism at various stages, and inadequate levels are linked to more insufficient recovery. In a comprehensive review, Colon evaluated the current literature regarding the protective properties of VD and its clinical relevance after traumatic brain injury, particularly for military personnel [13]. The included in vivo and in vitro studies support that VD modulates the immune responses to trauma, diminishes oxidative and toxic damage, and inhibits activation and progression of neuroinflammation.

Several observational studies suggested VD deficiency is common in patients after TBI (34–46·5%) [14, 15] and is associated with psychiatric deterioration (cognition, depression) [14] and possibly an unfavorable disease outcome [15]. However, the correlation between VD deficiency and worsening of psychiatric disorders may be an epiphenomenon since they are known to be related to VD deficiency independently of comorbid TBI [4].

There is no human research examining VD given prophylactically before TBI. Animal data suggests, however, that this strategy might be protective. Itho et al. observed that seven days of oral supplementation decreased the chances of neuronal damage after TBI in rodents [16]. Another animal study, performed by Wei et al., shows similar results, which are thought to be due to reducing the free radical damage and preventing apoptosis in damaged neurons [17].

For post-injury interventions, there are also experimental data. They suggest that VD treatment decreases brain edema, attenuates free radical damage, reduces neuronal loss in TBI animal models, reduces the inflammatory cytokines TNF-α, IL-6, and nitric oxide (NO), and attenuates neurological abnormalities after ischemia [18–20].

There are also a few human TBI trials. Lee et al. investigated in an open study the acute and long-term effects of VD supplementation on the recovery of patients with TBI [21]. When administering 100,000 IU cholecalciferol intramuscularly to 244 patients with deficiency (VD < 30 ng/mL) they found that 3 months outcomes assessing performance function (Extended Glasgow Outcome Scale: $p = 0.002$) and cognitive function (Mini Mental Status Examination; $p = 0.042$, and Clinical Dementia Rating; $p = 0.044$) were better than those of 64 non-deficient control patients. The initial low VD status measured when patients arrived at the hospital, however, was not found to be a risk factor for mortality. In a randomized placebo-controlled investigation by Sharma et al., 20 patients with moderate to severe TBI received 120,000 IU of VD orally [22]. They had a better overall clinical result than 15 placebo-treated patients, but no improvement in mortality rates (14.3% vs. 14.3%; $p = 0.79$). The better outcome was depicted by an increase in the level of consciousness from day 2 to day 7 (GCS scores: −3.86 vs. +0.19 points; p 0.0001), a shorter mechanical ventilation time (4.7 vs. 8.2 days, $p = 0.0001$), and a shorter ICU stay (6.19 vs. 9.07 days, $p = 0.003$). In addition, relative to the control group, there was a small rise in anti-inflammatory IFN- levels ($p = 0.65$) and a significant reduction in cytokines, which are key pro-inflammatory biomarkers for brain damage (IL-6: $p = 0.08$, TNF-: $p = 0.02$, IL-2: $p = 0.36$).

Despite promising experimental results, we are unaware of any clinical studies on primary (pre-trauma) or secondary (post-trauma) prophylaxis.

2.2 Vitamin D and neurovascular incidents

Stroke is the leading cause of disability and the second most common cause of death in the world, causing more than 10% or 5.7 million deaths per year [23]. Although relative stroke mortality has declined in the last decades, stroke prevalence is increasing due to the demographic shift towards a higher life expectancy [23, 24].

Brain tissue injury following stroke results from a complex series of pathophysiological events, including excitotoxicity, oxidative and nitrative stress, inflammation, and apoptosis [25]. VD is thought to have a beneficial impact on several of these factors. In a recently published comprehensive review Yarlagadda et al., based on experimental data, suggest several neuroprotective mechanisms of VD concerning vascular health: First, it can increase the expression of insulin-like growth factor 1 (IGF-1). IGF-1 can mitigate axon and dendrite degeneration, and by activating plasminogen, it also has antithrombotic effects [26]. Second, VD affects the vascular system by inducing vasodilation through nitric oxide synthase potentiation (NOS). As a result, it has the ability to decrease blood pressure, increase blood supply to neurons after an ischemic stroke, and relieve cerebral vasospasm after a subarachnoid hemorrhage. Third, VD stimulates the synthesis of stromal cell-derived factor 1α (SDF1α), vascular endothelial growth factor (VEGF), and endothelial NOS, thereby displaying an anti-inflammatory effect on myeloid and endothelial cells. Finally, VD protects cerebral endothelial cells from post-stroke blood–brain barrier (BBB) dysfunction. Relevant factors for this are its antioxidant properties, which include inhibiting the development of reactive oxygen species (ROS) production, and its ability to prevent tight junction proteins (occludin and claudin-5) expression from decreasing.

It is widely accepted that low plasma concentrations of VD are associated with an increased risk of symptomatic ischemic stroke in the general population. In a large population-based prospective study, Brøndum-Jacobsen et al. observed in 10,170 individuals from the general population a stepwise increasing risk of symptomatic ischemic stroke with decreasing plasma VD concentrations [27]. This finding was substantiated in a meta-analysis on prospective general population studies, including ten studies, 58,384 participants, and 2,644 events [27]. The odds ratio of ischemic stroke was 1.54 (1.43–1.65) when comparing the lowest versus highest quartile of VD concentrations [27].

Low serum VD levels are also thought to be significantly associated with poor prognosis in stroke patients. This has been confirmed by a recent meta-analysis by Liu et al. including ten studies and 6845 stroke patients indicating an increased risk of poor functional outcome (RR = 1.86; 95% CI = 1.16–2.98), all-cause mortality (RR = 3.56; 95% CI = 1.54–8.25), and recurrence of stroke (RR 5.49; 95% CI 2.69–11.23) [28].

While there is a significant body of randomized controlled trials examining vascular changes from VD treatment, there are only two on stroke outcome. In a non-blinded randomized controlled trial on 66 VD-deficient and -insufficient stroke patients, Narasimhan et al. tested the effects of administering single doses of Cholecalciferol (600,000 IU i.m.). The three months improvements of functional outcomes were significantly more prominent in the treatment group than in the control group (Scandinavian Stroke Scale: 6.39 ± 4.56 vs. 2.5 ± 2.20 points, $p < 0.001$) [29]. The randomized controlled trial by Gupta et al. tested VD-calcium supplementation in 25 out of 53 VD-deficient stroke patients (<75 nmol/L). After six months, patients in the treatment arm had a decreased mortality risk (HR = 0.26) and attained a better functional outcome (modified Rankin Scale score) (OR = 1.90) compared to those of the untreated group [30].

There are two recent studies to clarify the effects of oral VD supplementation on the outcomes in post-acute stroke patients in a rehabilitation setting. One randomized, double-blind placebo-controlled study by Sari et al. assessed if VD treatment (300,000 IU i.m.) affects the outcomes of rehabilitation and balance in 72 VD deficient hemiplegic stroke patients. By the end of the third month, activity levels (modified Barthel index scores) had significantly increased, and balance recovery (Berg balance scale) had accelerated in the supplementation group compared to the group of untreated patients [31]. Momosaki et al. conducted a multicenter, randomized, double-blind, placebo-controlled, parallel-group trial in 100 patients admitted to a convalescent rehabilitation ward after having an acute stroke [32]. After eight weeks of oral VD supplementation (2,000 IU/day), there were no between-group differences in Barthel Index scores, in Barthel Index efficiency, handgrip strength, and calf circumference. Thus, based on their findings and in contrast to those of the previous study, they cannot report on a positive effect of VD on rehabilitation outcomes.

2.3 Vitamin D and neurooncologic processes

Glioblastoma multiforme (GBM) is the most commonly occurring malignant primary brain tumor, representing 77–81% of all primary CNS malignancies [33]. The annual incidence rate is 0.59 to 5 per 100,000 persons. GBM is a grade IV diffuse astrocytic and oligodendroglial tumor with a poor prognosis. Despite recently improved standard of care treatment involving surgery, chemo, and radiation therapy, median survival is 14.6 months. Reasons for GBM development are presumably multifactorial, but exact pathomechanisms are not well understood. The inactivation of apoptotic pathways seems to play an essential role in facilitating tumorigenesis and –progression [34].

One of the risk factors to develop GBM is birth in the winter months, suggesting a VD association that goes back decades before disease onset [35]. Also, expression of Vitamin D Receptor (VDR) is associated with a good prognosis in GBM [36]. Zigmont et al. reported an inverse association between VD consumption and GBM risk among men aged 56 years and older. Levels of VD in men >56 were inversely related to the occurrence of high-grade glioma ($p = 0.04$), i.e., older men with high levels (>66 nmol/L) showing a reduced propensity. This association even existed in samples drawn premorbid i.e. from ≥2 yr. (OR = 0.59; 95% CI = 0.38, 0.91) to ≥15 yr. before diagnosis (OR = 0.61; 95% CI = 0.38,0.96) [37]. This temporal sequence is another piece of evidence for a causative relation.

Mulpur et al. explain possible mechanisms of VD as treatment option: [38]. First, There is direct cancer control by influencing the signaling of macrophages and dendritic cells of the immune system and activating the tumor suppressor p53. It is well known, for example, that in other malignancies like breast cancer, VD down-regulates Akt and MDM2 leading to TGFβ-1-dependent growth inhibition [34]. In GBM, VD can inhibit the hedgehog signaling pathway and disable brain tumor stem cells (BTSCs). Due to their importance in tumor formation, recurrence, and metastasis, BTSCs are considered to be the tumor's driving force. Then, adequate VD availability also has secondary benefits. The immune system's role is bolstered, which indirectly inhibits tumor cell growth. By reducing some of the unintended side effects of standard therapy, sufficient doses can be given, and treatment adherence can be improved [38].

There is but one published prospective open label study in humans that investigated in 470 newly diagnosed GBM-patients VD self-use, among other alternative medications. The sixty patients taking VD as an individual supplement had reduced mortality when compared with non-users (age-adjusted HR = 0.68; $p = 0.02$) [38].

VD has not yet been studied in a controlled clinical trial as a prophylactic or treatment in late-stage GBM or other primary brain tumors, as far as I am aware.

2.4 Vitamin D and infections

Meningitis and encephalitis, the infectious diseases of the brain tissue and the covering membranes, are endowed with substantial rates of mortality and with long-term sequelae in survivors. The WHO estimates the global incident cases to be 2.82 million and the death rate to be 318,400. Globally in 2016, 1.48 million YLDs and 21.87 million DALYs were due to meningitis [39]. Incidence, mortality and disability rates vary significantly according to region and pathogen. Bacterial infection is a major cause of meningitis, globally outnumbering other classes of organisms such as viruses, fungi, or parasites [39].

The mechanism of infection-induced brain cell damage is elaborately explained by Chaudhry, Hoffman and Weber [40]: They state that the cascade starts with pathogen invasion, which triggers activation of the immune system, including white blood cells, complement, and immunoglobulins. Immune cells and the damaged endothelial cells start to release cytokines, matrix metalloproteinases (MMPs), and nitric oxide (NO). While cytokines induce capillary wall changes in the blood–brain barrier, the MMPs, and NO, on the other hand, stimulate vasodilation that alters the cerebral blood flow. Cytokine release provokes the expression of more leukocyte receptors, which increases both white blood cell binding, i.e., adherence to capillary endothelium as well as extravasation. This then leads to further damage to the meninges and endothelial cells, thereby stimulating cytotoxic reactive oxygen species production and release of even more cytokines and chemokines. This coordinated assault aims to eliminate the invading pathogen, but it also harms and destroys nearby brain cells. Increased cytotoxic metabolite levels and permeability may further lead to cerebral edema and elevated intracerebral pressure. Those two factors, together with the altered blood flow, causes reduced perfusion pressure and possibly neural ischemia.

As Guevara et al. and Golpour et al. pointed out in their overviews, [41, 42]. VD exerts a wide range of effects on the very pathomechanisms implicated in brain infection. The targets of these actions can be both host cells by enhancing innate immunomodulatory activity as well as pathogen cells by displaying direct antibacterial and antimicrobial properties [41, 42]. The authors elucidate that VD, which is signaling through the VDR, stimulates innate immune cell functions, including phagocytosis, production of antimicrobial peptides (AMPs), and reactive oxygen species (ROS). It is also responsible for upregulation of the pattern recognition receptors (PRR) TLR2 and NOD2 and generation of TIMP-1, which downregulates matrix metalloproteinases (MMPs) [41]. Furthermore, VD inhibits the production of MMPs and proinflammatory cytokines. VD also deranges Th17 programming, which instead leads to the promotion of the regulatory T cell phenotype [41]. But, VD also directly impedes the growth, viability, and biofilm formation of various bacteria [41–43].

Infections with Streptococci and Mycobacteria, both not infrequently causing meningitis, have been shown to be repressed in the presence of adequate VD levels. In an in vitro experiment on isolated human neutrophils, Subramanian et al. found that VD boosts neutrophil killing of *S. pneumoniae* while also lowering inflammatory responses and apoptosis [44]. Rode et al. found in their experiments with naive human CD4+ T cells that in the defense against *M. tuberculosis*, there is an increased expression of VDR and an upregulation of VD-1 hydroxylase genes. VD blocks *M. tuberculosis*-induced cathelicidin downregulation and enables Th1 differentiation and IFN secretion, both of which are protective. These processes promoted *M. tuberculosis* intracellular death in human macrophages and monocytes [45].

While there is plenty of studies on lung, gut, or generalized infections in the form of sepsis [46], there is hardly any data on infections of the CNS. Regarding the effect of VD deficiency and meningitis outcome in adults, there is but one study on tuberculous meningitis (TBM). Dangeti et al. examined prospectively 40 HIV patients with tuberculous meningitis and found that there was but a trend for lower VD levels in patients with a poor compared to those with a good outcome (28.30 +/− 14.96 vs. 35.92 +/− 17.11 ng/ml, $p = 0.141$) [47].

Contrary to somewhat positive results of a meta-analysis including eight add-on supplementation studies to treat pulmonary tuberculosis, [46] there are no data on supplementing tuberculous meningitis patients. Neither are there any trials in the adult population on encephalitis or meningitis caused by other pathogens. There is also no study investigating prophylactic effects in highly exposed individuals.

2.5 Vitamin D and neuro-autoimmune processes

Multiple sclerosis (MS) is the most common inflammatory autoimmune disorder of the central nervous system, afflicting worldwide more than 2.8 million people, most of them young and of the female gender [48]. MS is a chronic, incurable condition that causes severe incapacity in one-third of patients after either a relapsing–remitting or gradual, steadily progressing disease path. It is also the most frequent cause of non-traumatic neurological disability among young adults in the Western Hemisphere [49].

The pathological hallmark, as the name implies, are multifocal demyelinated lesions, or "plaques", followed by gliosis. Perivascular inflammatory infiltration and focal blood–brain barrier breakdown can be seen in these plaques [50]. However, there is diffuse tissue damage even in the normal-appearing white and gray matter.

Here we find a low-grade diffuse inflammation with perivascular accumulation and parenchymal infiltration of lymphocytes, diffuse microglial activation, diffuse astrocytic gliosis, and diffuse neural or neuroaxonal loss and injury [50]. Different immunological mechanisms seem to be involved in the induction of tissue injury, but microglia activation associated with oxidative injury and mitochondrial damage appears to play a dominant role [50].

Several observational studies have shown that low serum VD levels are associated with an increased risk of developing MS, as well as increased disease activity and progression [51]. Miclea summarizes the various factors on how VD can positively influence MS pathology on a molecular level [51]: The ability of VD to suppress the progression of the experimental disease is attributed to its modulation of T cell trafficking into the CNS, its inhibition of Th1 cells, and its stimulation of IL-10 production. Demyelination is reduced via VD's activation of microglia resulting in the clearance of myelin debris and phagocytosis of pathological proteins such as amyloid-β peptides. Another supportive aspect is VD's ability to reduce the expression of inducible nitric acid synthase, a pro-inflammatory enzyme. Lastly, VD might induce remyelination by stimulating the maturation of oligodendrocytes and the activation of astrocytes.

There is no human study to examine the potential of VD to be used as a preventive therapy to control MS severity. Minura conducted a preclinical study in the MS animal model (EAE). Mice injected with VD but not those with VD analog had better outcomes. VD's down-modulatory potential was demonstrated in the histopathology of VD-treated animals, which showed reduced recruitment of inflammatory cells, mRNA expression of inflammatory parameters, and CNS demyelination.

Optic neuritis is an acute inflammatory and demyelinating disease of the optic nerve, of which at least half of monosymptomatic patients will eventually convert to clinically manifest MS. There is one double-blind, randomized, placebo-controlled pilot clinical trial examining the preventive effect of VD supplementation on conversion to MS [52]. When compared to the 15 patients in the placebo group, the fifteen VD deficient patients who received 50,000 IU of VD weekly for 12 months had a 68.4% lower risk of conversion to MS (relative risk = 0.316, p = 0.007) and a significantly lower incidence rate-ratio of demyelinating plaques in MRI (i.e., less cortical, juxtacortical, and corpus callosal plaques, less new T2 lesions, less new gadolinium-enhancing lesions, and less T1-weighted black holes) (p = 0.001 – 0.005).

Concerning supplementation of VD for patients with clinical manifest MS, there is a large number of studies and several meta-analyses. Overall results, however, were inconclusive. A Cochrane review pointed out that the unresolved nature of the final conclusion rests in great part in the low quality of included studies, but particularly in the heterogeneity of patient cohorts and the small sample size of most studies [53]. Taking this into consideration, Martínez-Lapiscina et al., in a most recent meta-analysis with 13 high-quality studies and 3,498 patients with early relapsing MS, showed that each 25 nmol/L increase in serum VD levels brings with it an average 10% decrease in new relapses and a 14–31% reduction in the risk of new radiological inflammatory activity [54].

The three most recent randomized controlled VD add-on trials published since 2019 that were not included in the previous meta-analyses showed mixed results. The SOLAR trial studied the effect of high-dose VD supplementation (14,007 IU/d) vs. placebo as an add-on therapy to interferon beta-1a. It demonstrated that at week 48 the 113 high-dose VD (14,007 IU/d) treated compared to 116 untreated patients had better MRI outcomes for combined unique active lesions (incidence rate ratio 0.68; 95% CI = 0.52–0.89; p = 0.0045) and for change from baseline in total volume of T2 lesions (difference in mean ranks: −0.074; p = 0.035). However, there was no difference regarding the development of the proportion of patients with no evidence of disease activity [55]. The CHOLINE trial reported in the VD group after 96 weeks a slower progression of disability (EDSS) (p = 0.026), better MRI outcomes with fewer new hypointense T1-weighted lesions (p = 0.025), and a lower volume of hypointense T1-weighted lesions (p = 0.031). However, there was only a marginal downward trend in the annualized relapse rate [56]. In the EVIDIMS trial, at the 18 months followups, there was no difference between high- (20,400 IU) and low-dose (400 IU) treatment arms regarding clinical outcomes (relapse rates, disability progression) and radiographical markers (T2-weighted lesion, contrast-enhancing lesion, brain atrophy) [57]. Unfortunately, only data on intergroup differences, not on intragroup shifts from baseline, were provided in this publication.

2.6 Vitamin D and toxic or metabolic encephalopathy

The National Institute of Neurological Disorders and Stroke (NINDS) defines encephalopathy as any diffuse disease of the brain that alters brain function or structure ... [in a way that it leads to an] altered mental status [58]. Patients can exhibit acute confusion, attention deficits, seizures, and coma, or more insidious chronic symptoms, such as mood disturbances and fatigue.

Even though toxic encephalopathy is a condition that can be coded in ICD 10, there is no sound data on its epidemiology, neither regionally nor internationally.

Encephalopathies can, according to etiology, be classified into toxic and metabolic and, according to disease course, into acute and chronic. Toxic causes are medications, illicit drugs, or toxic chemicals. Metabolic etiologies include electrolyte imbalance, organ failure (e.g., hepatic, renal), hypoxemia, sepsis, dehydration, hypertension, hereditary enzyme deficiencies, and vitamin deficiency (e.g., Wernicke: thiamine). Chronic encephalopathies are usually slowly progressing and lead to permanent, mostly irreversible, structural changes. Only rarely, depending on early detection and treatment, they may be halted or reversed. In contrast, acute encephalopathies often have a good outcome as soon as underlying abnormalities are corrected. Whereas many metabolic encephalopathies have an acute onset, toxic encephalopathies can have acute (e.g., CO) or chronic (e.g., heavy metals) disease courses.

Encephalopathies are morphologically characterized by cytotoxic cerebral edema (membrane damage), disruption of the membrane enzyme systems, axonal and neuronal injury, focal necrosis, and impairment of neurotransmitters secretion or receptor function [59]. Pathogenetic mechanisms include impairment of oxidative metabolism, protein synthesis, cytoskeletal structure, as well as the injury of capillaries and astroglial and microglial reactions [59].

There are but a few hints of an association of environmental toxins and VD, one of which concerns a patient's vulnerability to toxins. Studies using genetic markers of susceptibility suggest that genes can make specific individuals more vulnerable to environmental toxins. One of these candidates is the VDR gene. Recent findings suggest that VDR polymorphism influences, for example, the accumulation of lead in bones and could thus serve as a marker for lead-induced chronic encephalopathy [60].

Air pollutants and other environmental chemicals may trigger VD deficiency, either directly or indirectly. The exact mechanism is still not clear, but for heavy metals, it was suggested that it might be by increasing renal tubular dysfunction and downregulating the transcription of CYPs [61]. Endocrine-disrupting chemicals, on the other hand, may either directly inhibit the activity and expression of CYPs or can do this through indirect pathways [61]. Finally, carbon monoxide (CO) interferes with cytochrome-dependent cellular functions, but how it does this is not fully understood. It is known, however, that CO is released from CO-releasing molecules (CORM) and that CORM-2 decreases VD synthesis [62].

For metabolic encephalopathy, there is but one study. In this prospective investigation by Yousif et al. on 135 HCV-related liver cirrhosis patients, he detected significantly lower VD levels ((6.81 ± 2.75, vs. 16.28 ± 6.60; $p < 0.05$) in the 45 patients that developed hepatic encephalopathy (HE) [63]. HE patients with particularly severe deficiency had a significantly higher mortality rate (HR = 2.76, $p = 0.001$).

There are no retrospective or prospective controlled studies that have looked into the effect of VD as a treatment for encephalopathies.

2.7 Vitamin D and neurodegeneration

Neurodegeneration is characterized by selective dysfunction and progressive loss of synapses and neurons associated with pathologically altered proteins that deposit primarily in the human central nervous system [64]. Although each neurodegenerative disease is differentiated from the others by distinct protein accumulations and anatomic vulnerability of specific neuronal populations, they all share several fundamental mechanisms that are associated with progressive neuronal loss and death. These pathomechanisms include inflammation, apoptosis, oxidative stress, and proteotoxic stress linked to defects in the ubiquitin–proteasomal and autophagosomal/lysosomal systems [65].

In the following paragraphs, we will discuss the role of VD in Alzheimer's disease (AD) and Parkinson's disease (PD) as typical examples of neurodegenerative disorders.

2.7.1 Alzheimer's dementia

Dementia is a syndrome in which there is deterioration in memory, thinking, behavior and the ability to perform everyday activities. Globally, around 50 million people, of which 62% are women and 38% are men, have dementia, and there are nearly 10 million new cases every year. It is one of the major causes of disability and dependency among older people worldwide. Dementia, accounting for 2·4 million deaths is the fifth leading cause of death globally [66].

AD is the most common form of dementia, making up 60–70% of cases, [67] and is also the most common neurodegenerative disease. The cardinal pathological features of the disease are senile plaques and neurofibrillary tangles. Senile plaques consist of a central core of beta-amyloid, a 4-kD peptide. They are found outside of neurons and are typically surrounded by neurites that are abnormally configured [68]. Senile plaques are thought to contribute to the damage and death of neurons by interfering with neuron-to-neuron communication at synapses. Neurofibrillary tangles are made up of abnormally phosphorylated tau that accumulates in the perikaryal cytoplasm of specific neurons [68]. They block the intracellular transport of nutrients and other essential molecules [69]. Both senile plaques and neurofibrillary tangles activate microglia, with the aim of clearing toxic proteins and debris from dead and dying cells [69]. Chronic inflammation may set in when the microglia cannot keep up with all that needs to be cleared [69]. Brain function is further compromised by decreases in the brain's ability to metabolize glucose, its primary source of energy [69].

Based on experimental findings of treatment with the VD analog, Maxacalcitol, Saad El-Din suggested that VD may improve the histopathological picture of the brains of AD rats [70]. Also, it might significantly increase expression of Nrf2 and its downstream effectors (HO-1 and GSH), improve serum levels of calcium, decrease neuro-inflammation and Amyloid β load, as well as hyperphosphorylation of MAPK-38, ERK1/2, and tau proteins [70]. Masoumi was able to stimulate AD patients' macrophages with VD so that Aß phagocytosis and clearance increased while at the same time apoptosis decreased [71].

Cohort studies, including several meta-analyses, essentially indicate that VD deficiency is associated with a significantly increased risk of AD and all-cause dementia. There are three important prospective studies on the effect of VD to mitigate the risk of developing AD. Littlejohns et al. studied 1,658 older people (mean age 73.6 years), of which 102 developed AD after being observed for 5.6 years. VD deficiency, according to his results, is related to a substantially higher risk of AD. When compared to participants with adequate serum levels, the risk of developing AD was higher in severely (VD 25 nmol/L; HR = 2.22; 95 % CI = 1.02–4.83) and to a lesser extent also in moderately deficient (VD 50 nmol/L; HR = 1.69; 95 % CI = 1.06–2.69) patients [72]. Annweiler et al. investigating the effect of dietary VD intake in 498 older women followed for seven years, also confirmed that higher intake of VD (on average 2336.41 IU weekly) reduced AD risk (OR = 0.23; 95% CI = 0.08–0.67) compared to those with lower intake [73]. SanMartin et al. conducted a study to see whether VD might have properties that could prevent subjects with mild cognitive impairment (MCI) from deteriorating and thus converting to AD. After six months of VD supplementation, they found that correcting low VD levels would protect lymphocytes from oxidative death and increase Aβ1–40 plasma levels in 16 MCI patients. Aβ1–40 was monitored because it served as a marker for Aβ-amyloid clearance from the brain. Additionally, at the 18-month follow-up, cognitive status was assessed, and scores on the Clinical Dementia Rating (CDR), Montreal Cognitive Assessment (MoCA), and Memory Index Score improved [74].

Two trials looked at the effect of VD in patients with established AD. In a retrospective study by Chaves et al. on 202 patients with mild stage AD, the time of progression to severe stage of AD was shorter under VD compared with those without this treatment (5.4 ± 0.4 years vs. 4.4 ± 0.16 years, $p = 0.003$) [75]. The randomized, double-blind, placebo-controlled trial by Jingya Jia et al. on 210 AD patients suggests that daily oral VD supplementation (800 IU/day) over 12 months may improve cognitive function reflected by information retrieval, arithmetic, digit span, vocabulary, block design, and picture arrange scores ($p < 0.05$). It also had positive effects on the Aβ-related biomarkers in plasma Aβ42, APP, BACE1, APPmRNA, BACE1mRNA ($p < 0.001$) [76].

2.7.2 Parkinson's disease and other movement disorders

Parkinson's disease (PD) is a slowly progressing disabling disease characterized by bradykinesia, tremor, rigidity, and eventually postural instability. Furthermore, non-motor symptoms such as autonomic, sensory, or psychiatric symptoms also occur in most patients. PD is the second most common neurodegenerative disorder worldwide, with a prevalence of 1% in populations over 60 years of age in developed countries [77]. Males outnumber women one and a half to one [77]. In 2016 PD was affecting more than 6.1 million people globally and caused 3.2 million DALYs and 211,296 deaths [78].

PD is characterized by the loss of dopaminergic neurons in the substantia nigra pars compacta, but it also affects a variety of other brain regions. Lewy bodies are the histopathological hallmark of PD and are also held accountable for initiating and maintaining the pathological process [79]. They include several misfolded amyloid proteins such as alpha-synuclein (SNCA), phosphorylated tau (p-tau), and amyloid beta-protein (Aß). Although the exact mechanism of how misfolded proteins accumulate and cause neurodegeneration is unknown, mitochondrial damage, energy failure, oxidative stress, excitotoxicity, impaired protein clearance, and cell-autonomous mechanisms are all thought to play a role [79]. According to Braak's widely accepted theory, these processes are triggered by a "prion-like protein infection", starting in the gut or nasal mucosa and is then propagated via olfactory pulp or the vagal nerve to the brainstem. It then spreads to successive parts of the brain in a chronologically predictable rostrocaudal sequence [80].

VD has been linked to PD-pathology through its effects on L-type voltage-sensitive calcium channels (L-VSCC), nerve growth factor (NGF), matrix metalloproteinases (MMPs), prostaglandins (PGs), cyclooxygenase-2 (COX-2), reactive oxygen species (ROS), and nitric oxide synthase (NOS) [81]. VD has also been shown to play a role in dopamine synthesis by regulating the tyrosine hydroxylase gene [81].

Seven observational studies and a meta-analysis [82] have looked into the connection between VD and PD and, except for one, have consistently found low serum VD levels in PD patients. Like for other basal ganglia disorders [83], the prevalence of VD deficiency in PD is high (57% - 71%) [82]. However, data to tie this to a causal relationship have been controversial. Using the Finish National Drug-Reimbursement Database, Knekt et al. looked at the connection between VD levels in midlife and the risk of developing PD later in life. Throughout the 29-year follow-up period, 50 of the 3,173 men and women in the sample developed PD. Individuals with higher serum VD concentrations had a 65% lower PD risk than those with insufficient levels. After adjustment for confounding factors, the relative risk highest vs. lowest quartiles was 0.33 (95% CI = 0.14–0.80). Contrary to that, Shrestha et al. in their U.S. population-based prospective cohort study including 15,792 individuals aged 45 to 64 years, discovered no connection between serum VD concentrations and PD risk [84]. A total of 67 participants developed PD after a median of 17 years of follow-up. For those who developed PD and those who did not, the mean serum concentrations of VD were comparable (25.6 ± 8.4 ng/mL vs. 24.2 ± 8.5 ng/mL, $p = 0.24$).

Several meta-analyses have looked into the connection between VDR polymorphisms and PD risk. The most recent investigation by Wang et al. suggests that the SNP FokI is linked to a lower risk of PD in Asian but not in Caucasian populations [85].

There are three prospective PD supplementation studies and one small meta-analysis, but results are mixed [86]. Suzuki et al. randomized 114 PD patients to receive 1,200 IU of VD a day (n = 58) or a placebo (n = 56) for a period of 12 months [87]. The intervention group's serum VD level doubled, while the placebo group's level remained unchanged. At the same time, the intervention group's motor scores (H&Y stage, UPDRS) remained stable, while the placebo group's scores significantly deteriorated (difference between groups: $p = 0.005$). They concluded that VD supplementation might help stabilize PD motor aspects, at least for a short period [87]. Habibi et al. randomized 120 PD patients with levodopa-induced dyskinesia to receive either 1,000 IU of VD a day or a placebo [88]. At the 3-month follow-up, there was no difference in scores for levodopa-induced dyskinesia (UPDRS IV sub score) or motor function (UPDRS III motor score) [88]. Hiller et a. looked at balance problems and falls, [89] which are considered to be particularly frequent in PD [90], a major cause of morbidity and mortality, and challenging to treat, even with non-pharmacological therapies specifically designed to alleviate balance deficits [91]. They conducted a pilot (n = 58) randomized, double-blind intervention trial to measure the effects of 16 weeks of high dose VD (10,000 IU/day) on PD symptoms, but mainly on balance. Despite an increase in VD serum concentrations (30.2 ng/ml to 61.1 ng/ml), in the 27 VD treated patients, the Sensory Organization Test did not show a substantial improvement in balance ($p = 0.43$). A post hoc analysis comparing treatment effects in younger (age < 67 yrs.) and older (age ≥ 67 yrs.) participants, however, found a significant improvement in the SOT

Brain injury classification		VitD ≈ Risk	VitD ≈ outcome	experimental	prophylaxis	treatment early	treatment late
Aquired	Traumatic	D + *	D *	C +		B +	
	vascular	A + *	A + *	C +		C +	B +/–
	Neoplastic	D +				D +	
	Infectious					D -	
	Autoimmune	C + *	C + *	C +	C +	A +/–	
	Toxic-Metabolic			B +			
Degenerative	Alzheimer's D.	A ++/–			D +	C +	
	Parkinson's D.	B +/–				B (+)/–	

Study quality: D: observational studies only, C: one randomized controlled trial (RCT) or one representative cohort study (RCS), B: more than one RCT or RCS, A: one or more meta-Analysis.
*Study-outcome: Favorable +, very favorable ++, unfavorable - (*same study for two aspects).*

Table 1.
Characteristics of studies on vitamin D and neuropathological processes.

of 10.6 points in the group of younger PD patients ($p = 0.012$) [89]. There was, however, no effect on other PD symptoms.

In summary, there exist a large number of studies on VD and neurological diseases, but there is a broad variety of levels of evidence for individual neuropathological processes, and the result is not always favorable (**Table 1**). On epidemiological trials, the most widespread agreement is that VD deficiency is a risk factor for acquired and neurodegenerative nerve cell injury (Vit D ≈ risk) and a poor outcome (Vit D ≈ outcome) once the injury has occurred. Epidemiological studies with the highest degree of evidence (A) exist for stroke and AD, but there are none for brain infections and toxic-metabolic encephalopathy. VD as medication, particularly when used early in the process, has been extensively investigated in all categories with high-quality research for autoimmune diseases of the brain (A), neuro-trauma (B), and PD (B). VD was only studied as a late-stage treatment for stroke, with high-quality evidence (A) but mixed results, and as a prophylaxis for autoimmune diseases and AD, with medium to low-quality evidence (C and D) and positive results.

3. Conclusion

Going through the meanwhile numerous studies on the influence of VD in the various neuropathological processes, there is strong support that VD particularly plays a mitigating role in the development of chronic neurodegeneration and the measured response to acutely acquired nerve cell injuries and potential secondary damages. The mechanisms of cell afflictions and recovery are complex and not fully understood. However, despite the differences depending on the type of insult, there appear to be some common pathways in which VD is relevant. Adequate serum levels of VD prior to the initiation of these processes are now be thought to be neuroprotective. However, comprehensive data on using it as a treatment during the ongoing process or after the injury to neurons has been completed are much vaguer. (**Table 1**) There appears to be no evidence to support its use in patients who already have adequate levels in their system. Extremely high doses seem not to provide any added benefit but may increase the risk of VD intoxication [92].

There are a few other reviews on the link between VD and diseases of the brain. This work differs from these as it is currently the most up-to-date survey. But, more importantly, while most of them covered either specific subsections, for example, neurodegenerative [93] and psychiatric diseases [4], or disease groups like dementias [72] and movement disorders [83], this is one of the few articles that addresses the full spectrum of neurological conditions. Furthermore, it is the first to focus on the neuropathological process. This is significant because it refocuses attention on the basic science track, where there are still so many uncharted regions and where scientific advances can possibly have therapeutic implications.

Due to a vast body of evidence of recorded benefits, a consistent safety record, and low costs, VD deficiency should be assessed and corrected on a routine basis in all neurological disorders, regardless of the underlying neuropathological mechanism.

Author details

Carl Nikolaus Homann[1,2]

1 Department of Neurology, Medical University Graz, Austria

2 St. Elizabeth University of Health and Social Work, Bratislava, Slovakia

*Address all correspondence to: nik.homann@medunigraz.at

References

[1] Murray, G.D., et al., *The European Brain Injury Consortium survey of head injuries.* Acta Neurochir (Wien), 1999. **141**(3): p. 223-36.

[2] Hackman, H., et al., *Acquired brain injury in Massachusetts*. 2014, Massachusetts Department of Public Health and Massachusetts Rehabilitation Commission: Boston, MA.

[3] Moretti, R., M.E. Morelli, and P. Caruso, *Vitamin D in Neurological Diseases: A Rationale for a Pathogenic Impact.* Int J Mol Sci, 2018. **19**(8).

[4] Homann, C.N. and T. Urbanic, *Vitamin D und psychiatrische Erkrankungen [Vitamin D and psychiatric disorders]* in *Vitamin D-Mangel - Aktuelle Diagnostik und Prophylaxe in Fallbeispielen*, K. Amrein, Editor. 2018, UNI-MED Science: Bremen. p. 145-151.

[5] Stessman, L.E. and E.S. Peeples, *Vitamin D and Its Role in Neonatal Hypoxic-Ischemic Brain Injury.* Neonatology, 2018. **113**(4): p. 305-312.

[6] Tagliaferri, F., et al., *A systematic review of brain injury epidemiology in Europe.* Acta Neurochir (Wien), 2006. **148**(3): p. 255-68; discussion 268.

[7] Rutland-Brown, W., et al., *Incidence of traumatic brain injury in the United States, 2003.* J Head Trauma Rehabil, 2006. **21**(6): p. 544-8.

[8] Cremer, O.L., et al., *Prognosis following severe head injury: Development and validation of a model for prediction of death, disability, and functional recovery.* J Trauma, 2006. **61**(6): p. 1484-91.

[9] Myburgh, J.A., et al., *Epidemiology and 12-month outcomes from traumatic brain injury in australia and new zealand.* J Trauma, 2008. **64**(4): p. 854-62.

[10] *Socioeconomic Consequences of Traumatic Brain Injury: A Danish Nationwide Register-Based Study.* 2020. **37**(24): p. 2694-2702.

[11] Zhao, Z., et al., *Cellular microparticles and pathophysiology of traumatic brain injury.* Protein Cell, 2017. **8**(11): p. 801-810.

[12] Greve, M.W. and B.J. Zink, *Pathophysiology of traumatic brain injury.* Mt Sinai J Med, 2009. **76**(2): p. 97-104.

[13] Colon-Rosado, Y., *Vitamin D clinical relevance in the recovery from traumatic brain injury among the military population*, in *The Burnett Honors College*. 2016, University of Central Florida: Orlando, Florida. p. 84.

[14] Jamall, O.A., et al., *Prevalence and correlates of vitamin D deficiency in adults after traumatic brain injury.* Clinical endocrinology, 2016. **85**(4): p. 636-644.

[15] Toman, E., et al., *Vitamin D Deficiency in Traumatic Brain Injury and Its Relationship with Severity of Injury and Quality of Life: A Prospective, Observational Study.* J Neurotrauma, 2017. **34**(7): p. 1448-1456.

[16] Itoh, T., et al., *Neuroprotective effect of (–)-epigallocatechin-3-gallate in rats when administered pre- or post-traumatic brain injury.* Journal of Neural Transmission, 2013. **120**(5): p. 767-783.

[17] Wei, I.H., et al., *(-)-Epigallocatechin gallate attenuates NADPH-d/nNOS expression in motor neurons of rats following peripheral nerve injury.* BMC neuroscience, 2011. **12**: p. 52-52.

[18] Lin, A.M.Y., et al., *Zinc-induced apoptosis in substantia nigra of rat brain: neuroprotection by vitamin D3.* Free Radical Biology and Medicine, 2003. **34**(11): p. 1416-1425.

[19] Tang, H., et al., *Progesterone and vitamin D: Improvement after traumatic brain injury in middle-aged rats.* Hormones and behavior, 2013. **64**(3): p. 527-538.

[20] Cekic, M., I. Sayeed, and D.G. Stein, *Combination treatment with progesterone and vitamin D hormone may be more effective than monotherapy for nervous system injury and disease.* Frontiers in neuroendocrinology, 2009. **30**(2): p. 158-172.

[21] Lee, J.M., et al., *The Effect of Vitamin D Supplementation in Patients with Acute Traumatic Brain Injury.* World Neurosurg, 2019. **126**: p. e1421-e1426.

[22] Sharma, S., et al., *Neuroprotective Role of Oral Vitamin D Supplementation on Consciousness and Inflammatory Biomarkers in Determining Severity Outcome in Acute Traumatic Brain Injury Patients: A Double-Blind Randomized Clinical Trial.* Clin Drug Investig, 2020. **40**(4): p. 327-334.

[23] Kim, A.S. and S.C. Johnston, *Temporal and Geographic Trends in the Global Stroke Epidemic.* 2013. **44** (6_suppl_1): p. S123-S125.

[24] Feigin, V.L., B. Norrving, and G.A. Mensah, *Global Burden of Stroke.* 2017. **120**(3): p. 439-448.

[25] Khoshnam, S.E., et al., *Pathogenic mechanisms following ischemic stroke.* Neurological Sciences, 2017. **38**(7): p. 1167-1186.

[26] Yarlagadda, K., N. Ma, and S. Doré, *Vitamin D and Stroke: Effects on Incidence, Severity, and Outcome and the Potential Benefits of Supplementation.* 2020. **11**(384).

[27] Brøndum-Jacobsen, P., et al., *25-hydroxyvitamin D and symptomatic ischemic stroke: an original study and meta-analysis.* Ann Neurol, 2013. **73**(1): p. 38-47.

[28] Liu, H., J. Wang, and Z. Xu, *Prognostic utility of serum 25-hydroxyvitamin D in patients with stroke: a meta-analysis.* J Neurol, 2020. **267**(11): p. 3177-3186.

[29] Narasimhan, S. and P. Balasubramanian, *Role of Vitamin D in the Outcome of Ischemic Stroke- A Randomized Controlled Trial.* J Clin Diagn Res, 2017. **11**(2): p. Cc06-cc10.

[30] Gupta, A., et al., *Effect of Vitamin D and calcium supplementation on ischaemic stroke outcome: a randomised controlled open-label trial.* Int J Clin Pract, 2016. **70**(9): p. 764-70.

[31] Sari, A., et al., *A randomized, double-blind study to assess if vitamin D treatment affects the outcomes of rehabilitation and balance in hemiplegic patients.* Journal of physical therapy science, 2018. **30**(6): p. 874-878.

[32] Momosaki, R., M. Abo, and M. Urashima, *Vitamin D Supplementation and Post-Stroke Rehabilitation: A Randomized, Double-Blind, Placebo-Controlled Trial.* Nutrients, 2019. **11**(6): p. 1295.

[33] Grech, N., et al., *Rising Incidence of Glioblastoma Multiforme in a Well-Defined Population.* Cureus, 2020. **12**(5): p. e8195-e8195.

[34] Fulda, S., *Cell death-based treatment of glioblastoma.* Cell Death & Disease, 2018. **9**(2): p. 121.

[35] Efird, J.T., *Season of birth and risk for adult onset glioma.* International journal of environmental research and public health, 2010. 7(5): p. 1913-1936.

[36] Salomón, D.G., et al., *Vitamin D receptor expression is associated with improved overall survival in human glioblastoma multiforme.* J Neurooncol, 2014. **118**(1): p. 49-60.

[37] Zigmont, V., et al., *Association Between Prediagnostic Serum*

25-Hydroxyvitamin D Concentration and Glioma. Nutr Cancer, 2015. **67**(7): p. 1120-30.

[38] Mulpur, B.H., et al., *Complementary therapy and survival in glioblastoma.* Neuro-Oncology Practice, 2015. **2**(3): p. 122-126.

[39] Zunt, J.R., et al., *Global, regional, and national burden of meningitis, 1990–2016: a systematic analysis for the Global Burden of Disease Study 2016.* The Lancet Neurology, 2018. **17**(12): p. 1061-1082.

[40] Hoffman, O. and R.J. Weber, *Pathophysiology and treatment of bacterial meningitis.* Therapeutic advances in neurological disorders, 2009. **2**(6): p. 1-7.

[41] Guevara, M.A., et al., *Vitamin D and Streptococci: The Interface of Nutrition, Host Immune Response, and Antimicrobial Activity in Response to Infection.* ACS infectious diseases, 2020. **6**(12): p. 3131-3140.

[42] Golpour, A., S. Bereswill, and M.M. Heimesaat, *Antimicrobial and Immune-Modulatory Effects of Vitamin D Provide Promising Antibiotics-Independent Approaches to Tackle Bacterial Infections - Lessons Learnt from a Literature Survey.* European journal of microbiology & immunology, 2019. **9**(3): p. 80-87.

[43] Saputo, S., R.C. Faustoferri, and R.G. Quivey, *Vitamin D Compounds Are Bactericidal against <span class="named-content genus-species" id="named-content-1">Streptococcus mutans</span> and Target the Bacitracin-Associated Efflux System.* 2018. **62**(1): p. e01675-17.

[44] Subramanian, K., P. Bergman, and B. Henriques-Normark, *Vitamin D Promotes Pneumococcal Killing and Modulates Inflammatory Responses in Primary Human Neutrophils.* J Innate Immun, 2017. **9**(4): p. 375-386.

[45] Rode, A.K.O., et al., *Vitamin D Counteracts Mycobacterium tuberculosis-Induced Cathelicidin Downregulation in Dendritic Cells and Allows Th1 Differentiation and IFNγ Secretion.* Frontiers in immunology, 2017. **8**: p. 656-656.

[46] Wu, H.-x., et al., *Effects of vitamin D supplementation on the outcomes of patients with pulmonary tuberculosis: a systematic review and meta-analysis.* BMC Pulmonary Medicine, 2018. **18**(1): p. 108.

[47] Dangeti, G.V., et al., *Vitamin D deficiency in patients with tuberculous meningitis and its relationship with treatment outcome.* Int J Tuberc Lung Dis, 2018. **22**(1): p. 93-99.

[48] Walton, C., et al., *Rising prevalence of multiple sclerosis worldwide: Insights from the Atlas of MS, third edition.* Mult Scler, 2020. **26**(14): p. 1816-1821.

[49] Segal, B.M., *66 - Multiple Sclerosis*, in *Clinical Immunology (Fifth Edition)*, R.R. Rich, et al., Editors. 2019, Elsevier: London. p. 891-902.e1.

[50] Lassmann, H., *Chapter 1 - Multiple Sclerosis Pathology: Inflammation Versus Neurodegeneration*, in *Translational Neuroimmunology in Multiple Sclerosis*, R. Arnon and A. Miller, Editors. 2016, Academic Press: San Diego. p. 3-13.

[51] Miclea, A., et al., *A Brief Review of the Effects of Vitamin D on Multiple Sclerosis.* Frontiers in immunology, 2020. **11**: p. 781-781.

[52] Derakhshandi, H., et al., *Preventive effect of vitamin D3 supplementation on conversion of optic neuritis to clinically definite multiple sclerosis: a double blind, randomized, placebo-controlled pilot clinical trial.* Acta Neurol Belg, 2013. **113**(3): p. 257-63.

[53] Jagannath, V.A., et al., *Vitamin D for the management of multiple sclerosis.*

Cochrane Database Syst Rev, 2018. **9**(9): p. Cd008422.

[54] Martínez-Lapiscina, E.H., et al., *Associations of serum 25(OH) vitamin D levels with clinical and radiological outcomes in multiple sclerosis, a systematic review and meta-analysis.* Journal of the Neurological Sciences, 2020. **411**: p. 116668.

[55] Hupperts, R., et al., *Randomized trial of daily high-dose vitamin D(3) in patients with RRMS receiving subcutaneous interferon β-1a.* Neurology, 2019. **93**(20): p. e1906-e1916.

[56] Camu, W., et al., *Cholecalciferol in relapsing-remitting MS: A randomized clinical trial (CHOLINE).* Neurology - Neuroimmunology Neuro inflammation, 2019. **6**(5): p. e597.

[57] Dörr, J., et al., *High-dose vitamin D supplementation in multiple sclerosis - results from the randomized EVIDIMS (efficacy of vitamin D supplementation in multiple sclerosis) trial.* Mult Scler J Exp Transl Clin, 2020. **6**(1): p. 2055217320 903474.

[58] Slooter, A.J.C., et al., *Updated nomenclature of delirium and acute encephalopathy: statement of ten Societies.* Intensive Care Medicine, 2020. **46**(5): p. 1020-1022.

[59] Weis, S. and A. Büttner, *Chapter 14 - Neurotoxicology and drug-related disorders*, in *Handbook of Clinical Neurology*, G.G. Kovacs and I. Alafuzoff, Editors. 2018, Elsevier. p. 181-192.

[60] Onalaja, A.O. and L. Claudio, *Genetic susceptibility to lead poisoning.* Environmental Health Perspectives, 2000. **108**(suppl 1): p. 23-28.

[61] Mousavi, S.E., et al., *Air pollution, environmental chemicals, and smoking may trigger vitamin D deficiency: Evidence and potential mechanisms.* Environment International, 2019. **122**: p. 67-90.

[62] Feger, M., et al., *Effect of Carbon Monoxide Donor CORM-2 on Vitamin D3 Metabolism.* Kidney and Blood Pressure Research, 2013. **37**(4-5): p. 496-505.

[63] Yousif, M.M., et al., *Associated vitamin D deficiency is a risk factor for the complication of HCV-related liver cirrhosis including hepatic encephalopathy and spontaneous bacterial peritonitis.* Intern Emerg Med, 2019. **14**(5): p. 753-761.

[64] Kovacs, G.G., *Molecular pathology of neurodegenerative diseases: principles and practice.* 2019. **72**(11): p. 725-735.

[65] Dugger, B.N. and D.W. Dickson, *Pathology of Neurodegenerative Diseases.* Cold Spring Harbor perspectives in biology, 2017. **9**(7): p. a028035.

[66] Nichols, E., et al., *Global, regional, and national burden of Alzheimer's disease and other dementias, 1990–2016: a systematic analysis for the Global Burden of Disease Study 2016.* The Lancet Neurology, 2019. **18**(1): p. 88-106.

[67] WHO, in *Risk Reduction of Cognitive Decline and Dementia: WHO Guidelines*. 2019: Geneva.

[68] Perl, D.P., *Neuropathology of Alzheimer's disease.* The Mount Sinai journal of medicine, New York, 2010. **77**(1): p. 32-42.

[69] *2020 Alzheimer's disease facts and figures.* Alzheimer's & Dementia, 2020. **16**(3): p. 391-460.

[70] Saad El-Din, S., et al., *Active form of vitamin D analogue mitigates neurodegenerative changes in Alzheimer's disease in rats by targeting Keap1/Nrf2 and MAPK-38p/ERK signaling pathways.* Steroids, 2020. **156**: p. 108586.

[71] Masoumi, A., et al., *1alpha,25-dihydroxyvitamin D3 interacts with curcuminoids to stimulate amyloid-beta clearance by macrophages of Alzheimer's disease patients.* J Alzheimers Dis, 2009. **17**(3): p. 703-17.

[72] Littlejohns, T.J., et al., *Vitamin D and the risk of dementia and Alzheimer disease.* Neurology, 2014. **83**(10): p. 920-928.

[73] Annweiler, C., et al., *Higher vitamin D dietary intake is associated with lower risk of alzheimer's disease: a 7-year follow-up.* J Gerontol A Biol Sci Med Sci, 2012. **67**(11): p. 1205-11.

[74] Sanmartin, C., et al., *Vitamin D Increases Aβ140 Plasma Levels and Protects Lymphocytes from Oxidative Death in Mild Cognitive Impairment Patients.* Current Alzheimer Research, 2017. **15**.

[75] Chaves, M., et al., *[Treatment with vitamin D and slowing of progression to severe stage of Alzheimer's disease].* Vertex, 2014. **25**(114): p. 85-91.

[76] Jia, J., et al., *Effects of vitamin D supplementation on cognitive function and blood Abeta-related biomarkers in older adults with Alzheimer's disease: a randomised, double-blind, placebo-controlled trial.* J Neurol Neurosurg Psychiatry, 2019. **90**(12): p. 1347-1352.

[77] Portillo, M.C., A. Haahr, and M.V. Navarta-Sánchez, *Management, Levels of Support, Quality of Life, and Social Inclusion in Parkinson's Disease: Interventions, Innovation, and Practice Development.* Parkinson’s Disease, 2021. **2021**: p. 4681251.

[78] *Global, regional, and national burden of Parkinson's disease, 1990-2016: a systematic analysis for the Global Burden of Disease Study 2016.* Lancet Neurol, 2018. **17**(11): p. 939-953.

[79] Maiti, P., J. Manna, and G.L. Dunbar, *Current understanding of the molecular mechanisms in Parkinson's disease: Targets for potential treatments.* Translational neurodegeneration, 2017. **6**: p. 28-28.

[80] Braak, H., et al., *Staging of brain pathology related to sporadic Parkinson's disease.* Neurobiol Aging, 2003. **24**(2): p. 197-211.

[81] K, L.N. and L. Nguyễn, *Role of vitamin d in Parkinson's disease.* ISRN Neurol, 2012. **2012**: p. 134289.

[82] Rimmelzwaan, L.M., et al., *Systematic Review of the Relationship between Vitamin D and Parkinson's Disease.* J Parkinsons Dis, 2016. **6**(1): p. 29-37.

[83] Homann, C.N., et al., *Vitamin D and Hyperkinetic Movement Disorders: A Systematic Review.* Tremor and other hyperkinetic movements (New York, N.Y.), 2020. **10**: p. 32-32.

[84] Shrestha, S., et al., *Serum 25-hydroxyvitamin D concentrations in Mid-adulthood and Parkinson's disease risk.* Movement disorders : official journal of the Movement Disorder Society, 2016. **31**(7): p. 972-978.

[85] Wang, X., et al., *Vitamin D receptor polymorphisms and the susceptibility of Parkinson's disease.* Neurosci Lett, 2019. **699**: p. 206-211.

[86] Zhou, Z., et al., *The Association Between Vitamin D Status, Vitamin D Supplementation, Sunlight Exposure, and Parkinson's Disease: A Systematic Review and Meta-Analysis.* Medical science monitor : international medical journal of experimental and clinical research, 2019. **25**: p. 666-674.

[87] Suzuki, M., et al., *Randomized, double-blind, placebo-controlled trial of vitamin D supplementation in Parkinson disease.* Am J Clin Nutr, 2013. **97**(5): p. 1004-13.

[88] Habibi, A.H., et al., *Treatment of Levodopainduced dyskinesia with Vitamin D: A Randomized, double-blind, placebo-controlled trial.* Neurol Int, 2018. **10**(3): p. 7737.

[89] Hiller, A.L., et al., *A randomized, controlled pilot study of the effects of vitamin D supplementation on balance in Parkinson's disease: Does age matter?* PLOS ONE, 2018. **13**(9): p. e0203637.

[90] Homann, B., et al., *The impact of neurological disorders on the risk for falls in the community dwelling elderly: a case-controlled study.* BMJ Open, 2013. **3**(11): p. e003367.

[91] Steiger, L. and C.N. Homann, *Exercise therapy in Parkinson`s disease – An overview of current interventional studies.* Physiotherapy Research and Reports, 2019. **1**: p. 1-10.

[92] Feige, J., et al., *Vitamin D Supplementation in Multiple Sclerosis: A Critical Analysis of Potentials and Threats.* Nutrients, 2020. **12**(3).

[93] Koduah, P., F. Paul, and J.M. Dorr, *Vitamin D in the prevention, prediction and treatment of neurodegenerative and neuroinflammatory diseases.* EPMA J, 2017. **8**(4): p. 313-325.

Chapter 11

Vitamin D and Autism Spectrum Disorder

Maud Vegelin, Gosia Teodorowicz and Huub F.J. Savelkoul

Abstract

1,25(OH)2D is the hormonally active form of vitamin D known for its pleiotropic immunomodulatory effects. Via altering gene transcription, 1,25(OH)D exerts immunosuppressive effects and stimulates immune regulation. Recently, the interest in vitamin D in association with autism spectrum disorder (ASD) has been triggered. The prevalence of ASD has increased excessively over the last few decades, emphasizing the need for a better understanding of the etiology of the disorder as well as to find better treatments. Vitamin D levels in ASD patients are observed to be lower compared to healthy individuals and maternal vitamin D deficiency has been associated with an increased risk of ASD. Moreover, vitamin D supplementation improves ASD symptoms. These recent clinical findings strongly suggest that vitamin D is a factor in ASD onset and progression. Yet, possible mechanisms behind this association remain unknown. This review summarizes immunomodulatory properties of vitamin D and peripheral immune dysregulation in ASD, after which possible mechanisms via which vitamin D could rebalance the immune system in ASD are discussed. Although promising clinical results have been found, further research is necessary to draw conclusions about the effect and mechanisms behind the effect of vitamin D on ASD development.

Keywords: autism spectrum disorder, vitamin D, vitamin D receptor, vitamin D responsive element, immune system

1. Introduction

For many decades vitamin D has been known for its immunomodulatory effects. When metabolized into the active hormone calcitriol, it can bind to vitamin D receptors (VDRs). These VDRs are expressed by most cells in the human body, allowing vitamin D to have a broad range of functions. Upon binding of vitamin D to a VDR, gene transcription is altered. All types of immune cells in the human body express the vitamin D receptor, enabling vitamin D to alter immune responses [1]. In general, vitamin D has immunosuppressive properties and can therefore be beneficial in diseases characterized by inflammation and autoimmunity such as multiple sclerosis and inflammatory bowel disease [2]. Vitamin D deficiency is an increasing global problem with an estimated 30% of the population suffering from vitamin D deficiency and 60% being vitamin D insufficient [3]. Inadequate levels of vitamin D can have many adverse effects throughout the body due to the abundant expression of VDRs. Furthermore, maternal vitamin D deficiency has been suggested to affect development of the offspring. To date, the World Health

Organization does not recommend vitamin D supplementation to pregnant women. This illustrates the lack of awareness on the importance of vitamin D in health.

A disorder that recently received increased attention is autism spectrum disorder (ASD). ASD is a heterogeneous neurodevelopmental disorder, collectively describing autistic disorder, Asperger's syndrome and Pervasive Developmental Disorders Not Otherwise Specified (PDD-NOS). It is characterized by behavioral deficits, impaired communicative functioning and restricted and repetitive patterns of behavior [4]. ASD onset usually occurs in the first few years of life and proceeds into childhood and adulthood [5]. Genetics are of importance in the disorder – several studies show monozygotic twins share 60–90% of ASD symptoms [5, 6]. Additionally, ASD is four times more prevalent in boys, which is suggested to be due to the protective effects of estrogens in women [5, 7].

Despite the role of genetics, the prevalence of ASD has increased tremendously over the past few decades [8]. In the Netherlands, the prevalence of ASD increased from 90.000 to 190.000 cases between 2001 and 2009 [9]. More recently, the prevalence of ASD in the US was estimated at one in every 59 children aged eight years in 2014, which increased to one in every 54 children in 2016 [10]. Across all ages, the prevalence of ASD is estimated to be 1% of the worldwide population [11, 12]. Partially, this increase can be explained by improved diagnostics and increased awareness. However, the sudden and rapid increase also suggests the role of environmental factors in ASD onset. Research indicates that genetic predisposition predominates, requiring additional environmental triggers to develop ASD. Multiple environmental factors have been suggested, including antibiotic use, maternal infections during pregnancy and sun exposure. The strong increase in prevalence highlights the importance of understanding the role of environmental factors in the etiology of ASD [6].

The association between vitamin D and ASD was suggested in 2008 when it was observed that the increase in ASD prevalence coincides with the medical advice to avoid sun exposure [7]. Since then, clinical trials have been performed, trying to prove the association between vitamin D and ASD. UV-B is the most important source of vitamin D in humans, illustrating the requirement for sunlight. Research shows ASD prevalence is higher in countries at higher latitudes, coinciding with reduced UV-B intensity. Moreover, ASD patients consistently exhibit lower vitamin D levels than healthy individuals and studies have shown maternal vitamin D deficiency increases the risk of ASD. These findings encouraged scientists to study the effect of vitamin D supplementation on improving ASD symptoms, and thus far promising results have been found [7, 13]. Yet, the mechanisms behind the possible association between vitamin D and ASD remain unknown. Neuroinflammation, oxidative stress, autoimmunity and immune dysregulation are all observed in individuals with ASD [14]. Of these phenomena, immune dysregulation is the least well-described in literature. ASD patients suffer from chronic systemic inflammation, which is illustrated by a disbalance in cytokine expression and the presence of comorbidities such as gastrointestinal problems in a large fraction of ASD patients [15]. Increased immune activation is observed in ASD patients and is associated with more severe symptoms [16]. Taking into consideration the immunosuppressive properties of vitamin D, this suggests that perhaps vitamin D could play a role in rebalancing the dysregulated immune system in ASD patients and thereby reduce systemic inflammation. However, to date there is no recommendation for vitamin D supplementation in ASD patients.

Therefore, in this review the role of vitamin D in immune dysregulation in ASD patients is examined. First, immunomodulatory properties of vitamin D in general and peripheral immune dysregulation in ASD are described, with a focus on CD4+ T cell activity. Next, possible mechanisms behind this effect of vitamin D on immune dysregulation in ASD are discussed. This review is summarizing current knowledge on vitamin D and ASD and to examine possible mechanisms via which vitamin D might slow ASD development.

2. The immunomodulatory properties of vitamin D

2.1 Vitamin D: production and metabolism

Vitamin D is a steroid hormone with varying functions in the human body. Vitamin D precursors are extracted both from food and through the exposure to sunlight. Around 10% of the total amount of vitamin D in the body is provided by dietary sources and supplements [17]. There are two forms of vitamin D precursors: D2 (ergocalciferol) and D3 (cholecalciferol). Some plant products are rich in vitamin D2, whereas vitamin D3 is present in animal products, including fish and egg yolk [18]. Sunlight exposure accounts for about 90% of vitamin D and is thus the most important source of this vitamin [17]. When the human skin is exposed to UV-B, 7-dehydrocholesterol is converted into pre-vitamin D [19]. This process depends on factors such as UV-B intensity, skin color and coverage of the skin.

After the production of vitamin D3 in the body, it is first metabolized into the precursor 25-hydroxyvitamin D (25(OH)D). This reaction is performed in the liver by hydroxylases, of which CYP2R1 has the highest affinity for pre-vitamin D [20]. Vitamin D binding protein functions as a transporter of 25(OH)D to the kidney. Consequently, 1,25-dihydroxyvitamin D (1,25(OH)2D) is formed in the kidney by the enzyme CYP27B1. The activity of this enzyme is essential to produce bioactive vitamin D. 1,25(OH)2D is the hormonally active form of vitamin D [21]. In this review 1,25 (OH)2D reflects bioactive vitamin D. Besides renal CYP27B1, other cells in the human body can also express this enzyme. In this way, vitamin D can be directly synthesized not solely in the kidney but also in other tissues [20]. 1,25(OH)2D can be absorbed and then bind to the intracellular vitamin D receptor (VDR). Due to the lack of 1,25(OH)2D in its free form in the blood, vitamin D levels are based on 25(OH)D. This precursor is bound to vitamin D binding protein (DBP) in the circulation, allowing measurements to determine vitamin D levels [22, 23].

1,25(OH)2D can influence its own serum levels and binding to VDR. When serum 1,25(OH)2D levels are high, this enhances VDR expression. Moreover, 1,25(OH)2D has a negative feedback on CYP27B1, the enzyme involved in 1,25(OH)2D synthesis. Besides self-regulation, parathyroid hormone (PTH) and fibroblast growth factor 23 (FGF23) are important regulators of vitamin D metabolism. To sustain normal systemic vitamin D levels, CYP24A1 is stimulated by 1,25(OH)2D and degrades vitamin D. The CYP24A1 enzyme is present in all vitamin D target cells, resulting in the ability to regulate intracellular vitamin D levels [20].

2.2 Vitamin D: mode of action

By binding to VDR, which has a DNA-binding domain, 1,25(OH)2D can exert effects on the body through gene transcription. VDRs are located intracellularly in a wide range of cells. Due to this, vitamin D can exert effects on many different biological processes in the body [21, 24]. The regulation of genes by VDR is cell specific. After the binding of vitamin D to VDR, VDR interacts with the retinoic X receptor (RXR). The VDR/RXR heterodimer binds to vitamin D responsive elements (VDRE) in the promoter region of vitamin D responsive genes, influencing gene transcription [21, 25]. These VDREs are upstream of many genes and thereby exert an effect on different functions of the body. The most well-known activity of vitamin D in the body is its role in calcium homeostasis. By stimulating calcium absorption, vitamin D enhances bone density. However, vitamin D also plays a role in many other biological processes, including the control of cancer cell proliferation, skin function, cardiovascular disease and regulation of the immune system [20]. It has vasculo-protective roles, especially in blood vessels that are sensitive to inflammation [26]. Moreover, vitamin D is important in neurocognitive development through its stimulation of nerve growth factor production [27].

2.3 Vitamin D: modulating immune responses

Vitamin D has also been described to affect both innate and adaptive immunity and is therefore considered to be immunomodulatory, including control of effector functions, increasing barrier function and stimulating regulatory T cells [28]. 1,25(OH)2D binds to a VDR which is located intracellularly. Consequently, the VDR/RXR complex translocates to the nucleus and binds to a VDRE, thereby altering gene transcription [29]. Studies show that the required 1,25(OH)2D levels are likely to be higher than the average serum vitamin D levels to facilitate immunomodulation. To maintain bone health, 1,25(OH)2D serum levels should be around 20 ng/mL or higher [30]. In contrast, 1,25(OH)2D levels should approximately be 40–80 ng/mL to reach sufficient amounts necessary for immunomodulation. These high 1,25(OH)2D levels can be achieved by the autocrine and paracrine functions of immune cells regarding vitamin D [31]. As stated before, vitamin D exerts its effects through VDRs. These receptors are expressed in all immune cells, although in ranging amounts [31]. By binding of 1,25(OH)2D to VDRs, vitamin D can activate or suppress gene transcription. Additionally, 1,25(OH)2D can exert rapid non-genomic responses. In contrast to genomic responses which require hours to days to become apparent, these rapid responses take 1 to 45 minutes [32]. Unfortunately, the exact mechanism of how this works has yet to be discovered.

Interestingly, immune cells can also affect 1,25(OH)2D levels. Most immune cells, including macrophages and dendritic cells, express CYP27B1 and CYP24A1, the enzymes needed for active vitamin D synthesis and degradation respectively. This allows immune cells to directly control 1,25(OH)2D levels in their direct local microenvironment, exerting autocrine and paracrine effects [33, 34]. This contrasts with systemic 1,25(OH)2D levels, which are regulated by CYP27B1, PTH and FGF23. Previous studies show that the negative feedback loop present in renal CYP24A1 and 1,25(OH)2D does not apply to immune cell hydroxylases. Due to this, CYP24A1 is not activated by high levels of 1,25(OH)2D, resulting in increased vitamin D levels [35].

3. Peripheral immune dysregulation in ASD

ASD is characterized not only by behavioral deficits, but also by comorbidities, including gastrointestinal problems. In addition, there is an involvement of the immune system based on the increased inflammation, autoimmunity and oxidative stress in ASD patients compared to healthy individuals [36]. Additionally, the prevalence of allergies and infections among ASD patients is higher compared to healthy individuals [37, 38]. A recent study states that approximately 60% of all ASD patients suffers from immune dysregulation [39, 40].

3.1 Antigen presenting cells

Studies indicate that innate immune activation with activated antigen presenting cells and associated cytokine production is observed in ASD patients [41]. Increased numbers of monocytes with increased amounts of cytokines, with a shift towards pro-inflammatory cytokines are found in ASD patients compared to healthy individuals. IL-1β is one of these cytokines and is associated with more severe ASD symptoms. Upon TLR signaling, monocytes in ASD patients show increased activation and pro-inflammatory cytokine production [42, 43]. Macrophage or microglial activity associated with increased production of macrophage migration inhibitory factor (MIF) neuroinflammation in the brain is also altered in ASD patients [44]. MIF is a mediator of innate immunity by enhancing pro-inflammatory cytokine release and higher MIF levels result in less suppression of macrophage activity. Moreover, MIF levels are positively correlated with increased macrophage activity and thus ASD severity [45, 46]. Individuals with ASD show an increased number of dendritic cells, which is associated with more severe ASD symptoms [47]. These different findings thus illustrate increased innate immune activation in ASD patients.

Monocyte and macrophage activity are increased in ASD patients, both due to increased cell numbers and increased pro-inflammatory cytokine production. Contradictory, vitamin D suppresses pro-inflammatory cytokine release by M1 macrophages, while antimicrobial activities and differentiation into M2 macrophages are stimulated. Like a balance between Th1 and Th2 cells, a balance between M1 and M2 macrophages is required for immune homeostasis. An increase in both types of macrophages could thus be beneficial, if a balance is maintained [48, 49]. Altogether, vitamin D balances macrophage function and is thereby likely to positively affect macrophage function in ASD patients. The number of dendritic cells is also increased in individuals with ASD, resulting in increased T cell activation and, indirectly, development of more severe symptoms [47]. In contrast, vitamin D can induce a tolerogenic state in dendritic cells. The expression of surface molecules required for antigen presentation and T cell activation is inhibited and a shift from pro-inflammatory to anti-inflammatory cytokine secretion arises. Via these pathways, vitamin D could affect dendritic cells in ASD patients in such a way that it facilitates immunosuppression. Besides altered cytokine profiles that illustrate changes in CD4+ T cell differentiation, this shift in subsets is also shown by absolute cell numbers. Increased Th1 and Th17 populations are observed in ASD patients, combined with a decreased Treg population. Moreover, Tregs exhibit a reduced expression of Foxp3, CD25 and CTLA-4, which are all required for regulation of immune responses. Opposingly, vitamin D positively influences Th2 and Treg populations and hereby shifts immune responses to a more anti-inflammatory state [50, 51].

3.2 Pro-inflammatory cytokines

Altered cytokine expression has been observed in ASD patients with increased levels of pro-inflammatory cytokines IFN-y, IL-6, TNF-alpha, IL-8, IL-12, IL-17, IL-1ß, GM-CSF and MCP-1. IL-2 and IL-23. A meta-analysis described the strongest elevations were seen for IFN-y and thus Th1 cells stimulating inflammation and inhibiting Th2 proliferation in ASD patients compared to healthy individuals [52]. Besides, IL-6 is increased which as an important B cell activator enhances antibody production. In addition, IL-6 induces innate immune responses via the production of acute phase proteins [53]. Besides, IL-6 is important in signaling pathways in the central nervous system (CNS) by impairing synaptic plasticity and mediating behavioral deficits seen in ASD patients [54, 55]. IL-1ß has been shown to play a role in depression and anxiety through the hypothalamus-pituitary–adrenal (HPA) axis. Moreover, the role of IL-1ß has been suggested in training of the immune system. Upon excessive IL-1ß production, the immune system is characterized by less tolerance induction and increased prevalence of chronic inflammation [56]. However, a study reported no change in IL-1ß levels in ASD patients [57].

A study described significantly increased TNF-alpha, IL-6 and IL-17 levels and a decrease in IL-2 by peripheral blood samples of thirty ASD individuals compared to healthy controls [58]. Another study did not find significant alterations in IL-2 levels of ASD patients compared to healthy individuals [59]. TNF-alpha and IL-12 expression are consistently proven to be elevated in ASD patients [57, 60]. IL-17 expression is shown either to be increased [61–63] or similar in ASD patients compared to healthy individuals [64, 65]. Besides IL-17, IL-21 and IL-22 are two other important Th17 cytokines. These are both shown to be increasingly expressed in ASD patients [66]. Contradicting findings exist on the expression of IL-23, a cytokine important in Th17 differentiation [64, 65, 67]. GM-CSF is shown to be elevated in ASD patients. This cytokine is important in the activation of Th17 cells and hereby plays a role in autoimmunity [68]. Contradictory, GM-CSF is also suggested to have beneficial effects on ASD symptoms. For example, GM-CSF can cross the blood brain barrier and can act as neuronal growth factor [68]. GM-CSF was associated with improved development and behavior in ASD patients. Several chemokines, including IL-8 and MCP-1, are also elevated in ASD patients. These chemokines have the capacity to attract T cells to tissue inflammation sites [69].

3.3 Anti-inflammatory cytokines

Several studies observe alterations in anti-inflammatory cytokines in ASD patients, like reductions in TGF-ß expression [70, 71]. TGF-ß being involved in immune regulation and is associated with severity of ASD symptoms; the lower the TGF-ß status, the more severe ASD symptoms are [72]. The levels of IL-10 in ASD patients remain debatable. Some studies observed increased IL-10 levels [69], while others found similar IL-10 levels [73] or even lower IL-10 levels [71, 74] in ASD patients compared to healthy individuals. IL-10 modulates inflammatory response and thus the observed increased inflammation in ASD patients could be expected to be increased. Lack of this compensatory activity of IL-10 suggests immune dysregulation. Lastly, IL-35 is also connected to regulatory T cells and was found to be reduced in ASD patients [75]. Meta-analysis findings suggest that the changes in IL-4, IL-5 and IL-13 levels in ASD patients are insignificant [70]. On the other hand, multiple studies observe increased concentrations of IL-4, IL-5 and IL-13 in ASD patients [76]. In general, a decreased level of anti-inflammatory cytokines is found in ASD patients. This can result in chronic inflammation in ASD patients [6].

In summary, pro-inflammatory cytokines and chemokines are all increasingly expressed in ASD patients while anti-inflammatory cytokines are downregulated. Nevertheless, other studies showed an increased expression of anti-inflammatory cytokines combined with a decreased expression of pro-inflammatory cytokines upon vitamin D treatment. Upon exposure to vitamin D, immune cells secrete increased amounts of the anti-inflammatory cytokines IL-10 and TGF-ß. At the same time vitamin D suppresses the production of pro-inflammatory cytokines and chemokines. This cytokine expression profile indicates that vitamin D might have protective effects against ASD development.

3.4 CD4+ T cell populations

In general, an increase in inflammatory Th1 and Th17 cells can be observed in individuals with ASD and were directly correlated with severity of symptoms [71, 77]. In contrast, increased Th2 responses are associated with improved behavior in children with ASD [72]. This suggests also beneficial effects of a Th2-skewed immune system in ASD patients. While mostly an increased Th1/Th2 ratio is observed in ASD patients compared to healthy individuals [78], others describe increased Th2 relative to Th1 [72]. This contrast illustrates immune dysregulation in ASD patients [70]. In addition, a decreased Foxp3 expression positive Treg population is observed [] as well as decreased CTLA-4 expression [72]. Also, CD25 expression in activated CD4+ and CD8+ T cells is decreased [66, 71], while others showed a decreased ratio [79].

The observed dysregulation of the immune system in individuals with ASD is important not only for developing symptoms, but also affects the severity of the symptoms. In general, it can be concluded that ASD patients have increased Th1- and Th17-mediated immune responses and decreased Th2 and Tregs cytokines. Due to the increased immune activation, chronic inflammation can occur and worsen ASD symptoms. Children with genetic heritability have a higher chance of developing ASD, and the role of a disbalanced immune system in ASD development should be acknowledged.

3.5 Inflammation in ASD

In addition to peripheral immune dysregulation in ASD, other immunological dysfunctions in ASD are also of importance. The role of neuroinflammation, autoimmunity and oxidative stress have been investigated more widely in ASD patients and the importance of these processes should be noted. The difference between systemic inflammation and neuroinflammation is reflected by the fact that some cytokines are differentially expressed in the brain versus systemically. Increased TGF-ß levels are measured in the cerebellum of ASD patients, in contrast to decreased levels in the cerebrospinal fluid or the periphery [80]. Upon cell death, cells often secrete TGF-ß to reduce local inflammation. Neurons that showed degeneration were high in TGF-ß, suggesting the increased TGF-ß levels found in the brain of ASD patients are targeted at controlling neuroinflammation. Increased microglial activation, combined with increased pro-inflammatory cytokines and i-NOS activation results in neuroinflammation [41]. This is observed in a large fraction of all ASD cases and could lead to impaired connectivity in the CNS, resulting in the pathophysiology observed in ASD patients. Moreover, oxidative stress is increased in ASD patients, which is among others shown by increased i-NOS activation and the presence of reactive oxygen species. Oxidative stress can affect both immune cells and neurons, thereby causing neuroinflammation and neuron degeneration [36]. Vitamin D has been shown to increase glutamine, an antioxidant capable of counteracting the negative activities of free oxygen radicals, and to decrease nitric oxide. Via these ways, vitamin D could reduce oxidative stress in ASD patients [13].

Lastly, improving ASD symptoms is touched upon most in this review by discussing immune dysregulation in ASD, prevention of ASD is another topic that requires attention. While vitamin D is presumed to play a role in immune dysregulation, and thereby systemic inflammation in ASD patients, this is thought to be limited to the progression of ASD symptoms. ASD is a neurodevelopmental disorder, indicating the importance of the CNS in the etiology and pathophysiology of ASD. Considering the onset of ASD, neuroinflammation, rather than systemic inflammation, should be focused on. Vitamin D is proven to play an important role in neuronal development, which is also illustrated by the abundance of VDRs in the CNS [81]. Maternal vitamin D deficiency and risk of ASD have been commonly shown to be associated. When maternal vitamin D deficiency occurs, insufficient vitamin D impairs neurodevelopment in the infant [82] This illustrates the importance of adequate vitamin D levels during gestation. A recent study tested the efficacy of vitamin D supplementation in pregnant mothers of children with autism on reducing the risk of autism in the newborn sibling [83]. After maternal vitamin D supplementation and supplementation during the first three years of the newborn's lives, the risk of autism was shown to be reduced from 20% to 5%. This illustrates the importance of adequate maternal vitamin D status and the influence on ASD risk. Vitamin D supplementation is likely to be effective at reducing inflammation in ASD patients and improve symptoms of ASD. However, to prevent ASD it is more relevant to look at maternal vitamin D supplementation and the role of vitamin D in neurodevelopment. Therefore, further research should be performed to examine the possible mechanisms of vitamin D during gestation and the association with ASD development in the infant.

4. Vitamin D and ASD: clinical results

The possibility of an association between vitamin D and ASD was found when studies concluded that ASD prevalence is increased in high-latitude countries and with more cloud coverage, resulting in reduced UV-B intensity. Many studies observe the connection between low sun exposure and risk of ASD [84]. UV-B exposure is required for the conversion of 7-dehydrocholesterol into previtamin D underscoring the link between UV exposure, vitamin D generation and ASD development [85]. However, it was shown that vitamin D insufficiency in ASD patients is independent of sun exposure, ruling out the environmental factor causing vitamin D deficiency later in life. Moreover, ASD prevalence is suggested to be higher in dark skin-colored people compared to light skin-colored people [86]. It is suggested that increased skin pigmentation lowers the production of previtamin D, due to UV-B radiation that is absorbed by melanin and thereby less available for vitamin D synthesis [11]. For example, a study showed only 4.1% of the dark skin-colored pregnant women had sufficient vitamin D levels, compared to 37.3% in light skin-colored pregnant women [87]. However, other studies state skin pigmentation does not influence vitamin D synthesis and that a different lifestyle, i.e. less exposure to sunlight, could explain lower vitamin D levels in dark skin-colored people [88, 89]. Thus, common vitamin D deficiency in dark skin-colored people might explain the higher ASD prevalence among this group, however results are contradictory regarding the cause of lower vitamin D status.

4.1 Maternal vitamin D deficiency

ASD prevalence is increased in children of whom the mother was vitamin D deficient during gestation [87] and thus it is suggested that maternal vitamin D deficiency increases the risk of ASD in the infant [84, 90].

The possible role of maternal vitamin D deficiency is also illustrated by the influence of season of birth on ASD risk. Maternal vitamin D levels are often lowest in winter and spring months [91], which could be explained by differences in sun exposure and UV-B intensity [85, 91]. However, studies observe conflicting results regarding seasons most positively associated with ASD risk, questioning whether birth season is indeed a cofactor influencing the risk of ASD. Multiple studies observe highest ASD prevalence in children born in March [92]. These children have a higher risk of maternal vitamin D deficiency in the second half of gestation, since maternal 25(OH)D levels are lowest in winter and spring months. On the other hand, studies observing highest ASD prevalence among children born in May, July or August also exist [93–95]. Autumn months coincided with highest ASD prevalence, while birth in spring months reduced the risk of ASD [96]. Studies show that the first six months of gestation are most important for neurocognitive development in the infant, a process which is influenced by vitamin D [97, 98]. Therefore, it is suggested that maternal vitamin D deficiency increases the risk of ASD most when occurring in the first six months of gestation. As vitamin D levels are lowest in winter and spring, this would result in highest ASD prevalence among children who are born in summer. However, contradicting results on the association between birth season and ASD risk hinder a definite conclusion.

4.2 Vitamin D deficiency in ASD children

Studies show that children with ASD have lower vitamin D levels than healthy children. Since 2011, vitamin D insufficiency is classified as a 25(OH)D level between 20–30 ng/mL, whereas levels below 20 ng/mL are considered vitamin D deficient [3]. Individuals with ASD on average show 25(OH)D levels below 30 ng/mL [99–101]. In a recent study, 48% of the ASD cases was vitamin D insufficient and 40% vitamin D deficient, whereas none of the healthy children were deficient and only 20% was insufficient [101]. This study used different cut-off values, resulting in the fact that when using the standard cut-off of 20 ng/mL for vitamin D deficiency, the percentage of deficient children would even be higher than 40%. An average vitamin D level of 28.5 ng/mL was measured in ASD children, compared to 40.1 ng/mL in healthy children [102]. A significant negative correlation between vitamin D levels and severity of ASD symptoms was found, indicating low vitamin D levels can increase the severity of ASD [100]. When combining this finding with the previously mentioned association between season and vitamin D levels, this suggests the effect of season on ASD symptoms. Several case studies indeed observe that children with ASD experience less symptoms during summer compared to other seasons, which supports the plausible association between vitamin D and ASD [103].

In addition to the above-mentioned environmental factors that could cause vitamin D deficiency in ASD patients and are associated with progression of the disorder, genetics also play a role. In a study that compared vitamin D levels in ASD children and their healthy siblings, lower 25(OH)D levels were found in ASD children, suggesting genetics are upstream of vitamin D deficiency in ASD patients, rather than environmental factors [104]. Moreover, most studies on neonatal vitamin D levels and the association with ASD risk have found a negative correlation, illustrating that vitamin D deficiency presumably develops during gestation and is dependent on either or both genetics and maternal environmental factors [105, 106].

Furthermore, genetic polymorphisms are shown to be associated with impaired vitamin D metabolism and binding to VDR and can therefore predispose ASD. VDR gene polymorphisms were studied of which two were significantly associated with ASD [86]. Measured 25(OH)D serum levels did not significantly correlate with gene polymorphisms, suggesting vitamin D deficiency itself is not the cause of increased ASD risk, but rather genetic mutations. However, not all ASD patients suffer from these gene mutations and thus gene polymorphisms cannot explain all ASD cases [107]. To conclude, it is uncertain whether genetic or environmental factors alone predispose vitamin D deficiency in ASD patients. Nonetheless, clinical trials agree that reduced vitamin D levels are observed in ASD patients.

4.3 Vitamin D treatment in ASD patients

Due to the suggested association between vitamin D levels and ASD symptom severity, it is being investigated whether vitamin D supplementation could work as treatment to reduce ASD symptoms. The effect of vitamin D, n-3 fatty acids and the combination of the two were tested on ASD symptoms [108]. In the study, children with ASD received a daily dose of 2000 IU vitamin D3 for twelve months. This study did not find a positive effect of only vitamin D supplementation on reducing ASD symptoms. However, treatment with n-3 fatty acids only or the combined treatment with vitamin D and n-3 fatty acids did improve social awareness scores in children with ASD. In contrast, a positive effect of vitamin D treatment was observed on ASD symptoms [109]. Autism Behavior Checklist (ABC) and Childhood Autism Rating Scale (CARS) scores were used, two methods commonly used for scoring ASD symptoms. Children with ASD received one monthly dose of 150,000 IU vitamin D intramuscularly and daily doses of 400 IU vitamin D orally. After three months, both total ABC and total CARS scored were decreased significantly. These reductions were prominent in ASD children under the age of three compared to ASD children above the age of three, suggesting vitamin D treatment possibly is more effective at a younger age. Similarly, vitamin D treatment can be effective at reducing ASD symptoms. Upon receiving daily doses of 300 IU vitamin D3 per kg bodyweight orally, 67 out of 83 children with ASD experienced improved symptoms [110]. The positive effect of vitamin D was most prominent in the group with 25(OH)D levels above 40 ng/mL at the end of the study, suggesting higher vitamin D levels correlate with increased improvement of behavior. Although research is limited, recent studies on the effect of vitamin D treatment in ASD children show promising results.

A review supported the need of a high vitamin D dose for its efficacy [31]. Whereas the recommended daily intake of vitamin D is 30 ng/mL, a minimum dose of 40–80 ng/mL is suggested for vitamin D to exert its immunomodulatory effects in general. In ASD, most improved ASD symptoms upon vitamin D administration above 40 ng/mL. Worldwide it is estimated that 30% of all children and adults are vitamin D deficient, and around 60% has insufficient vitamin D levels [110]. This high percentage of insufficiency cases illustrates the need for vitamin D supplementation and/or increased sun exposure when the effect of vitamin D on the immune system is wished upon. Presumably, this would not cause adverse effects as studies on the toxicity of vitamin D have found little disease outcomes, except possibly hypercalcemia [111]. However, findings on hypercalcemia are inconsistent and it is thus not known whether hypercalcemia will indeed occur in the case of vitamin D levels above 40–80 ng/mL and most likely at a dose of 150 ng/mL [3, 91].

All in all, many clinical trials have been performed on the association between vitamin D and ASD. Low vitamin D levels are observed more often in ASD children compared to healthy children. Moreover, research indicates the role of maternal vitamin D deficiency in ASD is plausible and recent studies have illustrated the effectiveness of vitamin D treatment on improving ASD symptoms. Thus, clinical trials show promising results on the association between vitamin D and ASD and the effectiveness of vitamin D treatment in ASD patients. Lastly, rather than in ASD children there is still little research performed on immune functioning and vitamin D levels in adults with ASD as lower 25(OH)D levels were observed in adults with autistic disorder compared to healthy individuals [112]. The lack of research in this target group complicates extrapolation of the discussed results to adults. It is therefore uncertain whether vitamin D supplementation could improve ASD symptoms in adults.

5. Association vitamin D and ASD

The association between vitamin D and ASD is proven through clinical research. Clinical trials show promising results on vitamin D supplementation and the improvement of ASD symptoms. Characteristics of ASD, including behavioral deficits and impaired communicative functioning, impair the lifestyle of both patients and their close relatives – improvement of symptoms therefore would be highly beneficial [113]. Insights into the mechanisms would support a better understanding of the etiology of the disorder. Consequently, this can enhance the finding of better preventive measures and treatments. Besides the lack of research into the mechanisms behind the effect of vitamin D on ASD, further research is also required to better understand immunomodulatory properties of vitamin D in general, as well as immune dysfunction in individuals with ASD [31]. Similarly, there is a lack of research on several important cytokines in ASD patients, like IL-21, IL-22 and IL-35. Additionally, IL-10 expression in ASD patients remains debatable. Different studies have found either reduced, similar or increased IL-10 levels compared to healthy individuals. This suggests the high interpersonal variability between ASD patients and the heterogeneous etiology of the disorder, emphasizing the need for further research to determine possible subgroups on which tailored treatment design could be based [114]. In addition, the role of IL-2 in regulating immune responses in ASD remains elusive. IL-2 is a Th1 cytokine, important for T cell proliferation of effector T cells but also for regulatory T cells. Vitamin D is shown to reduce IL-2 levels. This implies a reduction in Th1 cytokines, but as IL-2 is required for TGF-ß-mediated induction of CTLA-4 and Foxp3 expression on Tregs this suggests that increased IL-2 expression would enhance immunosuppression [115–117].

Although research on the association between vitamin D and ASD is receiving increased attention, no causality has been proven. As discussed, it is unknown whether vitamin D deficiency is caused by genetic or environmental factors. The possibility of reduced endogenous vitamin D production in ASD patients raises the question whether vitamin D insufficiency is a cause or consequence of ASD. To date, it is uncertain whether vitamin D deficiency predisposes ASD onset or is developed because of ASD. Effectiveness of vitamin D supplementation is irrespective of the outcome of causality, as clinical trials have shown promising results on the positive effect of vitamin D on ASD symptoms. However, increasing sun exposure could be less effective in the case of impaired endogenous vitamin D production in ASD patients. Research on the mechanisms behind the role of vitamin D in ASD could support a better understanding of a possible causal relationship.

6. Conclusion

Vitamin D can have immunosuppressive effects on the immune system that could be of interest in ASD. By shifting immune responses away from Th1- and Th17-mediated towards Th2- and Treg-mediated, vitamin D promotes a tolerogenic state in the immune system. This could rebalance immune dysregulation in ASD, consequently reducing systemic inflammation among others. Clinical trials on the effect of vitamin D supplementation on improving ASD symptoms and reducing ASD risk are promising, highlighting the relevance of investigating vitamin D when studying ASD. This relevance is best illustrated by the finding that increased immune activity is positively correlated with severity of ASD symptoms, a process which could be counteracted by vitamin D. However, studies on the direct mechanisms of vitamin D on the immune system in ASD patients are absent. Therefore, further research is necessary to draw conclusions about a possible causal relationship. Moreover, further research into the mechanisms behind maternal vitamin deficiency and neuroinflammation are advised to investigate possible preventive actions of vitamin D in relation to ASD. Since vitamin D toxicity is rare, it is advised to increase vitamin D levels in pregnant women and ASD patients. However, insufficient research exists to state the effectiveness of vitamin D in regulating immune dysregulation in ASD patients with confidence.

Author details

Maud Vegelin, Gosia Teodorowicz and Huub F.J. Savelkoul*
Cell Biology and Immunology Group, Wageningen University and Research, Wageningen, The Netherlands

*Address all correspondence to: huub.savelkoul@wur.nl

References

[1] Mora, J. R., Iwata, M., & Von Andrian, U. H. (2008). Vitamin effects on the immune system: vitamins A and D take centre stage. Nature Reviews, Immunology, 8(9), 685-698. https://doi.org/10.1038/nri2378

[2] Cantorna, M. T., Snyder, L., Lin, Y. D., & Yang, L. (2015). Vitamin D and 1,25(OH)2D regulation of T cells. In Nutrients (Vol. 7, Issue 4, pp. 3011-3021). MDPI AG. https://doi.org/10.3390/nu7043011

[3] Holick, M. F. (2017). The vitamin D deficiency pandemic: Approaches for diagnosis, treatment and prevention. In Reviews in Endocrine and Metabolic Disorders (Vol. 18, Issue 2, pp. 153-165). Springer New York LLC. https://doi.org/10.1007/s11154-017-9424-1

[4] Kodak, T., & Bergmann, S. (2020). Autism Spectrum Disorder Characteristics, Associated Behaviors, and Early Intervention. Pediatr Clin N Am, 67, 525-535. https://doi.org/10.1016/j.pcl.2020.02.007

[5] Tchaconas, A., & Adesman, A. (2013). Autism spectrum disorders. Current Opinion in Pediatrics, 25(1), 130-144. https://doi.org/10.1097/MOP.0b013e32835c2b70

[6] Briceno Noriega, D., Savelkoul, H. F. J. (2014). Immune dysregulation in autism spectrum disorder. In European Journal of Pediatrics (Vol. 173, Issue 1, pp. 33-43). Springer. https://doi.org/10.1007/s00431-013-2183-4

[7] Cannell, J. J. (2008). Autism and vitamin D. Medical Hypotheses, 70(4), 750-759. https://doi.org/10.1016/j.mehy.2007.08.016

[8] Campisi, L., Imran, N., Nazeer, A., Skokauskas, N., & Azeem, M. W. (2018). Autism spectrum disorder. British Medical Bulletin, 127, 91-100. https://doi.org/10.1093/bmb/ldy026

[9] Gezondheidsraad. (2009). Autismespectrumstoornissen: een leven lang anders. Gezondheidsraad.

[10] Maenner, M. J., Shaw, K. A., Baio, J., Washington, A., Patrick, M., DiRienzo, M., Christensen, D. L., Wiggins, L. D., Pettygrove, S., Andrews, J. G., Lopez, M., Hudson, A., Baroud, T., Schwenk, Y., White, T., Rosenberg, C. R., Lee, L.-C., Harrington, R. A., Huston, M., ... Dietz, P. M. (2020). Prevalence of Autism Spectrum Disorder Among Children Aged 8 Years — Autism and Developmental Disabilities Monitoring Network, 11 Sites, United States, 2016. MMWR. Surveillance Summaries, 69(4), 1-12. https://doi.org/10.15585/mmwr.ss6904a1

[11] El-Ansary, A., Cannell, J. J., Bjørklund, G., Bhat, R. S., Al Dbass, A. M., Alfawaz, H. A., Chirumbolo, S., & Al-Ayadhi, L. (2018). In the search for reliable biomarkers for the early diagnosis of autism spectrum disorder: the role of vitamin D. Metabolic Brain Disease, 33(3), 917-931. https://doi.org/10.1007/s11011-018-0199-1

[12] Kim, Y. S., Leventhal, B. L., Koh, Y. J., Fombonne, E., Laska, E., Lim, E. C., Cheon, K. A., Kim, S. J., Kim, Y. K., Lee, H. K., Song, D. H., & Grinker, R. R. (2011). Prevalence of autism spectrum disorders in a total population sample. American Journal of Psychiatry, 168(9), 904-912. https://doi.org/10.1176/appi.ajp.2011.10101532

[13] Khamoushi, A., Aalipanah, E., Sohrabi, Z., & Akbarzadeh, M. (2019). Vitamin D and Autism Spectrum Disorder: A Review. International Journal of Nutrition Sciences, 4(1), 9-13. https://doi.org/10.30476/IJNS.2019.81436.1004

[14] Gładysz, D., Krzywdzińska, A., & Hozyasz, K. K. (2018). Immune Abnormalities in Autism Spectrum Disorder-Could They Hold Promise for Causative Treatment? Molecular Neurobiology, 55, 6387-6435. https://doi.org/10.1007/s12035-017-0822-x

[15] Nitschke, A., Deonandan, R., & Konkle, A. T. (2020). The link between autism spectrum disorder and gut microbiota: A scoping review. Autism, 136236132091336. https://doi.org/10.1177/1362361320913364

[16] Onore, C., Careaga, M., & Ashwood, P. (2012). The role of immune dysfunction in the pathophysiology of autism. In Brain, Behavior, and Immunity (Vol. 26, Issue 3, pp. 383-392). Academic Press. https://doi.org/10.1016/j.bbi.2011.08.007

[17] Lehmann, U., Hirche, F., Stangl, G. I., Hinz, K., Westphal, S., & Dierkes, J. (2013). Bioavailability of Vitamin D 2 and D 3 in Healthy Volunteers, a Randomized Placebo-Controlled Trial. The Journal of Clinical Endocrinology & Metabolism, 98(11), 4339-4345. https://doi.org/10.1210/jc.2012-4287

[18] Lamberg-Allardt, C. (2006). Vitamin D in foods and as supplements. In Progress in Biophysics and Molecular Biology (Vol. 92, Issue 1, pp. 33-38). Pergamon. https://doi.org/10.1016/j.pbiomolbio.2006.02.017

[19] Bikle, D. D. (2012). Vitamin D and the skin: Physiology and pathophysiology. In Reviews in Endocrine and Metabolic Disorders (Vol. 13, Issue 1, pp. 3-19). Springer. https://doi.org/10.1007/s11154-011-9194-0

[20] Pike, J. W., & Christakos, S. (2017). Biology and Mechanisms of Action of the Vitamin D Hormone. In Endocrinology and Metabolism Clinics of North America (Vol. 46, Issue 4, pp. 815-843). W.B. Saunders. https://doi.org/10.1016/j.ecl.2017.07.001

[21] Bikle, D. D. (2014). Vitamin D Metabolism, Mechanism of Action, and Clinical Applications. Chemistry & Biology, 21, 319-329. https://doi.org/http://dx.doi.org/10.1016/j.chembiol.2013.12.016

[22] Mondul, A. M., Weinstein, S. J., Moy, K. A., Männistö, S., & Albanes, D. (2014). Vitamin D-binding protein, circulating vitamin D and risk of renal cell carcinoma. International Journal of Cancer, 134(11), 2699-2706. https://doi.org/10.1002/ijc.28596

[23] Premer, C., & Schulman, I. H. (2018). Have we been measuring the wrong form of Vitamin D? Vitamin D as a prognostic biomarker for coronary artery disease mortality. In Circulation Research (Vol. 123, Issue 8, pp. 934-935). Lippincott Williams and Wilkins. https://doi.org/10.1161/CIRCRESAHA.118.313814

[24] Pike, J. W., & Meyer, M. B. (2010). The Vitamin D Receptor: New Paradigms for the Regulation of Gene Expression by 1,25-Dihydroxyvitamin D 3. Endocrinology & Metabolism Clinics of North America, 39, 255-269. https://doi.org/10.1016/j.ecl.2010.02.007

[25] Fraser, D. R. (2015). Vitamin D Deficiency and Energy Metabolism. Endocrinology, 156(6), 1933-1935. https://doi.org/10.1210/en.2015-1298

[26] Pilz, S., & Tomaschitz, A. (2010). Role of vitamin D in arterial hypertension. In Expert Review of Cardiovascular Therapy (Vol. 8, Issue 11, pp. 1599-1608). Expert Rev Cardiovasc Ther. https://doi.org/10.1586/erc.10.142

[27] Gezen-Ak, D., Dursun, E., & Yilmazer, S. (2014). The Effect of Vitamin D Treatment on Nerve Growth Factor (NGF) Release from

Hippocampal Neurons. Noropsikiyatri Arsivi, 51(2), 157-162. https://doi.org/10.4274/npa.y7076

[28] Dimeloe, S., Nanzer, A., Ryanna, K., & Hawrylowicz, C. (2010). Regulatory T cells, inflammation and the allergic response-The role of glucocorticoids and Vitamin D. In Journal of Steroid Biochemistry and Molecular Biology (Vol. 120, Issues 2-3, pp. 86-95). Elsevier Ltd. https://doi.org/10.1016/j.jsbmb.2010.02.029

[29] von Essen, M. R., & Geisler, C. (2018). VDR, the Vitamin D Receptor. In Encyclopedia of Signaling Molecules (pp. 5907-5914). Springer International Publishing. https://doi.org/10.1007/978-3-319-67199-4_287

[30] Bouillon, R., Van Schoor, N. M., Gielen, E., Boonen, S., Mathieu, C., Vanderschueren, D., & Lips, P. (2013). Optimal vitamin D status: A critical analysis on the basis of evidence-based medicine. Journal of Clinical Endocrinology and Metabolism, 98(8), E1283–E1304. https://doi.org/10.1210/jc.2013-1195

[31] Vanherwegen, A. S., Gysemans, C., & Mathieu, C. (2017). Regulation of Immune Function by Vitamin D and Its Use in Diseases of Immunity. Endocrinology and Metabolism Clinics of North America, 46(4), 1061-1094. https://doi.org/10.1016/j.ecl.2017.07.010

[32] Haussler, M. R., Jurutka, P. W., Mizwicki, M., Norman, A. W., Mizwicki, M., & Norman, A. W. (2011). Vitamin D receptor (VDR)-mediated actions of 1a,25(OH) 2 vitamin D 3 : Genomic and non-genomic mechanisms. Best Practice & Research Clinical Endocrinology & Metabolism, 25, 543-559. https://doi.org/10.1016/j.beem.2011.05.010

[33] Kongsbak, M., Levring, T. B., Geisler, C., & von Essen, M. R. (2013). The vitamin D receptor and T cell function. In Frontiers in Immunology (Vol. 4, Issue JUN). Frontiers Media SA. https://doi.org/10.3389/fimmu.2013.00148

[34] Sassi, F., Tamone, C., & D'amelio, P. (2018). Vitamin D: Nutrient, Hormone, and Immunomodulator. Nutrients, 10. https://doi.org/10.3390/nu10111656

[35] Van Etten, E., & Mathieu, C. (2005). Immunoregulation by 1,25-dihydroxyvitamin D3: Basic concepts. Journal of Steroid Biochemistry and Molecular Biology, 97(1-2), 93-101. https://doi.org/10.1016/j.jsbmb.2005.06.002

[36] Pangrazzi, L., Balasco, L., & Bozzi, Y. (2020). Oxidative Stress and Immune System Dysfunction in Autism Spectrum Disorders. International Journal of Molecular Sciences, 21(9), 3293. https://doi.org/10.3390/ijms21093293

[37] Xu, G., Snetselaar, L.G., Jing, J., Buyun Liu, Strathearn, L., Bao, W. (2018). Association of Food Allergy and Other Allergic Conditions With Autism Spectrum Disorder in Children/ JAMA Network Open. 1(2):e180279. doi:10.1001/jamanetworkopen.2018.0279

[38] Bjørklund, G., Saad, K., Chirumbolo, S., Kern, J. K., Geier, D. A., Geier, M. R., & Urbina, M. A. (2016). Immune dysfunction and neuroinflammation in autism spectrum disorder. In Acta Neurobiologiae Experimentalis (Vol. 76, Issue 4, pp. 257-268). Nencki Institute of Experimental Biology. https://doi.org/10.21307/ane-2017-025

[39] Careaga, M., Rogers, S., Hansen, R. L., Amaral, D. G., Van de Water, J., & Ashwood, P. (2017). Immune Endophenotypes in Children With Autism Spectrum Disorder. Biological Psychiatry, 81(5), 434-441. https://doi.org/10.1016/j.biopsych.2015.08.036

[40] Hughes, H. K., Mills Ko, E., Rose, D., & Ashwood, P. (2018). Immune Dysfunction and Autoimmunity as Pathological Mechanisms in Autism Spectrum Disorders. In Frontiers in Cellular Neuroscience (Vol. 12). Frontiers Media S.A. https://doi.org/10.3389/fncel.2018.00405

[41] Rodriguez, J. I., & Kern, J. K. (2011). Evidence of microglial activation in autism and its possible role in brain underconnectivity. Neuron Glia Biology, 7(2-4), 205-213. https://doi.org/10.1017/S1740925X12000142

[42] Enstrom, A. M., Onore, C. E., Van de Water, J. A., & Ashwood, P. (2010). Differential monocyte responses to TLR ligands in children with autism spectrum disorders. Brain, Behavior, and Immunity, 24(1), 64-71. https://doi.org/10.1016/j.bbi.2009.08.001

[43] Atri, C., Guerfali, F. Z., & Laouini, D. (2018). Role of human macrophage polarization in inflammation during infectious diseases. International Journal of Molecular Sciences, 19(6). https://doi.org/10.3390/ijms19061801

[44] Martinez, F. O., & Gordon, S. (2014). The M1 and M2 paradigm of macrophage activation: time for reassessment. F1000Prime Reports, 6(13). https://doi.org/10.12703/P6-13

[45] Ning, J., Xu, L., Shen, C. Q., Zhang, Y. Y., & Zhao, Q. (2019). Increased serum levels of macrophage migration inhibitory factor in autism spectrum disorders. NeuroToxicology, 71, 1-5. https://doi.org/10.1016/j.neuro.2018.11.015

[46] Grigorenko, E. L., Han, S. S., Yrigollen, C. M., Leng, L., Mizue, Y., Anderson, G. M., Mulder, E. J., De Bildt, A., Minderaa, R. B., Volkmar, F. R., Chang, J. T., & Bucala, R. (2008). Macrophage migration inhibitory factor and autism spectrum disorders. Pediatrics, 122(2). https://doi.org/10.1542/peds.2007-3604

[47] Saad, K., Zahran, A. M., Elsayh, K. I., Abdel-Rahman, A. A., Al-Atram, A. A., Hussein, A., & El-Gendy, Y. G. (2017). Frequency of Dendritic Cells and Their Expression of Costimulatory Molecules in Children with Autism Spectrum Disorders. Journal of Autism and Developmental Disorders, 47(9), 2671-2678. https://doi.org/10.1007/s10803-017-3190-5

[48] Song, L., Papaioannou, G., Zhao, H., Luderer, H. F., Miller, C., Dall'Osso, C., Nazarian, R. M., Wagers, A. J., & Demay, M. B. (2016). The Vitamin D Receptor Regulates Tissue Resident Macrophage Response to Injury. Endocrinology, 157(10), 4066-4075. https://doi.org/10.1210/en.2016-1474

[49] Zhang, X. L., Guo, Y. F., Song, Z. X., & Zhou, M. (2014). Vitamin D prevents podocyte injury via regulation of macrophage M1/M2 phenotype in diabetic nephropathy rats. Endocrinology, 155(12), 4939-4950. https://doi.org/10.1210/en.2014-1020

[50] Moaaz, M., Youssry, S., Elfatatry, A., Abd, M., & Rahman, E. (2019). Th17/Treg cells imbalance and their related cytokines (IL-17, IL-10 and TGF-β) in children with autism spectrum disorder. Journal of Neuroimmunology, 337. https://doi.org/10.1016/j.jneuroim.2019.577071

[51] Ahmad, Sheikh Fayaz, Zoheir, K. M. A., Ansari, M. A., Nadeem, A., Bakheet, S. A., AL-Ayadhi, L. Y., Alzahrani, M. Z., Al-Shabanah, O. A., Al-Harbi, M. M., & Attia, S. M. (2017). Dysregulation of Th1, Th2, Th17, and T regulatory cell-related transcription factor signaling in children with autism. Molecular Neurobiology, 54(6), 4390-4400. https://doi.org/10.1007/s12035-016-9977-0

[52] Masi, A., Quintana, D. S., Glozier, N., Lloyd, A. R., Hickie, I. B., & Guastella, A. J. (2015). Cytokine aberrations in autism spectrum disorder: A systematic review and meta-analysis. Molecular Psychiatry, 20(4), 440-446. https://doi.org/10.1038/mp.2014.59

[53] Tanaka, T., Narazaki, M., & Kishimoto, T. (2014). IL-6 in inflammation, Immunity, And disease. Cold Spring Harbor Perspectives in Biology, 6(10). https://doi.org/10.1101/cshperspect.a016295

[54] Wei, H., Chadman, K. K., McCloskey, D. P., Sheikh, A. M., Malik, M., Brown, W. T., & Li, X. (2012). Brain IL-6 elevation causes neuronal circuitry imbalances and mediates autism-like behaviors. Biochimica et Biophysica Acta - Molecular Basis of Disease, 1822(6), 831-842. https://doi.org/10.1016/j.bbadis.2012.01.011

[55] Wei, H., Zou, H., Sheikh, A. M., Malik, M., Dobkin, C., Brown, W. T., & Li, X. (2011). IL-6 is increased in the cerebellum of autistic brain and alters neural cell adhesion, migration and synaptic formation. Journal of Neuroinflammation, 8. https://doi.org/10.1186/1742-2094-8-52

[56] Jyonouchi, H., & Geng, L. (2019). Associations between monocyte and T cell cytokine profiles in autism spectrum disorders: Effects of dysregulated innate immune responses on adaptive responses to recall antigens in a subset of ASD children. International Journal of Molecular Sciences, 20(19). https://doi.org/10.3390/ijms20194731

[57] Ricci, S., Businaro, R., Ippoliti, F., Lo Vasco, V. R., Massoni, F., Onofri, E., Troili, G. M., Pontecorvi, V., Morelli, M., Rapp Ricciardi, M., & Archer, T. (2013). Altered cytokine and BDNF levels in autism spectrum disorder. Neurotoxicity Research, 24(4), 491-501. https://doi.org/10.1007/s12640-013-9393-4

[58] Eftekharian, M. M., Ghafouri-Fard, S., Noroozi, R., Omrani, M. D., Arsang-jang, S., Ganji, M., Gharzi, V., Noroozi, H., Komaki, A., Mazdeh, M., & Taheri, M. (2018). Cytokine profile in autistic patients. Cytokine, 108, 120-126. https://doi.org/10.1016/j.cyto.2018.03.034

[59] Ashwood, P., Krakowiak, P., Hertz-Picciotto, I., Hansen, R., Pessah, I. N., & Van de Water, J. (2011a). Associations of impaired behaviors with elevated plasma chemokines in autism spectrum disorders. Journal of Neuroimmunology, 232(1-2), 196-199. https://doi.org/10.1016/j.jneuroim.2010.10.025

[60] Ashwood, P., Krakowiak, P., Hertz-Picciotto, I., Hansen, R., Pessah, I., & Van de Water, J. (2011c). Elevated plasma cytokines in autism spectrum disorders provide evidence of immune dysfunction and are associated with impaired behavioral outcome. Brain, Behavior, and Immunity, 25(1), 40-45. https://doi.org/10.1016/j.bbi.2010.08.003

[61] Akintunde, M. E., Rose, M., Krakowiak, P., Heuer, L., Ashwood, P., Hansen, R., Hertz-Picciotto, I., & Van de Water, J. (2015). Increased production of IL-17 in children with autism spectrum disorders and co-morbid asthma. Journal of Neuroimmunology, 286, 33-41. https://doi.org/10.1016/j.jneuroim.2015.07.003

[62] AL-Ayadhi, L. Y., & Mostafa, G. A. (2012). Elevated serum levels of interleukin-17A in children with autism. Journal of Neuroinflammation, 9. https://doi.org/10.1186/1742-2094-9-158

[63] Suzuki, K., Matsuzaki, H., Iwata, K., Kameno, Y., Shimmura, C., Kawai, S., Yoshihara, Y., Wakuda, T., Takebayashi, K., Takagai, S., Matsumoto, K.,

Tsuchiya, K. J., Iwata, Y., Nakamura, K., Tsujii, M., Sugiyama, T., & Mori, N. (2011). Plasma Cytokine Profiles in Subjects with High-Functioning Autism Spectrum Disorders. PLOS ONE, 6(5). https://doi.org/10.1371/journal.pone.0020470

[64] Hashim, H., Abdelrahman, H., Mohammed, D., & Karam, R. (2013). Association between plasma levels of transforming growth factor-β1, IL-23 and IL-17 and the severity of autism in Egyptian children. Research in Autism Spectrum Disorders, 7(1), 199-204. https://doi.org/10.1016/j.rasd.2012.08.007

[65] Onore, C., Enstrom, A., Krakowiak, P., Hertz-Picciotto, I., Hansen, R., de Water, J. Van, & Ashwood, P. (2009). Decreased cellular IL-23 but not IL-17 production in children with autism spectrum disorders. Journal of Neuroimmunology, 216(1-2), 126-129. https://doi.org/10.1016/j.jneuroim.2009.09.005

[66] Ahmad, Sheikh F., Nadeem, A., Ansari, M. A., Bakheet, S. A., Attia, S. M., Zoheir, K. M. A., AL-Ayadhi, L. Y., Alzahrani, M. Z., Alsaad, A. M. S., Alotaibi, M. R., & Abd-Allah, A. R. A. (2017). Imbalance between the anti- and pro-inflammatory milieu in blood leukocytes of autistic children. Molecular Immunology, 82, 57-65. https://doi.org/10.1016/j.molimm.2016.12.019

[67] Enstrom, A., Onore, C., Hertz-Picciotto, I., Hansen, R., Croen, L., Van De Water, J., & Ashwood, P. (2008). Detection of IL-17 and IL-23 in plasma samples of children with autism. American Journal of Biochemistry and Biotechnology, 4(2), 114-120. https://doi.org/10.3844/ajbbsp.2008.114.120

[68] Sonderegger, I., Iezzi, G., Maier, R., Schmitz, N., Kurrer, M., & Kopf, M. (2008). GM-CSF mediates autoimmunity by enhancing IL-6-dependent Th17 cell development and survival. Journal of Experimental Medicine, 205(10), 2281-2294. https://doi.org/10.1084/jem.20071119

[69] Balestrieri, E., Cipriani, C., Matteucci, C., Benvenuto, A., Coniglio, A., Argaw-Denboba, A., Toschi, N., Bucci, I., Miele, M. T., Grelli, S., Curatolo, P., & Sinibaldi-Vallebona, P. (2019). Children with autism spectrum disorder and their mothers share abnormal expression of selected endogenous retroviruses families and cytokines. Frontiers in Immunology, 10(SEP). https://doi.org/10.3389/fimmu.2019.02244

[70] Masi, A., Glozier, N., Dale, R., & Guastella, A. J. (2017). The Immune System, Cytokines, and Biomarkers in Autism Spectrum Disorder. Neurosci. Bull., 33(2), 194-204. https://doi.org/10.1007/s12264-017-0103-8

[71] Moaaz, M., Youssry, S., Elfatatry, A., Abd, M., & Rahman, E. (2019). Th17/Treg cells imbalance and their related cytokines (IL-17, IL-10 and TGF-β) in children with autism spectrum disorder. Journal of Neuroimmunology, 337. https://doi.org/10.1016/j.jneuroim.2019.577071

[72] Ashwood, P., Krakowiak, P., Hertz-Picciotto, I., Hansen, R., Pessah, I. N., & Van de Water, J. (2011b). Altered T cell responses in children with autism. Brain, Behavior, and Immunity, 25(5), 840-849. https://doi.org/10.1016/j.bbi.2010.09.002

[73] Molloy, C. A., Morrow, A. L., Meinzen-Derr, J., Schleifer, K., Dienger, K., Manning-Courtney, P., Altaye, M., & Wills-Karp, M. (2006). Elevated cytokine levels in children with autism spectrum disorder. Journal of Neuroimmunology, 172(1-2), 198-205. https://doi.org/10.1016/j.jneuroim.2005.11.007

[74] Saghazadeh, A., Ataeinia, B., Keynejad, K., Abdolalizadeh, A.,

Hirbod-Mobarakeh, A., & Rezaei, N. (2019). Anti-inflammatory cytokines in autism spectrum disorders: A systematic review and meta-analysis. In Cytokine (Vol. 123). Academic Press. https://doi.org/10.1016/j.cyto.2019.154740

[75] Rose, D., & Ashwood, P. (2019). Rapid communication: Plasma interleukin-35 in children with Autism. Brain Sciences, 9(7). https://doi.org/10.3390/brainsci9070152

[76] Krakowiak, P., Goines, P. E., Tancredi, D. J., Ashwood, P., Hansen, R. L., Hertz-Picciotto, I., & Van de Water, J. (2017). Neonatal Cytokine Profiles Associated With Autism Spectrum Disorder. Biological Psychiatry, 81(5), 442-451. https://doi.org/10.1016/j.biopsych.2015.08.007

[77] Ahmad, Sheikh Fayaz, Zoheir, K. M. A., Ansari, M. A., Nadeem, A., Bakheet, S. A., AL-Ayadhi, L. Y., Alzahrani, M. Z., Al-Shabanah, O. A., Al-Harbi, M. M., & Attia, S. M. (2017). Dysregulation of Th1, Th2, Th17, and T regulatory cell-related transcription factor signaling in children with autism. Molecular Neurobiology, 54(6), 4390-4400. https://doi.org/10.1007/s12035-016-9977-0

[78] Li, X., Chauhan, A., Sheikh, A. M., Patil, S., Chauhan, V., Li, X. M., Ji, L., Brown, T., & Malik, M. (2009). Elevated immune response in the brain of autistic patients. Journal of Neuroimmunology, 207(1-2), 111-116. https://doi.org/10.1016/j.jneuroim.2008.12.002

[79] El-Aziz, S. A. A., & El-Din, R. A. A. (2012). Cellular-mediated and humoral immunity in children with autism. Egyptian Journal of Pediatric Allergy and Immunology, 10(1), 25-32. https://doi.org/10.4314/EJPAI.V10I1

[80] Vargas, D. L., Nascimbene, C., Krishnan, C., Zimmerman, A. W., & Pardo, C. A. (2005). Neuroglial activation and neuroinflammation in the brain of patients with autism. Annals of Neurology, 57(1), 67-81. https://doi.org/10.1002/ana.20315

[81] Eyles, D. W., Smith, S., Kinobe, R., Hewison, M., & McGrath, J. J. (2005). Distribution of the Vitamin D receptor and 1α-hydroxylase in human brain. Journal of Chemical Neuroanatomy, 29(1), 21-30. https://doi.org/10.1016/j.jchemneu.2004.08.006

[82] Jia, F., Shan, L., Wang, B., Li, H., Miao, C., Xu, Z., Lin, C.-P., & Saad, K. (2017). Possible role of vitamin D in autism spectrum disorder. Psychiatry Research, 260, 360-365. https://doi.org/10.1016/j.psychres.2017.12.005

[83] Stubbs, G., Henley, K., & Green, J. (2016). Autism: Will vitamin D supplementation during pregnancy and early childhood reduce the recurrence rate of autism in newborn siblings? Medical Hypotheses, 88, 74-78. https://doi.org/10.1016/j.mehy.2016.01.015

[84] Grant, W. B., & Soles, C. M. (2009). Epidemiologic evidence for supporting the role of maternal vitamin D deficiency as a risk factor for the development of infantile autism. Dermato-Endocrinology, 1(4), 223-228. https://doi.org/10.4161/derm.1.4.9500

[85] Saraff, V., & Shaw, N. (2016). Sunshine and Vitamin D. In Archives of Disease in Childhood (Vol. 101, Issue 2, pp. 190-192). BMJ Publishing Group. https://doi.org/10.1136/archdischild-2014-307214

[86] Dealberto, M. J. (2011). Prevalence of autism according to maternal immigrant status and ethnic origin. In Acta Psychiatrica Scandinavica (Vol. 123, Issue 5, pp. 339-348). https://doi.org/10.1111/j.1600-0447.2010.01662.x

[87] Bodnar, L. M., Simhan, H. N., Powers, R. W., Frank, M. P., Cooperstein, E., & Roberts, J. M.

(2007). High Prevalence of Vitamin D Insufficiency in Black and White Pregnant Women Residing in the Northern United States and Their Neonates 1. In J. Nutr (Vol. 137). https://doi.org/https://doi-org.ezproxy.library.wur.nl/10.1093/jn/137.2.447

[88] Bogh, M. K. B., Schmedes, A. V, Philipsen, P. A., Thieden, E., & Wulf, H. C. (2010). Vitamin D Production after UVB Exposure Depends on Baseline Vitamin D and Total Cholesterol but Not on Skin Pigmentation. Journal of Investigative Dermatology, 130, 546-553. https://doi.org/10.1038/jid.2009.323

[89] Mangin, M., Sinha, R., & Fincher, K. (2014). Inflammation and vitamin D: the infection connection. In Inflammation Research (Vol. 63, Issue 10, pp. 803-819). Birkhauser Verlag AG. https://doi.org/10.1007/s00011-014-0755-z

[90] Lee, B. K., Eyles, D. W., Magnusson, C., Newschaffer, C. J., McGrath, J. J., Kvaskoff, D., Ko, P., Dalman, C., Karlsson, H., & Gardner, R. M. (2019). Developmental vitamin D and autism spectrum disorders: findings from the Stockholm Youth Cohort. Molecular Psychiatry. https://doi.org/10.1038/s41380-019-0578-y

[91] Holick, M. F. (2007). Vitamin D Deficiency. In N Engl J Med (Vol. 357). www.nejm.org

[92] Hebert, K. J., Miller, L. L., & Joinson, C. J. (2010). Association of autistic spectrum disorder with season of birth and conception in a UK cohort. Autism Research, 3(4), 185-190. https://doi.org/10.1002/aur.136

[93] Ciéślińska, A., Kostyra, E., Chwała, B., Moszyńska-Dumara, M., Fiedorowicz, E., Teodorowicz, M., & Savelkoul, H. F. J. (2017). Vitamin D receptor gene polymorphisms associated with childhood autism. Brain Sciences, 7(9). https://doi.org/10.3390/brainsci7090115

[94] Cieslinska, A., Simmelink, J., Teodorowicz, G., Verhoef, H., Tobi, H., & Savelkoul, H. F. (2017). Distribution of Month of Birth of Individuals with Autism Spectrum Disorder Differs from the General Population in the Netherlands. In Autism - Paradigms, Recent Research and Clinical Applications. InTech. https://doi.org/10.5772/67205

[95] Shalev, H., Solt, I., & Chodick, G. (2017). Month of birth and risk of autism spectrum disorder: a retrospective cohort of male children born in Israel. BMJ Open, 7, 14606. https://doi.org/10.1136/bmjopen-2016-014606

[96] Lee, B. K., Gross, R., Francis, R. W., Karlsson, H., Schendel, D. E., Sourander, A., Reichenberg, A., Parner, E. T., Hornig, M., Yaniv, A., Leonard, H., & Sandin, S. (2019). Birth seasonality and risk of autism spectrum disorder. European Journal of Epidemiology, 34(8), 785-792. https://doi.org/10.1007/s10654-019-00506-5

[97] Samuelsen, G. B., Larsen, K. B., Bogdanovic, N., Laursen, H., Graem, N., Larsen, J. F., & Pakkenberg, B. (2003). The Changing Number of Cells in the Human Fetal Forebrain and its Subdivisions: A Stereological Analysis. Cerebral Cortex, 13(2), 115-122. https://doi.org/https://doi.org/10.1093/cercor/13.2.115

[98] de Graaf-Peters, V. B., & Hadders-Algra, M. (2006). Ontogeny of the human central nervous system: What is happening when? Early Human Development, 82(4), 257-266. https://doi.org/10.1016/j.earlhumdev.2005.10.013

[99] Cannell, John J., & Grant, W. B. (2013). What is the role of vitamin D in autism? Dermato-Endocrinology,

5(1), 199-204. https://doi.org/10.4161/derm.24356

[100] Feng, J., Shan, L., Du, L., Wang, B., Li, H., Wang, W., Wang, T., Dong, H., Yue, X., Xu, Z., Staal, W. G., & Jia, F. (2017). Clinical improvement following vitamin D3 supplementation in Autism Spectrum Disorder. Nutritional Neuroscience, 20(5), 284-290. https://doi.org/10.1080/1028415X.2015.1123847

[101] Mostafa, G. A., & AL-Ayadhi, L. Y. (2012). Reduced serum concentrations of 25-hydroxy vitamin D in children with autism: Relation to autoimmunity. Journal of Neuroinflammation, 9. https://doi.org/10.1186/1742-2094-9-201

[102] Meguid, N. A., Hashish, A. F., Anwar, M., & Sidhom, G. (2010). Reduced Serum Levels of 25-Hydroxy and 1,25-Dihydroxy Vitamin D in Egyptian Children with Autism. The Journal of Alternative and Complementary Medicine, 16(6), 641-645. https://doi.org/10.1089/acm.2009.0349

[103] Cannell, J.J. (2017). Vitamin D and autism, what's new? Reviews in Endocrine and Metabolic Disorders, 18(2), 183-193. https://doi.org/10.1007/s11154-017-9409-0

[104] Fernell, E., Bejerot, S., Westerlund, J., Miniscalco, C., Simila, H., Eyles, D., Gillberg, C., & Humble, M. B. (2015). Autism spectrum disorder and low vitamin D at birth: A sibling control study. Molecular Autism, 6(1), 3. https://doi.org/10.1186/2040-2392-6-3

[105] Schmidt, R. J., Hansen, R. L., Hartiala, J., Allayee, H., Sconberg, J. L., Schmidt, L. C., Volk, H. E., & Tassone, F. (2015). Selected vitamin D metabolic gene variants and risk for autism spectrum disorder in the CHARGE Study. Early Human Development, 91(8), 483-489. https://doi.org/10.1016/j.earlhumdev.2015.05.008

[106] Wu, D. M., Wen, X., Han, X. R., Wang, S., Wang, Y. J., Shen, M., Fan, S. H., Zhuang, J., Li, M. Q., Hu, B., Sun, C. H., Bao, Y. X., Yan, J., Lu, J., & Zheng, Y. L. (2018). Relationship Between Neonatal Vitamin D at Birth and Risk of Autism Spectrum Disorders: the NBSIB Study. Journal of Bone and Mineral Research, 33(3), 458-466. https://doi.org/10.1002/jbmr.3326

[107] Schmidt, R. J., Niu, Q., Eyles, D. W., Hansen, R. L., & Iosif, A. M. (2019). Neonatal vitamin D status in relation to autism spectrum disorder and developmental delay in the CHARGE case–control study. Autism Research, 12(6), 976-988. https://doi.org/10.1002/aur.2118

[108] Mazahery, H., Conlon, C. A., Beck, K. L., Mugridge, O., Kruger, M. C., Stonehouse, W., Camargo, C. A., Meyer, B. J., Tsang, B., Jones, B., & von Hurst, P. R. (2019). A Randomised-Controlled Trial of Vitamin D and Omega-3 Long Chain Polyunsaturated Fatty Acids in the Treatment of Core Symptoms of Autism Spectrum Disorder in Children. Journal of Autism and Developmental Disorders, 49(5), 1778-1794. https://doi.org/10.1007/s10803-018-3860-y

[109] Feng, Y., Qiu, T., Chen, H., Wei, Y., Jiang, X., Zhang, H., & Chen, D. (2020). Association of serum IL-21 and vitamin D concentrations in Chinese children with autoimmune thyroid disease. Clinica Chimica Acta, 507, 194-198. https://doi.org/10.1016/j.cca.2020.04.030

[110] Saad, K., Abdel-rahman, A. A., Elserogy, Y. M., Al-Atram, A. A., Cannell, J. J., Bjørklund, G., Abdel-Reheim, M. K., Othman, H. A. K., El-Houfey, A. A., Abd El-Aziz, N. H. R., Abd El-Baseer, K. A., Ahmed, A. E., & Ali, A. M. (2016). Vitamin D status in autism spectrum disorders and the efficacy of vitamin D supplementation in autistic children. Nutritional Neuroscience, 19(8), 346-351.

https://doi.org/10.1179/14768305
15Y.0000000019

[111] Vieth, R. (2007). Vitamin D toxicity, policy, and science. Journal of Bone and Mineral Research, 22(SUPPL. 2), V64–V68. https://doi.org/10.1359/jbmr.07s221

[112] Humble, M. B., Gustafsson, S., & Bejerot, S. (2010). Low serum levels of 25-hydroxyvitamin D (25-OHD) among psychiatric out-patients in Sweden: Relations with season, age, ethnic origin and psychiatric diagnosis. The Journal of Steroid Biochemistry and Molecular Biology, 121(1-2), 467-470. https://doi.org/10.1016/j.jsbmb.2010.03.013

[113] Lord, C., Elsabbagh, M., Baird, G., & Veenstra-Vanderweele, J. (2018). Autism spectrum disorder. The lancet, 392, 508-520. https://doi.org/10.1016/S0140-6736(18)31129-2

[114] Marchezan, J., Winkler dos Santos, E. G. A., Deckmann, I., & Riesgo, R. dos S. (2018). Immunological Dysfunction in Autism Spectrum Disorder: A Potential Target for Therapy. Neuroimmunomodulation, 25(5-6), 300-319. https://doi.org/10.1159/000492225

[115] Apert, C., Romagnoli, P., & Van Meerwijk, J. P. M. (2018). IL-2 and IL-15 dependent thymic development of Foxp3-expressing regulatory T lymphocytes. Protein Cell, 9(4), 322-332. https://doi.org/10.1007/s13238-017-0425-3

[116] Jeffery, L. E., Burke, F., Mura, M., Zheng, Y., Qureshi, O. S., Hewison, M., Walker, L. S. K., Lammas, D. A., Raza, K., & Sansom, D. M. (2009). 1,25-Dihydroxyvitamin D 3 and IL-2 Combine to Inhibit T Cell Production of Inflammatory Cytokines and Promote Development of Regulatory T Cells Expressing CTLA-4 and FoxP3. The Journal of Immunology, 183(9), 5458-5467. https://doi.org/10.4049/jimmunol.0803217

[117] Jeffery, L. E., Qureshi, O. S., Gardner, D., Hou, T. Z., Briggs, Z., Soskic, B., Baker, J., Raza, K., & Sansom, D. M. (2015). Vitamin D Antagonises the Suppressive Effect of Inflammatory Cytokines on CTLA-4 Expression and Regulatory Function. PLOS ONE, 10(7), e0131539. https://doi.org/10.1371/journal.pone.0131539